P9-DTI-679

WITHDRAWN
UTSA Libraries

DATE DUE

Hospital Structure and Performance

The Johns Hopkins Series in Contemporary Medicine and Public Health

CONSULTING EDITORS

Samuel H. Boyer IV, M.D.   Albert H. Owens, Jr., M.D.
Gareth M. Green, M.D.   Edyth H. Schoenrich, M.D., M.P.H.
Richard T. Johnson, M.D.   Jerry L. Spivak, M.D.
Paul R. McHugh, M.D.   Barbara H. Starfield, M.D., M.P.H.
Edmond A. Murphy, M.D.

Ann Barry Flood and W. Richard Scott

Hospital Structure and Performance

with Byron W. Brown, Jr., Donald E. Comstock, Wayne Ewy, William H. Forrest, Jr., and other members of the staff of the Stanford Center for Health Care Research

The Johns Hopkins University Press
Baltimore and London

© 1987 The Johns Hopkins University Press
All rights reserved
Printed in the United States of America

The Johns Hopkins University Press
701 West 40th Street
Baltimore, Maryland 21211
The Johns Hopkins Press Ltd., London

∞ The paper used in this publication meets the minimum requirements of
American National Standard for Information Sciences—Permanence of Paper
for Printed Library Materials, ANSI Z39.48-1984.

Library of Congress Cataloging-in-Publication Data

Flood, Ann Barry, 1944–
    Hospital structure and performance.

    (The Johns Hopkins series in contemporary medicine and public health)
    Bibliography: p.
    Includes index.
    1. Hospital care—United States—Evaluation. 2. Hospitals—United
States—Administration. 3. Hospital care—Evaluation. 4. Hospitals—
Administration. I. Scott, W. Richard. II. Title. III. Series. [DNLM: 1.
Hospital Administration—United States. 2. Hospitals—standards—
United States. WX 150 F631h]
RA981.A2F58   1987   362.1′1   86–21139
ISBN 0-8018-3360-4 (alk. paper)

Library
University of Texas
at San Antonio

To Irma D. Barry and to the memory of W. Larkin Barry and
of Hildegarde and Charles H. Scott, in appreciation of a lifetime
of support and examples of the pursuit of quality

Contents

$233.^{90}_{75}$

List of Figures

List of Tables

Preface

This volume brings together for the first time the work by members of the Stanford Center for Health Care Research concerning the relations between hospital structure and performance based on three separate but interrelated data bases. We believe that our findings and methodologies have important implications for today's health care delivery in hospitals and should be accessible to a wide variety of readers. Although some of the major findings have been published in professional journals, heretofore the reader interested in the overall conceptual and methodological approach, the relationship of the studies, and the more detailed results was obliged to reconstruct them from a variety of journal articles and three very aptly named "technical reports." Only those most desperate for knowledge or most challenged by puzzles could successfully manage this maze.

Included in this volume are new chapters describing the conceptual and methodological issues that confront those who study the determinants of hospital performance, reviewing previous research focused on cost and quality of care in hospitals, and presenting our theoretical framework and methodological approach for addressing the issues we raise. Other new chapters summarize and integrate our overall findings in the three studies. Edited and revised versions of previously published articles reporting specific measures and findings are also included.

Our intended audience is multiple. Health services researchers—including social scientists from a variety of different disciplines—will be interested in both our theoretical and our methodological designs for assessing hospital performance and for studying the organizational and professional staff factors that affect its cost and quality. Health policy makers may well consider the implications of many of our findings on quality of care and the potential use of our methods for assessing performance in U.S. hospitals. Health administrators and health professionals will be interested in the practical implications of our findings concerning the factors within hospitals associated (or not associated) with the quality of care. Finally, students of organizations and the professions should find our approach of value in studying any settings where professionals make up a major share of the staff. We have attempted to avoid statistical, organizational, or sociological jargon in describing our theoretical approach and methods, as well as our findings, in order to make these accessible to people in different disciplines and with varying perspectives and interests.

The original Center team and their contributions are described more fully in the Introduction, where we also give an overview of the theoretical framework and methodological approach to each study. In addition to Center members whose roles are described in the Introduction, Curtis S. Engelhard, M.A., assisted Brown and Ewy with statistical procedures. Flood and Scott received aid from a number of other sociologists, including Joan R. Bloom, R.N., Ph.D.; Donald E. Comstock, Ph.D.; Mary L. Fennell, Ph.D.; Thomas G. Rundall, Ph.D.; and Claudia Bird Schoonhoven, Ph.D. Schoonhoven took a leading role in conducting the survey of surgical complexity. On-site data on hospital and staff characteristics were collected (for the Intensive Study) by a field team of four interviewers: Sharon Fox, R.N.; David O'Brien; Donald Pepper; and Judy Stott, R.N. Forrest was assisted in his staging work by Gordon Taylor, M.D., and Gordon Campbell, M.D. Research assistants included Terry Amburgey, Polly Hildebrand, Linda R. Pearline, Gary D. Sandefur, and William Siegle. Programming support was provided by Paul Goldstein, Jerry Halpern, Anne Harrington, David Harris, John S. James, and James Sharp. Finally, Maxwell was assisted in data management and clerical support by Jane Ann Davis, Eileen Gray, Consuelo Martinez, Stephen Maxwell, Julie Pechota, Gary Reid, Hay Chan Sargent, Elizabeth Wahlquist, and Alison Walsh.

This work has benefited from the guidance, suggestions, and efforts of many others as well. Over the years many colleagues at Stanford University have influenced our conceptualizations and methods. Although we admit that the list is incomplete, we want to mention several colleagues who have been especially helpful and who deserve special recognition for their efforts. John P. Bunker, M.D., of the Stanford Medical School, was an enthusiastic supporter of the Center who contributed both helpful critiques and suggestions for appropriate medical expertise and also supplied needed encouragement to continue the work during its infancy and its heyday and after its official demise. Helpful comments on the design and methodological issues raised by our studies were provided by Michael T. Hannon, Ph.D., and John W. Meyer, Ph.D., in sociology; Alain C. Enthoven, Ph.D., Victor R. Fuchs, Ph.D., and Harold S. Luft, Ph.D., in economics; and Lincoln Moses, Ph.D., in statistics. In medicine, many physicians from the Stanford Medical School and the Palo Alto

Medical Clinic contributed to the development of the staging and physical status measures. These individuals are acknowledged by name in our 1974 technical report. We also owe a special thanks to the staffs at the four nearby hospitals in which our pilot work took place: Stanford Hospital, French Hospital in San Francisco, Memorial Hospital in San Leandro, and Alexian Brothers Hospital in San Jose. El Camino Hospital in Mountain View provided the basic information for computing costs of specific medical services.

Others have also contributed by reading drafts and commenting on our work, including anonymous reviewers for our earlier work as well as this manuscript. A partial list of such contributors would include Mark S. Blumberg, M.D., Avedis Donabedian, M.D., Stephen M. Shortell, Ph.D., Duncan Neuhauser, Ph.D., J. Joel May, Ira M. Rutkow, and Austin Ross.

In a study of this magnitude and duration, it is difficult to list all of the people who have contributed to its success. Even a list of the major cast and the organizations in which they worked is long. Names of individuals in each of the organizations listed below can be found in our three technical reports; here we acknowledge groups and organizations whose support and work was crucial to the success of this project.

First, for providing data for the study, we thank the many staff members at the Commission on Professional and Hospital Activities in Ann Arbor, Michigan, who aided in work involving patient abstract data; the technicians at each of the hospitals who collected patient-level on-site data for the Intensive Study and the staff at each hospital who cooperated in their collection; the American Medical Association, which cooperated in providing information on each participating surgeon and anesthesiologist; and the several hundred surgeons and nurses across the country who participated in the study to rank surgical procedures according to the complexity and uncertainty involved in performing them. Staff at each of the hospitals in the Intensive Study deserve special praise and much gratitude for their cooperation and contributions to this study. (These hospitals are listed in appendix B.)

Several organizations provided policy guidance and/or financial support to the team performing this work: the Policy Committee of the National Academy of Sciences; the Ad Hoc Planning Group and Committee of Principal Investors for the Institutional Differences Study (our first project); the National Center for Health Services Research and Health Care Technology, Department of Health and Human Services; the Kaiser Family Foundation; the National Institutes of Mental Health Training Grant on Organizations and Mental Health at Stanford University; the Department of Anesthesia, Stanford School of Medicine; and the Research Board of the University of Illinois at Urbana-Champaign. In each case, several members have been especially instrumental in providing valuable guidance in our research or contractual advice; they are acknowledged by name in our reports.

For work completed at the University of Illinois, several students have served ably as research assistants: Michael T. Bishop, M.D., M.B.A.; Janet L. Lauritsen, M.A.; Kimberly Sharp, M.D., Ph.D.; and Michael T. Witkowsky, M.A. Many colleagues in the sociology department and the Medical Humanities and Social Sciences Program at the College of Medicine provided helpful reviews and suggestions of the recent work presented here. We are especially indebted to Denice A. Wells, secretary for the Medical Humanities and Social Sciences Program of the College of Medicine, who provided almost all of the clerical support in preparing this manuscript, processing and reprocessing each change in wording with great patience and skill.

After noting the many people and organizations who have contributed to this work, we reiterate that the views, interpretations, and conclusions presented throughout this manuscript are the authors' own and should not be considered as representative of the organizations or people acknowledged here.

We would also like to thank each of the publishers for permission to include edited or revised versions of our previously published work. In particular, chapter 2 is an edited version from *Administrative Science Quarterly* 22(1977): 177–201. Earlier versions of chapters 7 and 11 and selected tables from chapter 6 appeared in *Medical Care* 17, no. 11 (1979): 1088–1102; 22, no. 2 (1984): 98–114, 115–25; and 22, no. 10 (1984): 967–69. Chapter 8 is an edited version of an article that appeared in *Health Services Research* 17, no. 4 (1982): 341–66; and chapter 9, of an article in *Journal of Health and Social Behavior* 19 (1978): 240–54. An earlier version of chapter 10 appeared in *Memorial Fund Quarterly/Health and Society* 57 (1979): 234–64.

Hospital Structure and Performance

Introduction: Overview of a Research Program

This volume assembles in one place some of the products of a research program conducted over more than a decade. The principal object of our work has been to describe and explain differences in the performance of hospitals in the United States. As is well known, hospitals are complex organizations and perform many types of functions. Our research has placed prime emphasis on the work that hospitals do in caring for inpatients, especially patients undergoing surgery. Two features characterize our research design: (1) the use of outcome indicators to assess the quality of hospital performance and (2) an effort to represent and measure the complex structural and personnel components that make up the modern hospital.

In this introduction, we provide a brief history of the Stanford Center for Health Care Research, the host organization under whose auspices the research was conducted. What is most important, we describe the three major data sets on which all of our studies are based. (App. A lists all of the reports, dissertations, and publications to date based on these data.)

This work has been supported by PH 43-63-65, under the sponsorship of the National Academy of Sciences; by HRA 230-75-0169 and 230-75-0173 under the National Center for Health Services Research; and by the Research Board of the University of Illinois. Basic data utilizing information from the Professional Activity Study reported in this book were supplied by the Commission on Professional and Hospital Activities of Ann Arbor, Michigan. For the IS and SIS, data were released by the seventeen participating hospitals. For the ES, the identities of individual hospitals were not revealed. CPHA performed the analyses based on individual records and reported information to us in such a way that no patient, physician, or hospital could be identified. Any analysis, interpretation, or conclusion based on these data is solely that of the authors, and CPHA specifically disclaims any responsibility for any such analysis, interpretation, or conclusion.

THE STANFORD CENTER FOR HEALTH CARE RESEARCH

The Stanford Center for Health Care Research (SCHCR) had its roots in the National Halothane Study, an investigation of the relation between halothane anesthesia and postoperative hepatic necrosis (Bunker et al. 1969). The halothane study was designed by J. Weldon Bellville, Byron W. Brown, Jr., John P. Bunker, and William H. Forrest, Jr., and managed by Forrest. In addition to the findings with regard to halothane toxicity, the study results pointed up the large differences in postsurgical mortality among the thirty-four hospitals studied. In a paper discussing this result, Moses and Mosteller (1968) called for further study of these differences among hospitals in the quality of surgical care as measured by patient outcomes.

Under the sponsorship of the National Research Council of the National Academy of Sciences, a portion of the remaining halothane study monies was set aside to pursue the question of whether hospitals did differ in their surgical outcomes by more than could be explained by differences in the patient populations they served, and if so, by how much. Further, were such differences discovered, what characteristics of hospitals might help to account for them?

The SCHCR, funded by contract to the National Academy of Sciences and administered by the National Center for Health Services Research, came into existence in June 1971 to conduct this study of *institutional differences* (IDS) in postoperative mortality (SCHCR 1974). Following the completion of this project, two related studies were carried out, both under contract to the National Center for Health Services Research. The first of these added measures of *service intensity* to enable us to relate outcome differences to the quantity and cost of services received (Forrest et al. 1977). The second added measures of *length of stay,* allowing us to further specify the relation between quality and the cost of care in hospitals (Forrest et al. 1978).

The principal investigators for all three of these projects were: William H. Forrest, Jr., associate professor in the Department of Anesthesia, Stanford University School of Medicine; Byron W. Brown, Jr., professor in the Department of Family, Community and Preventive Medicine, Stanford University School of Medicine; and W. Richard Scott, professor of sociology, Stanford University. Forrest served as director of the SCHCR. Ann Barry Flood was first associated with the project as a research assistant, and she completed her dissertation in sociology in connection with the project. She remained at the SCHCR as a research associate, taking major responsibility with Scott for designing the instruments associated with gathering data on hospital and physician staff organization and conducting analyses of the relation between hospital characteristics, costs, and patient outcomes. She is currently assistant professor of health services research in the program of Medical Humanities and Social Sciences (College of Medicine), the Department of Health and Safety Studies

(College of Applied Life Studies), and the Department of Sociology (College of Liberal Arts and Sciences) at the University of Illinois at Urbana-Champaign. Wayne Ewy began work as a research associate in biostatistics and eventually became the assistant director. Together with Brown, Ewy developed the statistical approach employed in adjusting measures of outcome and service intensity for differences in patient condition and was largely responsible for implementing these procedures. In addition to his coordinating responsibilities as director of the SCHCR, Forrest took primary responsibility for enlisting the assistance of other physicians to stage all of the operative procedures investigated. He is now manager of Preclinical Biometrics, Warner-Lambert/Parke-Davis Pharmaceutical Research Division, at Ann Arbor, Michigan. Betty Maxwell provided expert administrative support (as well as psychological counseling and group therapy to the research staff) for all of the studies. Numerous others who contributed importantly to one or another of these projects are acknowledged in the Preface.

In 1978, after the final report for the third project was completed, the SCHCR was formally dissolved. Although it was originally intended to provide a focus for continuing studies of health care systems, changes in the research priorities of some of the principal staff members, together with competing job opportunities for others, suggested that it was prudent to dissolve the Center as a formally constituted entity. In spite of the disappearance of a research base, a number of the original investigators have continued to conduct studies based on the data sets assembled to explore the relation between the characteristics of hospitals and the patient care they provide.

MAJOR DATA SETS

The Extensive Study

Two samples of hospitals constitute the basic data sets. The first, called the Extensive Study (ES), involved the use of summary data from 1,224 short-term hospitals in the United States that participated during the base study year 1972 in the Professional Activity Study (PAS) of the Commission on Professional and Hospital Activities (CPHA). CPHA performs a data collection and statistical analysis service for its subscribers based on the abstracting of information from patient records on all patients discharged from each facility. All data on patient characteristics, length of stay, and outcomes, principally mortality, were obtained from PAS patient abstracts. In order to ensure the anonymity of each of the reporting hospitals, CPHA performed some of the required analyses under the direction of Center staff.

For most of the ES studies, attention was focused on a subset of approximately 300,000 surgical patients categorized into fifteen surgical diagnostic categories. Categories were chosen to include a broad range of ages, both sexes, a variety of organ systems, a variety of surgical specialties among physicians, and surgical disease amenable to staging. Another consideration was to select categories containing a large enough number of patients who experienced death inhospital to allow estimation of outcome based on this measure. This criterion of sufficient numbers of deaths supported the inclusion of diseases either having a high mortality or occurring frequently among patients. Specific surgical procedures are listed in tables 5.1 and 11.1. The original design included several additional categories of patients to be studied in detail, but because of time and financial considerations, they were never fully implemented.

Also of interest were two additional categories of 225,000 nonsurgical patients having diagnoses similar to some of the patients treated surgically. These two groupings (surgical and nonsurgical) were regarded as the "study patients" in the ES. For these patients, data indicating the physical status of the patient on admission were obtained from the PAS abstract. The items included age, sex, several routine admission findings such as urinalysis and white blood count, and diagnosis or operation codes additional to the qualifying diagnosis and operation. Using predetermined weights, these data were used to quantify the extent of the surgical disease and the initial health status of each patient. This information was then employed to adjust subsequent measures of hospitalization outcomes, such as length of stay and death inhospital.

Finally, some much less detailed analyses were conducted utilizing all other ("nonstudy") patients discharged from the ES hospitals during 1972. Approximately 11 million patients were included in this set.

Data to characterize the organizational features of the 1,224 hospitals came from three sources. First, information was obtained on each hospital from the annual survey for 1972 conducted by the American Hospital Association (AHA 1973). This survey contains detailed information on beds, utilization, facilities and services, types of personnel, management, and financing. The second source of information was the American Medical Association's *Consolidated List of Hospitals with Approved Graduate Training Programs,* revised to 1 July 1973, listing the level of affiliation and the number of approved training programs for interns and residents, as well as the numbers of foreign and U.S. physicians enrolled in them for each hospital (AMA 1973). Third, we were able to use the PAS data to devise a variety of measures concerning the types of patients seen and the types of treatments provided in each hospital, as well as to characterize the specialties and experience of the attending physician and primary surgeon. (Additional details concerning the data assembled in connection with the ES, together with analyses based on them, are presented in chap. 5, 6, 11, and 12.)

The Intensive Study

The second sample of hospitals was a small subset of the ES hospitals. This sample, called the Intensive Study (IS), contained seventeen hospitals. From the total roster of over 1,300 hospitals participating in CPHA, we screened to obtain those voluntary or nonfederal, not-for-profit hospitals that provided short-term care for a variety of medical and surgical diagnoses, had at least 3,000 annual discharges, and had participated in PAS for at least three years. This subset of 742 hospitals was then stratified by size, the ratio of expenses to occupied beds, and teaching status, and a random sample of 300 hospitals was selected. These hospitals were then contacted to solicit their collaboration in the research. Of the 270 that responded affirmatively, a set of 32 was selected on the basis of previous stratification variables, the frequency of certain operative procedures, geographic region, and a very simply adjusted mortality rate. Of these, sixteen hospitals agreed to participate in the proposed study, which involved extensive on-site data-collection activities. In addition, one hospital administratively linked to a study hospital entered at its own expense. Although the original plan had been to select sixteen representative hospitals from the set of thirty-two, the seventeen hospitals in effect selected themselves in terms of their willingness to cooperate in the research. (The participating hospitals are listed in app. B.)

While the final sample can not be strictly described as having been randomly selected from either all U.S. hospitals or even all those participating in the ES, it contained substantial variation in both structural and performance characteristics. IS hospitals ranged in size from 149 to 634 beds, and in annual expenses per occupied bed from $28,000 to $56,000; six of the hospitals were affiliated with a medical school or had an approved and active house staff program; and they ranged in location across eleven states and all major regions of the country.

A variety of techniques and sources were exploited in order to assemble a rich assortment of data on the IS hospitals. Principal objects of study included patients; the organization of the hospital, including characteristics of its managers and employees; the organization of the medical staff; individual surgeons; and the social and economic features of the area in which the hospital was located. We briefly discuss each.

Two sets of patients were studied. The first were patients undergoing surgical treatment in the same diagnostic categories employed in the original design of the ES (or at least categories as comparable as could be devised). However, unlike all of the other patient data utilized in our research, these data were collected directly from the hospital during the time when the patient was undergoing treatment. Rather than relying on PAS patient abstracts, we had information on these patients collected by a technician employed and trained by the SCHCR staff but located on site in each study hospital. Most technicians were trained nurses, and some were members of the nursing administration in the host hospital. In addition, a highly placed liaison person was designated in each hospital to assist with the solution of any data-gathering problems, and a coordinator located at the Center supervised all phases of data collection. A manual prepared and pilot-tested prior to the onset of the study contained detailed definitions and protocols for patient selection and data recording. Center staff worked closely with the technicians throughout the ten-month study period, forwarding lists of patients' forms due and overdue, returning forms for correction, and providing assistance and direction by letter and phone.

The technicians gathered data from a number of sources within the hospital, including patient interviews; forms filled out by the patient's anesthetist, surgeon, and nurse in the postsurgery ward; chart reviews; and a follow-up patient questionnaire. In all, seven types of forms were completed on each study patient at varying time points from the evening prior to surgery to forty days following surgery, whether or not the patient had been discharged.

Each technician selected potential study patients—patients scheduled for one of the fifteen operative procedures or for relevant exploratory procedures— by examining the hospital's surgical log. The log itself was copied and mailed to the Center, permitting the correction by phone of errors of exclusion. Of the 10,563 cases qualifying for study during the ten-month period of data collection, about 80 percent, 8,593, actually were included. Losses were due chiefly to patient refusal (12 percent), surgeon refusal (3 percent), lack of critical information on disease stage or outcome (2 percent), and difficulties of classification due to multiple operative procedures (1 percent). The distribution of study patients across surgical procedures, together with other descriptive statistics, can be found in table 6.1.

This first set of patient-level data for the IS varied in a number of important ways from the patient data obtained from PAS. It was prospective rather than retrospective; it was obtained from multiple, varying sources rather than simply by abstracting from the patient's chart; it contained more complete outcome information, including assessments of morbidity at seven and forty days postsurgically as well as mortality; and it provided information on health status following discharge from the hospital for up to forty days.

One important use made of these data was to compare them with data recorded on the same patients in PAS and to contrast analytic results based on the IS and ES approaches. The results of this comparison (called the Little ES study) are reported in chapter 6.

A second study, called the Service Intensity Study (SIS), was conducted within the seventeen hospitals of the IS. The patients in the SIS overlapped somewhat with the IS patients, but the SIS relied on PAS data in order to study virtually all of the patients discharged from these hospitals during the period

May 1970–December 1973. PAS abstracts were available on approximately 670,000 patients; however, the final set of patients studied numbered 603,580. The great majority of those excluded were newborns, so that the final sample consisted of 98 percent of all other patients. Data assembled on these patients included measures of outcome, principally death inhospital; intensity of services utilized, including specific diagnostic tests such as blood chemistry tests, the use of the intensive-care unit, and the number of types of drugs received; and measures of patient condition at the time of admission.

Information on hospital characteristics and the organization of the medical staff for the IS and the SIS was obtained in a manner different from that used to collect patient data. Two teams of two interviewers each were employed and trained by Center staff to conduct interviews and distribute questionnaires in each study hospital. These data-collection activities averaged approximately two weeks per site. All interview guides and questionnaire forms were pretested in two nonstudy hospitals. Interviews were conducted with key personnel who acted as expert informants describing the characteristics and activities of their units. Personnel interviewed within each hospital included the hospital administrator, the director of the operating room, the supervisor of the recovery room, the director of the nursing service, the head nurses of patient-care units (including intensive-care units [ICUs] and wards receiving twelve or more surgical patients per year), ward supervisors, the director of pathology services, the director of radiology, the manager of the blood bank, the chiefs of surgical services, and the chiefs of anesthesia.

Types of personnel receiving questionnaires and average return rates for each category were: surgical ward and ICU staff, 75 percent ($N = 2,494$); operating-room staff, 84 percent ($N = 348$); pathologists, 59 percent ($N = 96$); radiologists, 68 percent ($N = 93$); anesthetists, 50 percent ($N = 110$); and surgeons, 56 percent ($N = 518$).

In addition to these data gathered on site, we obtained other types of information for each of the seventeen hospitals from the annual survey of the American Hospital Association for the years 1970–73. Having this information (e.g., staffing, occupancy rate, and types of facilities) available for multiple years allowed us to take into account any important changes occurring during the time of the study.

In addition to the questionnaire information noted above, which was available for about half the surgeons in the study hospitals, other sources of data were employed in order to characterize physicians treating study patients. We obtained data from the records of study hospitals or from the American Medical Association concerning the qualifications of all surgeons treating the set of IS study patients—those undergoing one of the fifteen selected surgical procedures. Working with a number code to ensure the surgeons' anonymity, we obtained information on education and board certification for virtually all of these surgeons. We used data from the PAS records to characterize the experience of all the surgeons in the study hospital, and each surgeon was asked by the technician to report the percentage of his or her practice that occurred at the study hospital. The major specialties excluded were ophthalmological and dental surgery.

It should be noted that two hospitals were dropped from analyses involving the level of training and qualifications of surgeons. One was dropped because it did not provide the requested information. The other was removed because in its use of the medical staff it differed from all of the other study hospitals: it was the only hospital in which care was provided primarily by residents and interns under the supervision of physicians in a nearby medical school; thus it was not possible to determine who the "real" attending physician for any given patient was.

The final type of data assembled for the IS and SIS concerned the characteristics of the community within which the hospital was located. Hospitals are known to vary considerably in the size of area served. In order to determine the appropriate boundary of the service area for each hospital, we asked the administrator to provide a geographic description of the area from which most of its patients were drawn. These descriptions ranged from the downtown section of the city (one hospital), to the city and surrounding county (eleven hospitals), to the city and county together with several other contiguous counties (five hospitals). Using the designated boundaries for each hospital, we assembled several types of data.

U.S. census data were employed to measure the size, median income and education level, and percentage of nonwhite residents of the population (U.S. Bureau of the Census 1973b). For the hospital that specified its community as a portion of the city, the U.S. census of housing block statistics were used (U.S. Bureau of the Census 1970). For hospitals serving more than one county, these statistics were averaged after being weighted by population size. Information on the community's age distribution was obtained from the 1970 census (U.S. Bureau of the Census 1973a), and in order to have a measure of change, information on population size and income were obtained from the 1960 census (U.S. Bureau of the Census 1962).

Information on the number of physicians and registered nurses in each service area per 100,000 population was obtained from the county and metropolitan area data on health manpower collected by the National Center for Health Statistics (U.S. Department of Health, Education, and Welfare 1971). Information on other hospitals located in the same service area was obtained from the AHA annual survey for the year 1973 (AHA 1974a). After excluding any long-term, federal, and specialized hospitals, we used selected information on the characteristics of other area hospitals to assess the degree of competition present for the study hospitals. (Additional details regarding the data assembled for the IS, as well as analyses of these data, are to be found in chaps. 2, 5, 6, 8, and 9; and for the SIS, in chaps. 5, 6, 7, and 10.)

The Surgeon and Postsurgical Nurse Survey

The third and final data set utilized in these studies was a set of scores designed to assess the perceived level of difficulty represented by the surgical work—both operations and postoperative care—performed. To obtain these judgments, a set of scales was developed to assess the relative complexity and uncertainty of selected procedures as perceived by surgeons and nurses. It was desirable to obtain these measures from a sample independent of the participants in the study hospitals—both ES and IS hospitals—so two national samples, one of surgeons and one of nurses, were drawn and asked to serve as expert raters of these variables. A list of seventy-one surgical procedures was selected to represent the full range of complexity/uncertainty and to include operations most frequently performed. Six indicator questions were developed for each group of expert raters—three to assess complexity and three to assess uncertainty—and each rater was asked to distinguish among the seventy-one procedures, on a scale from one to nine, on one of the six questions. For example, as an indicator of uncertainty, some surgeons were asked to order the procedures in terms of "the extent to which the surgeon's work is standardized." The surgeons were asked to consider their work limited to the time in the operating suite, and the nurses, to the first seven days postsurgically.

As noted, two samples of raters were selected. All surgeon raters were members of the American College of Physicians and Surgeons and were selected by a stratified random-sampling procedure taking into account geographic region, community versus medical school practice, and type of surgical specialty. A sample of 1,200 surgeons produced usable responses from 623, a return rate of 52 percent. Nurse raters were selected by a two-step procedure. First, a national sample of hospitals was selected using size, teaching status, and geographical region as stratifying variables. Then, with the cooperation of the director of nursing in each hospital, a sample was drawn of ward nurses with more than one year of nursing experience in care for postsurgical patients, as well as experience with a broad range of postsurgical cases. Of a total sample of 545 nurses contacted, 354 produced usable responses, a return rate of 65 percent.

Returns indicated a very high degree of consensus among both nursing and surgeon raters as well as between the two panels in judgments of the relative difficulty of surgical treatment and care. Although we had hoped for theoretical reasons to distinguish between surgical complexity and surgical uncertainty, the indicator questions were not successful in this regard: correlations of indicators were as large across as within the two dimensions. Intercorrelations for the six indicators among surgeon raters ranged from an r (Pearson product-moment correlation) of .53 to an r of .98, with a mean r of .82. Among the nursing panel the consensus was even higher, with r ranging from .96 to .99. (A more complete description of the scales for measuring surgical difficulty, together with descriptions of the complexity and uncertainty scores assigned by surgeon and nurse raters to all seventy-one procedures, is reported by Schoonhoven and associates at the SCHCR [Schoonhoven et al. 1980]. Additional information and analyses utilizing these measures of surgical complexity are found in chaps. 2 and 11.)

PART I
Hospital Structure

1 · Conceptualizing Hospital Structure

W. Richard Scott and Ann Barry Flood

The structural features of organizations vary greatly, and students of organizations are interested in understanding both the determinants and the consequences of this variation. Of course, the greatest variations occur between differing types of organizations—between, for example, shoe factories and airline companies—but even within a given type, considerable variation may exist. This volume focuses attention on hospitals in the United States during the decade of the 1970s. In this place and time, hospitals exhibited great diversity—in size, in complexity of facilities, in qualifications of staff, and in variety of goals, such as inpatient and outpatient care, prevention, teaching, and research.

In this chapter, we seek to develop a conception of hospital structure. What are the major components or elements of these organizational forms? Along what dimensions do they vary? The conceptual model to be developed should take into account the purpose of our research. Organizations are complex systems, and which parts or aspects are salient varies with the types of questions to be addressed.

As described in the Introduction, the primary focus of interest in most of the studies conducted by the Stanford Center for Health Care Research (SCHCR) has been to discern and explain variations in hospital performance, in particular the quality of inpatient care for surgical patients. This interest has shaped our conception of hospital characteristics—the features selected for analysis, as well as arguments concerning the way these features act to influence performance. Had we elected to examine research productivity or training quality within hospitals, we would have developed a different model of hospital structure. From our perspective, the quality of patient care is an aspect of organizational *effectiveness*. As we discuss in detail in chapter 4, effectiveness, like structure, is a complex concept, with many meanings and many possible measures. In chapter 5 we detail our own definitions and describe and defend our reliance on outcome measures to assess quality of surgical care.

In addition to assessing and measuring the effectiveness of performance and examining its relation to characteristics of hospital structure, we are also interested in other relationships. Some of our analyses examine, for a given level of quality, what features of hospitals are associated with a higher intensity of services or with longer lengths of stay (and hence higher costs for patient care). Such studies focus on the relative *efficiency* of the hospital. Both of these concerns are similar in that they emphasize the *consequences* of organizational structures. In analyses of this type we use the structural characteristics of hospitals as independent variables that are viewed as influencing hospital performance, its effectiveness, and its efficiency. In other studies hospital structure is viewed as a dependent variable. We seek to identify the determinants of structural variation. In doing so, we place explanatory emphasis on the *environment* within which the hospital is situated or on the characteristics of its *technology*—the nature of the work being performed.

All of our studies, however, share in common a view of the hospital as a place where complex work is performed. While such a view may seem commonplace to many, it is only one of many approaches available when examining organizations. Organizations provide, among other things, a setting where persons compete for status and resources, where symbols are developed and borrowed, where power is generated and employed, where participants teach and learn, and where knowledge is created. To focus on organizations as settings for work is to explore an important but limited part of the complex reality that is organizational structure.

We begin by examining the characteristics of hospital structure, since they may help us to account for variations in performance, especially effectiveness. We then consider more briefly factors that we expect to help us to account for variations in hospital structure. In both sections we describe hypotheses that have guided the collection and analyses of our data. Then, in a final section, we note connections between these two interests.

STRUCTURE AND EFFECTIVENESS

If hospitals are found to differ in terms of the effectiveness of their performance, how are such differences to be explained? Our theoretical approach emphasizes organizational differences, but what kind of organization is a hospital? On the one hand, it is a *bureaucratic* structure characterized by a highly developed horizontal division of labor, a hierarchical authority system, and an elaborate structure of roles and rules for controlling behavior. The two clusters of bureaucratic variables to which we gave primary attention were (1) differentiation, or the division of labor among participants and subgroups; and (2) coordination, which includes measures of personal and impersonal control systems, such as rules, as well as communication.

In addition to being a complex bureaucratic structure, a hospital is a *professional* organization. Professional participants, especially physicians, take responsibility for and execute some of the most fateful tasks relating to the quality of patient care. Professionals undergo long periods of training and socialization designed to enable them to perform complex work responsibly. In addition, in a hospital, physicians organize themselves as a medical staff to secure an arena of professional decision making and activity independent of the domains within which administrators and others such as nurses hold power and to promote fidelity to professional standards among their own members. The professional character of hospital organization adds two additional clusters of variables: (3) the qualifications of professional staff participants, as assessed by training and experience; and (4) the power of the medical staff, both in relation to other groups exercising control in the hospital and in terms of its ability to select and control its members.

In an important sense, bureaucratic and professional structures represent alternative arrangements for the performance of complex tasks (see Freidson 1973; and Scott 1981, 153–56, 222–24). From this perspective, individual professionals may be viewed as miniature organizations, each equipped with general principles providing internalized controls that guide the application of a broad repertory of skills to a range of specific problems. This approach to rationalizing work differs from that of the conventional bureaucratic solution which subdivides work among many participants and coordinates and controls their activities through externally imposed rules and hierarchies.

These contrasting approaches to complex work come together in varying combinations in professional organizations (see Scott 1982). In some types, individual practitioners, although subject to some external constraints, exercise a large amount of discretion as they independently carry on their professional work. Such organizations operate as little more than collections of facilities and general managerial services to support the efforts of individual practitioners. In the past, some hospitals have operated primarily as "the doctor's workshop," giving practitioners virtually free rein in performing their medical tasks (see Somers and Somers 1961, 67–72). In other types, administrators tend to dominate professional work, subordinating professional activities to administrative requirements and permitting individual practitioners, particularly nonphysician health professionals in hospitals, such as nurses, social workers, or technicians, to exercise relatively little discretion. In still other types, professionals organize themselves, as in a hospital medical staff, to oversee and coordinate the performance of individual professionals. These professional control systems vary greatly in their influence on practitioner behavior.

Since our primary objective was to examine the effect of hospital characteristics on the quality of patient care, attention was concentrated on those participants and units most directly and most centrally involved in patient-care activities—in what may be termed the "technical core" of the hospital (see Thompson 1967). The proposed dimensions and units of hospital structure were selected to emphasize those features that had a direct or at least strong indirect impact on patient care. The skill and experience of certain participants, such as physicians and nurses providing care, are factors of obvious importance, but no less critical are those work arrangements and facilities that facilitate or inhibit their decisions and actions.

Keeping in mind the dual nature of hospitals as both bureaucratic and professional organizations, we discuss in more detail the four clusters of structural variables as well as three classes of variables used primarily as controls. Following this, we argue that most of these distinctions can usefully be applied to a variety of types of units within hospitals.

Dimensions of Structure

Four major dimensions of hospital structure* have been identified:

differentiation, the extent to which separate functions, goals, or tasks are assigned to different organizational subunits or to different participants

coordination, the extent to which organizational resources are expended to integrate the activities of subunits or members of the organization

power, the extent to which members or subunits can influence organizational decisions or exert control over other subunits or their own members

staff qualifications, the level of education, training, and work experience of hospital employees and medical staff

Each of these dimensions has been further defined by the identification of a number of variables focusing attention on different aspects of the dimension. For example, within the dimension of differentiation, we have measured such variables as the division of labor (e.g., occupational specialization), the variety of services offered, and subunit specialization; and within the dimension of staff qualifications are included the level of training for differing types of personnel, the duration of work experience, and professional orientation or commitment. Some measures within dimensions may be expected to correlate highly, while others are likely to be independent or even negatively associated. For example, various mechanisms of coordination, such as frequency of supervision or the extensiveness of rule manuals, may represent alternative modes of control, so that the presence of one reduces the likelihood of the other.

Three additional structural dimensions are of somewhat less interest the-

*Portions of the remaining sections of this chapter are adapted from Scott, Forrest, and Brown 1976.

oretically but were expected to have significant effects on other structural variables as well as on hospital performance:

size, the scale of the hospital or its subunits
resources, hospital assets and expenditures on patient care
teaching status, the extent to which the hospital is linked to a medical school or conducts approved training programs for residents and interns

Measures for all of the structural variables, although of varying detail and complexity, were obtained for all hospitals in both studies—the 17 hospitals in the Intensive Study (IS) and the 1,224 hospitals in the Extensive Study (ES). They are defined more fully in subsequent chapters as appropriate, and detailed descriptions of the measures developed for the IS are contained in SCHCR 1974 (173–89) and Forrest et al. 1977 (116–45), and for the ES in SCHCR 1974 (48–56) and Forrest et al. 1978 (66–96).

Organizational Units

In addition to identifying multiple dimensions and multiple variables within each dimension, we also recognize the presence of multiple types of organizational units within hospitals. More so than most organizations, hospitals are made up of several types of units whose structural features may not closely correspond. Many such units might be distinguished, but our purposes were served by the identification of six types:

1. *hospitalwide organization,* those features that characterize the hospital organization as a whole or refer to those structures relevant to the functioning of the entire organization, such as the central hospital administration;
2. *surgical ward organization,* characteristics of all patient-care wards or intensive-care units servicing twelve or more surgical patients within a calendar year;
3. *operating room organization,* characteristics of the operating room, defined to include the recovery room, isolated for attention because of its central role in the treatment of surgical patients;
4. *ancillary service unit organization,* characteristics of three units—radiology and nuclear medicine, clinical and anatomical pathology, and the blood bank—assumed to be critical to the treatment of surgical patients, particularly for the subset selected for detailed study;
5. *medical staff organization,* the arrangements developed by the medical staff for admitting new physicans, controlling the activities of its members, and collaborating with those who manage the hospital; and
6. *individual surgeons,* whose individual characteristics may have an independent impact on hospital performance, in particular the quality of patient care, since individual professional practitioners perform somewhat autonomously of hospital or medical staff structures.

Each of these organizational units may exhibit differing values on the primary structural dimensions identified. This possibility is illustrated by analyses of the intercorrelation of similar structural variables across multiple units. Such data were reported in Scott, Forrest, and Brown 1976 (83, table 6), where measures of differentiation are shown to vary widely across such units as surgical wards, the operating room, and the medical staff within the same hospital.

Data on all six types of units were collected in the IS. However, reliance on existing data sources for the ES restricted studies based on these data to hospitalwide measures and some medical staff characteristics.

Structure and Performance

In our examination of the relation between hospital structure and performance, many hypotheses were generated and explored. Many of these hypotheses rest on arguments contained in the general organizational literature, as well as on previous studies of health care organizations. Here we attempt to describe and illustrate only the types of hypotheses guiding our research. Throughout our work we assume *ceteris paribus* for each hypothesis. More specific discussions are to be found in the empirical chapters of this volume. (A comprehensive review of studies relating hospital structural features to both cost and quality is contained in chap. 3.)

One general line of argument relates the extent of differentiation to the effectiveness of performance. While previous analysts, such as Blau and Schoenherr (1971), have identified several varieties of differentiation, including horizontal, vertical, and spatial, we focus only on the horizontal—the extent to which different types of goals or tasks are assigned to different units or members of the organization.

Differentiation can occur within an organization at both the departmental and the individual level. Measures of departmental differentiation include the number of different patient-care services and facilities provided at the hospital and the division of the medical staff into specialized components. Individual differentiation can refer either to the subdivision of work within a task or to the specialization of workers by types of tasks. Since we are dealing with professional performers, we emphasize the latter, measuring the extent to which individual physicians specialized in one or another type of patient care. Using these types of measures of differentiation, our expectation would be that

H1: The greater the differentiation among subunits and among professional providers, the greater the level of organizational effectiveness.

Several studies of hospitals have emphasized the importance of coordination and control as factors affecting the quality of care. In their study involving ten hospitals, Georgopoulos and Mann (1962) placed primary emphasis on mechanisms of coordination. They found a wide range of indicators of coordination activities as reported by hospital staff members—including preventive, regulatory, and promotive coordination—to be associated with high-quality nursing care and with overall hospital care as assessed by staff participants. These results were largely replicated in a second study of ten hospitals by Longest (1974). And research by Shortell, Becker, and Neuhauser (1976) in forty-two acute-care hospitals showed an association among measures of coordination between nursing care and support departments such as radiology and the laboratory and the quality of care.

Two studies suggest that coordination among physicians may also be conducive to higher-quality care. A study by Neuhauser (1971) of thirty community hospitals reported positive correlations between the number and frequency of various reports by means of which medical work is controlled and coordinated and several measures of the quality of care. And a study by Rhee (1977) of medical care in Hawaii reported that quality was higher in more highly organized medical settings.

These and related studies only underline the general proposition from organizational theory concerning the importance of coordination when complex tasks are being performed (see, for example, Lawrence and Lorsch 1967; and Galbraith 1973). Thus, our general prediction is that

H2: The greater the resources devoted to coordination, the greater the level of organizational effectiveness.

Organizational theorists also have argued that the dimensions of differentiation and coordination are connected. Differentiation is expected to be an organizational response to complexity of work; and the higher the level of differentiation, the more effort needs to be devoted to coordination (see Lawrence and Lorsch 1967). Indeed, it is possible that the advantages that accrue to organizations from specialization are only reaped when such differentiation is matched by adequate levels of coordination. Thus, a "contingency" prediction would be that

H3: When the differentiation among organizational units is high, the more effort expended to coordinate those units, the greater the level of organizational effectiveness.

Obviously, this general proposition is relevant to and can be tested utilizing various organizational units within the hospital setting. We expect not only amount but also type of coordination to have important effects, and the appropriateness of various mechanisms of coordination will vary depending on the nature of the work within and the interdependencies among organizational units (see Thompson 1967; and Neuhauser 1971). Where interdependence is not high and many of the activities can be routinized, administrators and clerical personnel can manage the necessary coordinating tasks. We did not attempt to develop measures of effectiveness for the performance of the more routine hospital tasks (e.g., record keeping, laboratory testing, dietary services, and housekeeping) but would expect them to be better performed under conditions of high levels of differentiation and of administrative coordination. Our expectation would be that

> H4: When the differentiation among hospital units performing routine tasks is high, the greater the ratio of hospital managerial and coordinative staff to other types of workers, the greater the level of effectiveness for these services.

Like many other types of organizations, hospitals depend on hierarchical controls and vertical linkages for the coordination and control of routine tasks, but like other kinds of professional organizations, they rely heavily on lateral modes of coordination. Such linkages are particularly crucial for units whose work activities are highly interdependent, as may be the case for surgical wards and the operating suite. Thus, our expectations would be that

> H5: The greater the frequency of horizontal contacts between the operating suite personnel and the surgical ward personnel, the better the quality of surgical care.

Turning to the dimension of power, two types of arguments relating to effectiveness can be illustrated. First, following Tannenbaum (1968), we argue that organizations vary in the total amount of power that all groups of participants exercise over one another. In some organizations little influence is exerted by any group of participants, while in others many groups exercise high levels of influence. Previous research in a variety of types of organizations suggests that the more total power exercised within an organization by its participants, the more effective that organization. Thus

> H6: The greater the overall levels of power exercised by various groups of hospital participants over decisions, the higher the level of hospital effectiveness.

Second, following the work of Roemer and Friedman (1971), we expect the nature of the medical staff organization to have important effects on the quality of care. We focus, naturally, on staff control of surgeons and surgical work. The relative power of the staff to exercise control over surgeons can be assessed using such indicators as the stringency of admissions procedures for staff membership and surgical privileges and the types of peer review mechanisms employed. We expect that

> H7: The greater the power of the surgical staff organization over its members, the better the quality of surgical care.

The qualifications of hospital participants can be viewed as both an individual-level and an organizational variable. While individual workers, not hospitals, have training and experience, hospitals do have influence over the characteristics of their personnel. Hospitals recruit and either retain or lose staff members, both employees and physicians. Overall levels of staff training and experience are important characteristics of hospital structure. Thus, at the hospital level, we would expect that

H8a: The higher the average qualifications of hospital staff, the better the quality of care.

And, at the individual physician level,

H8b: The higher the level of relevant training and experience possessed by the individual surgeon, the higher the average quality of care experienced by his or her patients.

ENVIRONMENT, TECHNOLOGY, AND STRUCTURE

In some analyses, we treat the characteristics of hospital structure as dependent variables—as features to be explained. For these studies, the principal types of independent variables used are characteristics of the environment or context within which the hospital operates and characteristics of the technology employed by the hospital.

Environment and Structure

Organizations are open systems, strongly shaped by the characteristics of their environment. The demographic and socioeconomic structure of population in the area served, the number and types of physicians and other types of health care providers, and the number and types of competing facilities are expected to influence the structural features of hospitals. We also expected various types of connections between hospitals and their environments to influence hospital structure. For example, hospitals seek various types of accreditations from external review bodies as a form of legitimation. Some hospitals are affiliated with medical schools, and others are part of a larger hospital system.

Previous organizational research suggests that hospitals serving a more varied group of patients and a more diverse set of physicians will exhibit a more differentiated structure (see Aiken and Hage 1968). Consistent with this general perspective, Comstock and Schrager (1979) proposed hypotheses of the following sort:

H9: The more diverse the education level or age distribution and the greater the proportion of nonwhites in a community, the more varied the demands for health care services and thus the greater the differentiation of services provided by hospitals in that community.

H10: The greater the variety of physician specialties in a community, the greater the differentiation of hospital services.

The structural characteristics of hospitals are expected not only to reflect such "demand" characteristics of environments but also to be responsive to salient "supply" features. Thus, we would expect hospitals to be responsive to such community resources as financial support and the availability of skilled health care personnel, in particular the number of physicians and registered nurses in the community. This suggests that

H11: The greater the financial and personnel resources available to hospitals in a community, the greater the differentiation of hospital services.

Finally, it is also possible to examine the effect of resources on the extent of duplication of services among hospitals.

These and related hypotheses were tested by Comstock and Schrager (1979) with data from the seventeen IS hospitals and their associated service areas. Because their focus was on the environmental impact on the structure of services in an area, Comstock and Schrager augmented the basic IS data set with information on the types of facilities found in all area hospitals, information available from the American Hospital Association's *Guide to the Health Care Field* (AHA 1974a). Differentiation of hospital services was defined as simply the number of different types of hospital services provided by community hospitals. The AHA data were also used to compute a measure of service duplication within each area.

Comstock and Schrager found, as expected, that differentiation of services within an area was strongly associated with population diversity (with the exception of percentage of nonwhites) and physician specialization, the latter variable having the strongest association. Area financial and personnel resources were also strongly associated with service differentiation. Finally, contrary to expectation, they found that the higher the ratio of physicans to population, the greater the extent of duplication of service facilities across hospitals in the service area.

Although as just illustrated, environmental characteristics can be employed as independent variables in order to examine their impact on structural features of hospitals, in most of the research reported in this volume they are used primarily as contextual measures, and we seek to control for their effects in order to examine other variables of interest. For example, in many of the studies, we control for hospital size (a feature of ambiguous meaning, since it reflects both environmental demand and organizational response [see Scott 1981, 235]) and for affiliation with a medical school. And in studies involving measures of service intensity and costs, we control for the effects of region of the country, since this variable has been shown to influence length of stay and, hence, consumption of services.

Membership in a hospital system is one of the most publicized developments on the contemporary hospital scene. Although most hospitals in the United States have been and continue to be independent or "free-standing" organizations, an increasing number have become affiliated with corporate systems managing more than one hospital (Starr 1982). The American Hospital Association conducted a special survey on system membership at the time of our study (AHA 1974b) and found that about 15 percent of community hospitals were members of hospital systems. Of these system hospitals, about 30 percent were religious chains, almost 25 percent were mergers, and altogether about 25 percent were investor-owned. By the early 1980s over 30 percent of all acute-care hospitals in the United States had entered into some kind of formal system (see Goldsmith 1981; and Ermann and Gabel 1984); of these, about 40 percent were investor-owned (AHA 1985).

Our own analyses, however, do not place great emphasis on system membership. There are several reasons for this. System membership was not a highly salient issue during the 1970s, when most of our data were collected. While we have information on whether hospitals in our samples were affiliated with a system (two of the seventeen hospitals in the IS shared a common medical staff organization, but none was in a true hospital system at the time of our study), we lack detailed information on the structural characteristics of these systems, which are known to vary widely, from loose consortiums to tightly coupled units (see Zuckerman 1979; and Brown and McCool 1980). Further, survey results reported by Alexander and Cobbs (1984) based on data from over 160 multihospital systems revealed that only 16 percent of these forms had developed an integrated medical staff by 1983; that is, in 84 percent of the systems recently surveyed, each member hospital had its own separate medical staff organization. Given our primary interest in the quality of inpatient care, we have placed great stress on the characteristics of medical staff organization. Moreover, as we describe in chapters 8 and 9, these characteristics were found to be among the most important predictors of this measure of performance. These results suggest that even in a population increasingly comprising multisystem forms, as the more peripheral structures have been transformed, the internal "technical-core" features of hospitals may not have undergone as substantial changes. Thus, our lack of attention to system membership of the hospitals studied in most of the analyses reported in this volume, while certainly a drawback, probably has had little impact on the results observed and the conclusions drawn.

Technology and Structure

Technology refers broadly to the nature of the work performed by an organization, and it has been shown to be a major factor in determining the characteristics of organizational structure, including the qualifications of the participants who occupy the structure (see Woodward 1965; and Perrow 1967). We emphasize particularly the kinds of demands the work poses for those who carry out the principal tasks. Complex organizations like hospitals carry on many types of work, but we focus attention on professionals caring for patients—in particular the work involved in treating surgical patients.

Two dimensions of technology that are widely recognized as important are complexity and uncertainty. We defined *complexity* as the extent to which work activities or materials are characterized by many and intricately related tasks or parts and *uncertainty* as the extent to which work activities or materials are characterized by a lack of predictability. As described in the Introduction (and in more detail in Schoonhoven et al. 1980), we obtained ratings on each of these dimensions for a large number of surgical procedures from a national sample of surgeons and surgical nurses. As another indicator of the complexity/uncertainty of surgical work, we assessed the risk level associated with the selected types of surgical procedures by measuring the probability of death associated with each type of operation.

These measures of technology can be applied either to work performed by an individual participant or to work carried on by an organizational unit. For example, hypotheses such as the following can be tested at the level of the individual worker:

H12: The greater the uncertainty/complexity of work performed, the higher the qualification of individual participants.

And at the level of the organizational subunit, we can examine hypotheses such as the following:

H13: The greater the predictability of the workflow for an organizational unit, the greater the standardization of policies and procedures within the unit.

H14: The greater the predictability of the workflow for an organizational subunit, the greater the centralization of decision making within the unit.

These and similar hypotheses illustrate the kinds of arguments we examine to account for differences in the structural features of hospitals (see chap. 2). A final set of hypotheses, described below, considers both technical and structural features in combination in order to account for differences in performance.

Technology, Structure, and Performance

The hypotheses described below are labeled contingency predictions because they take into account the match between structure and technology in predicting hospital performance. Previous theoretical and empirical work on organizational effectiveness by Woodward (1965), Lawrence and Lorsch (1967), and others suggests that structures well suited to one type of task may be poorly suited to another, so that the nature of the work being performed should be taken into account in predicting performance by type of structure. To the extent that hospitals or their subunits perform surgical work varying in difficulty, structural units of a given configuration may be expected to vary in their success depending on the nature of the fit or match.

An earlier prediction was that higher staff qualifications were associated with better-quality care. This hypothesis implies a monotonic relationship between the two variables. However, Roemer and Friedman (1971) have argued that the relationship is contingent instead. When the task is complex or uncertain, higher staff qualifications are a necessity; however, when the task is easy, less qualified physicians may perform as well as the highly qualified. This suggests that

> H15: For the performance of tasks that are more complex or more uncertain, the higher the level of qualifications of the staff, the better the quality of care.

Structural differentiation may be viewed as an important organizational response to work complexity—one that enhances effectiveness. We can reformulate our earlier hypothesis to incorporate performance as follows:

> H16: When the complexity of the technology is high, the greater the differentiation of structure, the better the quality of care.

Although these and a number of other contingent predictions are tested in the following chapters, it is important to recognize the potential complexity of these relations, which, as our colleague Schoonhoven (1981) has argued, assert the presence of an interaction effect but usually fail to specify the functional form it may take. Schoonhoven's work illustrates some of the problems and possibilities of contingency analyses by examining a variety of possible types of contingent relations between hospital structure and technology and the quality of surgical care.

A SYNTHETIC MODEL

If we collect and abstract from the general arguments made regarding both the determinants and the consequences of organizational structure, we arrive at

Figure 1.1. Synthetic model of hospital structure and performance

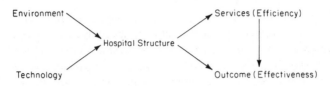

the diagram depicted in figure 1.1. This model provides a good vehicle for synthesizing and summarizing our interests and for introducing the analyses reported in this volume. At the center of all of our studies is the structure of the hospital and its associated medical staff organization. We view this structure as multidimensional and multilayered, and we are interested in describing and analyzing the manner in which work is divided and coordinated, the kinds of personnel that participate, and the manner in which they exert influence over one another.

The structural features of hospitals are seen as partially determined by the environment within which the hospital operates—by the demographic and social and medical features of the community within which it is located. A related determinant is the technology, defined as the types of demands made upon the organization by the complexity/uncertainty of the problems posed by the types of patients treated. While organizations do not invariably adapt to the conditions of their environments and the demands posed by their technologies, we assume that most attempt to do so, in part for reasons of self-interest and survival.

While determinants of structural features of hospitals are likely to be of interest primarily to students of organization and practicing administrators, a concern for the consequences of hospital structure is likely to be more widely shared. Health care providers, patients, and those with more general interests in planning and policy issues are all likely to be interested in hospital effectiveness and efficiency, their correlates and causes.

In our studies, efficiency is assessed primarily in terms of measures of service intensity and the length of patient stay. The principal outcome of interest is the patient's condition following treatment, measured in terms of morbidity and mortality in the IS and mortality in the ES. We are interested in determining which characteristics of hospitals are associated with observed differences in services and outcomes. (Of course, other factors, principally the patient's condition on admission, also determine service levels and outcomes, so that we must take such effects into account before we can evaluate hospital factors [see chap. 4].) Both classical microeconomic and contingency theory arguments suggest that assuming competition, there are pressures on organizations to reduce costs and increase quality. While it is not obvious that hospitals in the mid-1970s were subject to strong market pressures, most of our predictions presume that hospitals do attempt to adapt their structures so as to improve the quality of care.

Finally, we are interested in determining whether there is an association between the intensity of services provided and the effectiveness of the treatment as assessed by patient outcomes. Some health economists have argued that once a given level of health care has been attained, there is little or no association between levels of services and health outcomes (see, for example, Fuchs 1974, 16). We can assess this relationship using detailed measures of service intensity available in the IS (see chap. 7).

All of the chapters contained in this volume probe one or another of the relationships depicted in figure 1.1. Using a variety of data sources and a variety of techniques, we attempt to improve our understanding of the manner in which environmental context and technology help to account for differences in the structural features of hospitals and how, in turn, these features help to account for differences in the performance of hospitals. We argue that the results of testing our hypotheses, although based on data characterizing hospitals in the 1970s, have important implications for current theoretical, policy, and management concerns regarding the relations between hospital structure and performance.

2 · Technology and the Structure of Hospital Subunits: Distinguishing Individual and Workgroup Effects

Donald E. Comstock and W. Richard Scott

It seems clear that work that is more routine can be done effectively and efficiently by bureaucratic organizations, whereas less routine work requires more flexible, less hierarchical, and less formalized organizations. Although this view relating technology and structure has manifold roots, its origin can be clearly seen in March and Simon's (1958, 141–50) discussion of the use of performance programs—detailed rules for determining what an individual does and how he or she is to do it—as an organizational device to overcome the cognitive limits on rationality. When work is predictable, effectiveness and efficiency are enhanced by the development of clear decision rules and operating procedures that allow minimal discretion to individuals. But when work is not predictable, performance programs cannot be developed, and individuals must be called upon to make the best judgments of which they are capable. Later theoretical and empirical work (Burns and Stalker 1961; Litwak 1961; Woodward 1965; Perrow 1967) focused less on the situation of the individual and more on the structural features of organizations (e.g., division of labor, span of control, formalization, and centralization) as these relate to the work being performed.

Nevertheless, after two decades of research, we still cannot evaluate the importance of technology as a determinant of organizational structure. As the number of empirical studies examining the relation between an organization's technology and its social structure grows, so does the confusion about how these variables are related. While several studies report strong correlations between technology and various components of social structure (Woodward 1965; Hage and Aiken 1969; Khandwalla 1974), others show no strong associa-

For an earlier version of this chapter see Comstock and Scott 1977.

tions (Hickson, Pugh, and Pheysey 1969; Mohr 1971; Child and Mansfield 1972).

PREVIOUS STUDIES

Some of the confusion in research findings stems from the somewhat misplaced creativity of researchers who seem reluctant to replicate definitions or measures. Thus, current measures of technology rest on different conceptions. Some, for example, emphasize the nature of the materials, some the operations employed, and others the knowledge used in the work process (Hickson, Pugh, and Pheysey 1969; Lynch 1974). Also some concentrate on different phases of the work process, either inputs, throughputs, or outputs (Scott 1975), and some focus on different dimensions of the concept, for example, task difficulty and task variability (Van de Ven and Delbecq 1974), hardness of materials (Rushing 1968), manageability of tasks and materials (Mohr 1971) or workflow integration (Hickson, Pugh, and Pheysey 1969). Similarly, many different structural factors have been examined, ranging from the use of sophisticated controls (Khandwalla 1974) to the style of supervision (Mohr 1971). Even when similar variables have been used, such as formalization or centralization, they are seldom operationalized to maximize comparability.

Such problems, while annoying, are fairly visible and so subject to correction. A source of confusion that is less apparent is the variation in the organizational level at which concepts of technology and structure are applied (Grimes and Klein 1973), although there does appear to be growing recognition of the importance of distinguishing among at least three possible levels: (1) that of the individual participant, (2) that of the workgroup or subunit, and (3) that of the larger organization (Udy 1965).

It is, of course, desirable to be able to assess technology and structure at the organizational level, but such efforts are extremely hazardous. Most research rests on an implicit assumption of homogeneity (Scott et al. 1972), positing uniformity of work and structural forms across participants and departments, although we know that differentiation is characteristic of complex organizations. Large variations in structural units within organizations have been documented by Hall (1962) and Lawrence and Lorsch (1967), among others, yet attempts to develop overall measures of technology and structure by averaging the characteristics of subunits have continued. Thus, Hickson, Pugh, and Pheysey (1969) combined data gathered by interviews with chief executives and a number of department heads into a single measure—workflow integration—for the organization as a whole. And Hage and Aiken (1969), while careful to give greater weight to the reports of the supervisory staff, combined worker and supervisor responses across departments to arrive at a single measure of routineness of work in health and welfare agencies. Similarly, structures that are likely to exhibit considerable diversity in centralization or in formalization, for example, are characterized by an average score reported for the organization. In our view, it would be more appropriate to conceive of organizational structure as an overarching framework of relationships linking subunits of considerable diversity and to attempt to develop measures that capture the distinctive characteristics of this suprastructure.

Two analysts have attempted to deal specifically with the problem of technological variation within organizations and still focus on the organizational level. Woodward (1965) avoided the issue somewhat by restricting attention to the "production system" of the organization and confining her research to a sample of manufacturing concerns. Even so, she found that in a sample of 100 organizations, 8 had two systems of production, while 4 others eluded categorization because their production systems were "extremely mixed" (38–40). Khandwalla (1974, 81) likewise focused on the operations performed by the production units of manufacturing firms but explicitly recognized that "most manufacturing firms of any size operate not one but several technologies." To capture this variation, Khandwalla allowed respondents to rate the extent to which each of five major types of technologies was used in the manufacturing processes of their organizations but then largely lost this variety through a crudely weighted scale combining scores into a general index. In general, however, Khandwalla's choice of structural variables—the extent of vertical integration and decentralization of top decision making—seems better calculated than most to measure general features of organizational structure.

Other analysts have examined the relation between technology and structure at the level of the workgroup or department, both within single organizations (Bell 1967; Grimes and Klein 1973; Hrebiniak 1974; Van de Ven and Delbecq 1974) and across organizations (Hall 1962; Kovner 1966; Mohr 1971; Simpson 1972). Although it was recognized in these studies that organizations may be composed of subunits with different technologies, measures were often based on the characteristics of tasks performed by individual workers. Such summary measures, again, require the assumption of homogeneity. While this assumption is more tenable at the subunit level than at the organizational level, it may still lead to distortion, since many workgroups and most departments include different types of work. In addition, concentrating on the characteristics of individual tasks so as to arrive at some modal task measure may lead the analyst to overlook those characteristics of technology distinctive to the subunit level, such as measures of variety of work or characteristics of workflow.

Finally, a few studies have focused on the relation between task characteristics and work arrangements at the level of the individual participant. Hrebiniak (1974) performed analyses at both the individual and the workgroup level, while Dornbusch and Scott (1975) concentrated on the individual level. Indeed, the latter study, recognizing that individual workers may perform a variety of tasks that are in turn associated with varied structural arrangements, focused on selected types of tasks carried out by individuals. For example, research tasks carried out by a faculty member within a university were shown to be associated with a different set of control arrangements than were teaching tasks performed by the same person (Dornbusch and Scott 1975, 232–42).

These different research approaches suggest that it is useful to distinguish among at least three levels of organizational analysis: individual, subunit, and organization. Characteristics of technology at one level may not be reflected directly at some other level. Thus, it is quite possible for individual workers to be performing complex tasks in the framework of a relatively simple administrative system, for example, physicians working in a group-practice clinic. Conversely, individual workers may carry out a few simple tasks as part of a technology that is highly complex when viewed at the departmental or organizational level, as in the case of workers on an assembly line (Mohr 1971).

Even at the same organizational level, predictions linking technology and structure should take into account the nature of the variables. Measures at the workgroup or subunit level may involve aggregation of the characteristics of individuals or their tasks—what Lazarsfeld and Menzel (1961) refer to as analytic variables—for example, the average level of difficulty of work performed within a subunit. Although clearly a measure at the subunit level, this type of variable should relate more closely to aggregated characteristics of individuals, such as average qualifications, than to more global characteristics of the workgroup such as the centralization of decision making. The research reported in this paper concentrated attention on the level of the workgroup or subunit. Within this level, however, we attempted to differentiate those variables that summarized characteristics of individual work from those that described the work of the subunit as whole. Like many previous discussions, we focused on the extent to which the tasks and workflows were predictable. While other aspects of technology, such as complexity, analyzability, or even noise level, might have important implications for structure, our concern was not to develop comprehensive measures of technology but to test the thesis that measures taken at different levels of organization may reveal different relationships.

A MODEL

Many labels have been suggested for the dimension of work that we refer to as predictability, including "uncertainty" (March and Simon 1958), "uniformity" (Litwak 1961), "number of exceptions" (Perrow 1967), and "variety" (Rackham and Woodward 1970). Predictability is based on a knowledge of work processes and materials. We define *technological predictability* as the degree to which raw materials and transformation processes are well understood, so that they present few unexpected contingencies for qualified performers.[1] *Task predictability* refers to the extent to which raw materials and task activities associated with the performance of a particular job are well understood and nonproblematic for individuals in that position. *Workflow predictability* refers to the extent to which raw materials and transformation processes associated with the combination of tasks carried on by an organizational subunit are well understood and nonproblematic for individuals in the unit.

Measures of technology such as that developed by Hickson, Pugh, and Pheysey (1969) confound this distinction by combining into a single scale measures of task predictability (e.g., the level of automaticity of the hand tools and machines used) and measures of workflow predictability (e.g., whether workflow stops immediately in the event of a breakdown, the use of buffer stocks, and the possibility of rerouting work).

The Effects of Task Predictability

We expected task predictability to have its principal effects on the qualifications and specialization of the subunit staff. Tasks that are highly predictable permit the extensive subdivision of work among staff members. Among the efficiencies associated with such differentiation are short training periods, replaceability of participants, increased skills through frequent repetition of activities, and ease of observation and control (Gulick 1937). By contrast, work on less predictable tasks cannot be easily subdivided. They are more likely to be assigned to workers having sufficient general training and experience to be able to act effectively in uncertain situations. Thus, we expected the qualifications of staff members to decrease, and role specialization to increase, as the level of task predictability increased.

There is relatively little empirical support for these relationships except the study by Hage and Aiken (1969), who reported that organizations carrying on more routine work (as measured at the level of the tasks performed by individual workers) were less likely to have well-trained or professional staffs. Other studies, such as Hall's (1968), have reported a negative correlation between the average level of professional training and the division of labor but have not presented data directly linking task characteristics to either variable.

The following hypotheses summarize the effects of task predictability:

H1: The greater the predictability of tasks, the lower the qualifications of staff members.

---

1. While recognizing that all performers are not equally qualified and so do not understand the materials and processes to the same degree, our approach focused, not on such individual differences, but on the general adequacy of the knowledge base underlying work activities. We assumed that such differences were taken into account by organizational decision makers as they designed control systems or determined staffing patterns.

H2: The greater the predictability of tasks, the greater the differentiation of staff roles.

The Effects of Workflow Predictability

Workflow predictability, in contrast to task predictability, was expected to have its major influence on the control system of the subunit. Both standardization of policies and procedures and the centralization of decision making within the subunit were expected to increase as the flow of work became more predictable.

More predictable workflows permit greater reliance on rules and other formalized procedures as a means of control and coordination. Pugh et al. (1969) reported a positive relation between their complex index of workflow integration and a scale reflecting the "structuring of activities," consisting of indicators measuring specialization, standardization, and formalization. However, this relationship was tested at the organizational rather than the subunit level. The reports by Pugh and associates (Hickson, Pugh, and Pheysey 1969; Pugh et al. 1969) that the influence of technology was overwhelmed by the effects of size have proved to be controversial (Aldrich 1972). At the subunit level, Hrebiniak (1974) found an association between technology (measured by complexity, uniformity, and analyzability) and the extent of rule usage within workgroups, after controlling for supervisory style. We also expected workflow predictability to be related to the centralization of decision making within the subunit. Unpredictable workflows—for example, uncertainties as to the mix of tasks from one work period to another—create strategic contingencies that tend to lead to the decentralizing of power within units (Hickson et al. 1971). The more predictable the workflow at the subunit level, the more centralized we would expect decision making to be within the subunit. Most empirical studies have focused attention on centralization at the organizational level; however, Mohr (1971) reported a small negative correlation between "manageability," or predictability of work, for a sample of workgroups and "participativeness," or decentralization of decision making. He found a slightly stronger association between participativeness and workgroup interdependence, a characteristic that we would regard as an aspect of workflow predictability. Our expectations are summarized in the following hypotheses:

H3: The greater the predictability of the workflow for a subunit, the greater the standardization of policies and procedures within the subunit.

H4: The greater the predictability of the workflow for a subunit, the greater the centralization of decision making within the subunit.

The Effects of Subunit Size

Size has been a principal rival to technology for many researchers concerned with explaining the structure of organizations and their subunits. As with technology, most empirical research on size has dealt with the organization rather than the subunit. A number of studies at the organizational level have reported a strong positive association between size and structural differentiation, as measured by both work roles and specialized work units (Hall, Haas, and Johnson 1967; Pugh et al. 1969; Blau and Schoenherr 1971; Child 1973). Blau and Schoenherr (1971, 183, 214–15) also examined the effect of subunit size on the division of labor and reported a strong positive effect after controlling for other contextual variables, such as agency size and community environment. Several of these studies also reported that size was positively related to formalization or standardization, but Child (1973) rather convincingly demonstrated that differentiation ("complexity" in his terms) was more strongly related to standardization than size and that the association between size and standardization disappeared when the effect of differentiation was controlled. Our expectation was, then, that subunit size would affect staff differentiation but would have no direct effect on standardization.

Previous research has also consistently reported a negative relation between the size of an organization and the centralization of decision making (Pugh et al. 1969; Blau and Schoenherr 1971; Child 1973). Blau and Schoenherr (1971, 193–204) did not report data relating size of local office directly to centralization, but they did note that office size was positively associated with the span of control and negatively related to supervisory ratio, two variables that may relate to centralization. We expected subunit size to be negatively associated with centralization. Finally, we expected subunit size to be negatively related to the average level of staff qualifications. The general rationale supporting this prediction was that of economies of scale: a given level of technical expertise is required to perform certain work, but larger units can spread their qualified staff more thinly, using them in consultative roles with less qualified participants. Again, Blau and Schoenherr (1971, 247–48) reported that at the subunit level, controlling for several aspects of community environment and agency context, larger local offices had less highly educated staff employees. The following hypothesis is therefore offered concerning the effects of subunit size:

> H5: The greater the size of the organizational subunit, (*a*) the greater the differentiation of staff roles, (*b*) the lower the centralization of decision making within the subunit, and (*c*) the lower the average level of qualifications of staff members.

Staff Characteristics and Subunit Structure

The work of many researchers has indicated that the four dimensions we used as dependent variables in the above hypotheses—qualifications, differentiation, centralization, and standardization—are likely to be interrelated. Although most of these researchers have focused on organizations rather than subunits (and thus their findings might be less relevant to our setting), we have used their studies as a general guide for some predictions about the interrelations between staff and subunit characteristics.

We expected that the higher the qualifications of staff employed within a given subunit, the lower the levels of role differentiation, centralization, and standardization. Such predictions are consistent with the general view of professional work organizations (Scott 1966; Bucher and Stelling 1969; Freidson 1970) and are supported by empirical findings on the structural characteristics of both professional organizations and professional departments (Hall 1968). The report by Child (1973, 177–78) of a positive relation between specialist qualifications and role differentiation is only seemingly contradictory, because Child's measure assessed the highest level of expertise present rather than the average level of qualification of staff members.

An expectation that differentiation is positively related to standardization is consistent with most of the research that has been reviewed. Blau and Schoenherr (1971) emphasized that structural differentiation engendered problems of communication and coordination. Others have noted that when the work involved is relatively routine and predictable, such coordination is likely to take the form of the development of standardized procedures and formal rules (March and Simon 1958; Thompson 1967).

Finally, we expected centralization of decision making at the subunit level to be associated with greater standardization. Since both are viewed as effects of workflow predictability, on this basis alone they would be expected to covary. It also seems that standardization of policies and procedures is necessary if centralized decisions are to be implemented at the subunit level. It should be noted that this prediction is inconsistent with findings at the organizational level, where standardization and centralization have been found to be negatively related (Pugh et al. 1969; Blau and Schoenherr 1971; Child 1973). In explanation, Blau and Schoenherr (1971, 121) argued that standardized personnel policies make decentralization of decisions about work less precarious for management. However, such an argument seems more applicable at the overall organizational level, where generalist managers attempt to exercise broad controls over specialized subunits, rather than within subunits, where we would expect managers making decisions about work-related activities to attempt to ensure the compliance of their staff. Indeed, the finding that the decentralization of decision making and the standardization of work procedures are negatively associated at the organizational level is completely consistent with the

Figure 2.1. Predicted relations between technology and structure in wards

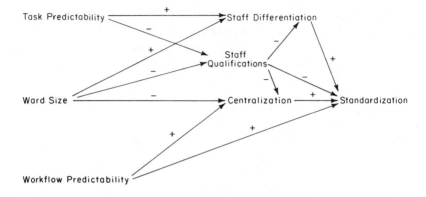

expectation that standardization of work procedures is associated with the centralization of decision making at the subunit level.

Our predictions relating staff characteristics and subunit structure are summarized by the following hypotheses:

H6: The higher the qualifications of the subunit staff, (*a*) the lower the extent of staff differentiation, (*b*) the lower the centralization of decision making, and (*c*) the lower the standardization of procedures and policies.

H7: The greater the extent of role differentiation within the subunit, the higher the standardization of procedures and policies.

H8: The higher the centralization of decision making within the subunit, the greater the standardization of procedures and policies.

Among the four staff member and subunit characteristics, staff qualifications were assumed to be the primary determinant. Task predictability was expected to affect staff qualifications, as previously noted, so that staff members would be assigned to organizational subunits in response to the types of tasks allocated to each subunit. Although this line of reasoning should be applicable to all types of organizations, it was especially appropriate for general hospitals—the type of organization in which this study was carried out. There is a close association between type of task, occupational specialty, and level of training in medicine, and decisions about staffing hospital wards are made on the basis of the types of patients assigned to each ward. At the level of the subunit or ward, we expected a better-trained and more professionally oriented staff to result in lower differentiation of roles, less centralization of decisions, and less standardization of policies and procedures. In turn, we expected higher levels of differentiation and centralization to result in greater standardization, since both increase the need for controls to ensure that activities are coordinated and decisions carried out. The predicted interrelationship of these dimensions, together with expectations relating to the direct effects of task predictability, workflow predictability, and subunit size, are summarized by the causal diagram in figure 2.1.

DATA AND METHODS

Our model was tested on data from 142 patient-care wards in sixteen of the acute-care general hospitals in the Intensive Study. (The seventeenth hospital was dropped due to incomplete data on our technology measures.) Within this sample of hospitals, our study focused on those wards that had cared for at least twelve surgical patients during the year preceding the study. Although the rationale for this decision rested on our related study of the quality of surgical care, it was very pertinent to this research, since our measure of task predictability was based on the care of surgical patients. This selection criterion did not prove to be very restrictive: 82 percent of all wards in the sixteen hospitals were included in the study. The number of wards studied in each hospital ranged from three to fifteen and varied according to the size of the hospital. Types of wards included were intensive-care, surgical, medical, combined medical and surgical, orthopedic, pediatric, obstetrical, and mental health.

Five principal sources of data were used in the analysis: (1) a questionnaire completed by each hospital administrator with the assistance of his or her staff, together with a follow-up interview of the administrator; (2) interviews with the head nurse of each ward; (3) questionnaires administered to all registered and practical nurses on each ward, with a return rate averaging more than 75 percent; (4) a weekly census of patients in different categories of surgical and medical care for each ward for a four-month period; and (5) independent ratings from nurses of the predictability of postsurgical care for patients in the categories of surgical operations used for the ward census.

The first three types of data were collected by one of two teams, each composed of two interviewers, who spent from one to two weeks in each study hospital conducting interviews and administering questionnaires. The patient census was conducted throughout the study by part-time technicians located in each hospital. Although their primary activity was to gather information on individual patients for the study on the quality of surgical care, they were also asked to gather organizational data requiring extended periods of collection, such as the ward census. Both the interviewers and the technicians used detailed schedules and structured instruments in their data collection, received extensive training before going to the hospitals, and were in constant communication with the staff of the Stanford Center for Health Care Research (SCHCR), who supervised and coordinated all phases of the data collection. The final source of data was a nationwide sample of nurses used as a panel of "expert" judges to evaluate the relative predictability of the nursing tasks associated with seventy-one surgical operations. This panel was used for this judgment task only and was independent of the nurses involved in the study of wards.

Measures

Our measure of task predictability combined information on the types of surgical patients being treated on each ward with scores assessing the predictability of nursing-care tasks for each type of surgical operation. This approach assumes that the type of operation performed on each patient determines the predictability of care tasks confronting the nursing staff. (See SCHCR 1974 [733–47] or Schoonhoven et al. 1980 for a list of the seventy-one operations and the indicator questions asked of the expert panel.)

Every eighth day over a four-month period a census in each ward receiving surgical patients was made by classifying each patient under one of seventy-one surgical categories and recording the number in each category. The seventy-one operations were selected with the assistance of surgeon and anesthesiologist consultants to best represent the range of common surgical operations. A three-day sample of operations performed in the hospitals studied indicated that the seventy-one operations accounted for 59–93 percent of the operations performed in these hospitals. The remaining patients were classified into one of four residual categories: medical, obstetrical, presurgical, or other postsurgical patients not included in the seventy-one specific types. An eight-day sampling period was designed to avoid any bias in patient types that might be associated with a specific day of the week. The census yielded a distribution of patients across seventy-one operations for each ward. To these distributions we assigned a set of task predictability scores derived from the judgments of the panel of nurses.

Nurse raters on the panel were selected by a two-step procedure. First, a national sample of forty-eight general, acute-care hospitals were selected using size, teaching status, and geographic region as stratifying variables. Directors of nursing in thirty-five of these hospitals agreed to cooperate, and with their assistance, 542 ward nurses with more than one year of nursing experience caring for postsurgical patients and experience with a broad range of postsurgical cases were selected. Each was asked to assess the relative predictability or complexity of the nursing tasks associated with each of the seventy-one surgical operations by responding to one of six questions. Three questions were used to assess the relative complexity of nursing care, and three to assess the relative predictability.

To assess predictability, each respondent was asked to rate each operation on a nine-point scale on the "extent to which the postsurgical nursing care for 71 operations differs" on one of the following criteria: (a) "the extent to which contingencies arise which require the nurse to exercise judgment during the care

Table 2.1. Measures of ward technology and structure

	Mean	Standard Deviation	Range Low	Range High	N
Technology					
Task predictability	4.71	1.19	0.85	7.7	136
Workflow predictability	3.37	1.90	1.0	8.0	123
Structure					
Staff qualifications					
RN ratio	0.48	0.18	0	1.0	142
Professional activities	−0.06	2.02	−6.7	7.2	142
Staff differentiation	0.77	0.07	0.46	0.87	142
Centralization					
Routine decisions	−0.06	2.51	−5.4	5.9	139
Policy decisions	0.85	0.44	−0.44	2.18	140
Standardization	−0.12	5.23	−13.6	11.6	123
Ward Size	23.96	8.98	6.3	50.8	142

routine," (*b*) "how standardized the care routine is for each operation," and (*c*) "the number of alternatives there are to choose among for any given procedure in the nursing care routine for each operation."

The rating task was obviously a somewhat tedious one, but for the six questions a total of 354 nurses produced usable responses for a return rate of 65 percent. Approximately half of these, or 175 nurses, scored the surgical operations in terms of their predictability. Intercorrelations among the predictability measures based on the three criteria listed were all above .97, indicating nearly perfect agreement among nursing raters. These data were therefore combined into one overall task predictability scale. Unfortunately, our measures of predictability were also correlated almost as highly with our measures of the complexity of care, indicating either that these dimensions are highly correlated for this type of work or that we failed to construct questions that permitted our raters to distinguish between the two dimensions. Average scores on the nine-point scale ranged from a low of 1.26 for the predictability of the nursing tasks associated with the surgical category "open heart surgery for valvular or vascular disease with cardiopulmonary bypass" to a high of 7.72 for the category "proctoscopy and sigmoidoscopy without biopsy." Our measure of task predictability for each ward was obtained by simply applying the appropriate scale scores to the distribution of patients for that ward and dividing by the total number of patients in each ward. The mean, standard deviation, and range for this and other ward level measures are reported in table 2.1.

Unfortunately, our index of workflow predictability was as crude as our measure of task predictability was elaborate! It was derived from the identification by the head nurse of the type of care predominating on each ward: intensive, surgical, medical, combined surgical and medical, orthopedic, pediatric, obstetrical, and mental health. Based on our estimate of the variety, timing, and ordering of care tasks on each type of ward, we ranked them in the order given above, assigning a score of 1 to intensive-care wards as experiencing the least predictable level of workflow and a score of 8 to mental health wards as the most predictable in their workflow.

For surgical patients, and especially for those with very acute conditions requiring intensive care, not only is the timing and order of tasks less predictable but the patient turnover is more rapid than that in medical wards, resulting in a greater variety of cases. Wards providing more specialized care (orthopedic and obstetrical) and more extended care (mental health) were assigned scores indicating relatively higher workflow predictability. Based on discussions with nurses, we concluded that the order and timing of nursing care were more predictable for pediatric than for orthopedic patients largely because pediatric wards usually serve few acute cases, children who are seriously ill being placed in intensive-care units or on surgical wards. Similarly, the order and timing of care tasks were more predictable for obstetrical than for any other type of care except mental health. This last type of ward was placed at the high end of the workflow predictability scale, even though the therapeutic tasks posed by these patients are highly unpredictable. Our focus was on workflow at the ward level, and turnover for this patient group was relatively low. Furthermore, since most general hospitals care only for the less serious psychological problems and patients are often ambulatory, nursing-care tasks often consist of custodial care and general patient supervision.

If differences in ward type have a significant effect on the control systems of these subunits or if the scores have been inappropriately assigned to these types of wards, we would expect to observe significant nonlinear effects in the subsequent analysis. In our analysis, therefore, whenever this measure of workflow predictability was used, we conducted tests for linearity.[2] In each case, the nonlinear component of variance proved not to be significant. These results

2. In order to test for nonlinear effects for these dependent variables, we used a slightly altered version of a test suggested by Johnston (1972, 146–47) based on the increase in the multiple correlation coefficient obtained by going from the continuous variable to a set of dummy variables representing the categories of the variable. The technique is similar to Blalock's (1970, 410ff.) suggested test for the difference between E^2 and R^2 but is more applicable to multiple regressions. The difference between the R^2 for the dummy regression and the R^2 for the continuous variable regression is the amount of variance explained by the nonlinear relation between workflow predictability and each dependent variable. An F-test for the significance of this remainder is given by the formula

$$F(k - q, n - k - 1) = \frac{(R^2_d - R^2_c)/(k - 1)}{(1 - R^2_d)/(n - k - 1)},$$

give some support to the validity of our attempt to order these wards on workflow predictability based on our assessment of task variety and patient turnover, though we recognize the need for the development of more systematic measures of these variables at the subunit level.

Our measure of subunit size was the total number of full-time-equivalent staff members employed on each ward. The zero-order correlations of size with task predictability and workflow predictability were $-.20$ and $-.10$, respectively. Task predictability and workflow predictability had a correlation of .36. These levels of association indicated that subsequent regression analyses would be free of problems of multicollinearity.

Our measures of staff qualifications focused on the nursing staff as the largest and most significant component of the ward staff. One assessed initial level of training, and the other measured the extent to which this training was being supplemented and maintained by current professional activities. The first measure, the RN ratio, was based on the proportion of the ward's total staff, excluding clerical personnel, who were registered nurses. These data were obtained during interviews with the head nurses. The extent of current professional activity was measured by three indicators: (1) staff nurses' (including the practical nurses') membership in professional associations; (2) the number of professional courses taken during the past year for which certification was received or which significantly enhanced professional knowledge, exclusive of in-service training;[3] and (3) the number of articles in professional journals read per month. Indices of professional activity were obtained by averaging responses from nurses in each ward. Although these indices were not highly correlated (associations with courses, .12; courses with articles, .19; and associations with articles, .22), since these activities could reflect alternative approaches to professional enhancement, we decided to convert them to standard scores and combine them into a single index of professional activity.

An index of staff differentiation was developed from data obtained from organizational charts constructed during interviews with the head nurses. The charts contained current information on the various job categories utilized on each ward, together with the number of staff members in each position. These data were used to calculate an index of differentiation developed by Gibbs and Martin (1962): $D = 1 - [\Sigma X^2 / (\Sigma X)^2]$, where X is the number of staff members in each position present on the ward, and the summations are taken across all job titles. The larger the number of positions and the more even the distribution

---

where R^2_d is the squared multiple correlation coefficient for the regression with dummy variables, R^2_c is the same for the regression with the continuous independent variable, k is the number of variables in the dummy-variable regression, q is the number of variables in the regression with the continuous variable, and n is the number of observations.

3. For this indicator only, attention was restricted to the responses of day-shift nurses, since opportunities to attend courses were regarded as much greater for staff members on the evening and night shifts.

of persons among them, the higher the score of a ward on this index, which has a possible range from zero to one. As reported in table 2.1, the mean value of staff differentiation was .77, with a standard deviation of .07. The small variance for this measure indicates that there was little difference among wards in staff differentiation. To us this indicated that job titles and assignments were fairly standard across different types of wards and in different hospitals and regions of the country. This may be an example of an industry effect in the definition of occupational roles within hospitals.

To compute a measure of centralization of decision making for each ward, we used a two-step procedure. First, influence scores for the position of staff nurses and the position of head nurses were calculated; then the centralization of influence was determined by subtracting the mean score of the staff nurses in each ward from the score of their head nurse.

We defined organizational influence as the ability of members occupying positions in the organization to affect organizational decisions, for example, decisions about goals, policies, personnel, or the work of the organization. To assess relative influence, we asked members of each ward to rate on a five-point scale the influence of the positions of staff nurse and head nurse, as well as other hospital positions, on each of four types of ward-level decisions: (1) hiring a replacement staff nurse for the ward, (2) adding a new staff nurse position to the ward staff, (3) determining the appropriate disciplinary action for a staff nurse who had committed a serious medication error, and (4) changing the nursing-care system on the ward, for example, adopting team nursing. This set was designed to cover a range of decisions affecting the operation of the ward, from routine administration through the setting of general policy. These four ward-level decisions were selected from a pretest sample of approximately twenty different decisions. We attempted to select decisions that maximized variance along three dimensions: (1) the organizational space affected, (2) the time for which they would hold, and (3) their level of abstraction (Katz and Kahn 1966, 259).

The ratings of influence by staff nurses on a ward were averaged and then combined with those of each head nurse, giving a weight of four to the staff nurse ratings and a weight of one to the ratings by the head nurse. These weights represent a compromise between (*a*) giving equal weight to the ratings of all ward participants, thus possibly undervaluing the head nurse's judgments, and (*b*) weighting the head nurse's judgments equally with the average of the rest of the staff, risking too much emphasis on the perceptions of the head nurse. In general, more attention needs to be devoted to determining appropriate weighting schemes for combining data from different organizational positions (Scott et al. 1972, 141), but in this specific case the weighting scheme had little effect on the results because of the high consensus between staff nurses and head nurses in their judgments of influence (Comstock 1980).

An index of centralization for each of the four decisions was calculated for each ward by subtracting the weighted influence score for the staff nurses from the weighted influence score for the head nurse. It appears that our items tapped two points along the range of decisions, each associated with a different distribution of influence. Ward-centralization scores based on the first three items, dealing with more routine decisions, were highly intercorrelated (.55, .60, .74); therefore, the differences in weighted influence scores for the head nurse and staff nurses were converted to standard scores and summed to provide a measure of centralization of routine administration decisions for each ward. The fourth item, dealing with a major policy decision, produced ward-centralization scores that were not highly correlated with the first three items (.11, .28, and .35); it was therefore left to stand alone as an indicator of the centralization of policy decisions.

The level of standardization of ward procedures and policies was measured by asking the staff nurses (by questionnaire) and each head nurse (by interview) to rate the extent of explicitness of the following policies: (1) dress or attire on the ward, (2) returning to work after an illness, (3) conditions under which staff may be requested to work overtime, (4) arrangements under which nurses can accept verbal orders from physicians, (5) the time by which patients' baths must be completed, (6) the range of time allowed for passing out patients' medication, (7) information and format for charting nurses' notes, and (8) the administration of enemas. Most of these items were related to the conduct of the activities of the ward as a whole rather than to the performance of an individual's tasks. The individual's tasks selected were those thought likely to be interdependent with the work of others, such as charting nurses' notes and the timing of baths and medications. As with the decisions measuring ward centralization, these items were taken from a much longer list explored in pilot work. The final set was selected to represent a range of work-related issues familiar to nurses on the various wards surveyed.

We believe that our approach, which focused on participants' perceptions of explicitness, provides a more accurate reflection of standardization than the more commonly used measures based on the extent to which rules and regulations are written. There may be a large discrepancy between such written codes and the effective determination of staff members' behavior. By focusing on the extent to which participants perceive that rules have been explicitly formulated to govern specified areas of conduct, we hoped to assess more accurately the degree to which rules, whether written or unwritten, guided behavior.

In scoring the responses of participants on standardization, as with centralization, we assigned weights of one to four for the head nurse's responses as compared with those of the staff nurses. All eight items were then combined to provide a single measure of standardization for a ward. The reliability coefficient, calculated from correlating odd with even items and corrected with the Spearman-Brown prophesy formula, was .827, indicating this to be a highly reliable measure.

Validity Assessment

In addition to the test for nonlinearity in our measure of workflow predictability, each measure of ward structure or a characteristic of the staff based on the aggregation of responses of individual staff nurses was tested to determine whether there were significant differences among wards. In all such tests for ward effects, the F-ratio for a one-way analysis of variance was significant at the .001 level or less. The beta-squared values were: .20 for professional activity, .25 for standardization, .29 for centralization of routine decisions, and .18 for centralization of policy decisions. In each case we appear to have a reasonably valid measure of a ward characteristic.

FINDINGS

The analysis relied primarily on multiple regressions for each staff and ward characteristic and is therefore arranged by dependent variable. Before turning to the tests of specific hypotheses, we wish to report data bearing on a central assumption underlying our approach.

Separating the Effects of Task and Workflow Predictability

In our theoretical formulation, we argued for the utility of distinguishing measures of work that involve the aggregation of individual task characteristics from measures that describe the characteristics of the workflow at the subunit level. Implicitly, our formulation was as much concerned with absent relationships as with present ones. We assumed that the more "analytic" variable, task predictability, would not be highly related to standardization, a measure of the structure of control at the ward level. Similarly, we assumed that the more "global" variable, workflow predictability, would not be highly related to qualifications or differentiation, variables measuring characteristics of staff (Lazarsfeld and Menzel 1961).

Following the suggestion of Blalock (1963, 64ff.), we computed partial correlations for each of these pairs of variables, controlling for all other variables regarded as causal (see fig. 2.1). If there were no causal relationship between them, then these partial correlations would be 0. The partial correlation between task predictability and ward standardization was .05, while those for workflow predictability with RN ratio and with professional activity were −.08 and −.11 respectively; and the partial correlation between workflow predictability and staff differentiation was −.03. Since none of these correlations was significantly different from 0, they provide support for our position that the effects of task and workflow technologies can be distinguished. Thus, task predictability has no direct effect on subunit standardization, and workflow predictability does not affect either the qualifications or the specialization of staff members. All other prediction equations generated by the model presented in figure 2.1 were also examined. None of the correlations was significant except that between task predictability and centralization, and this has been added to the subsequent analysis.

Regression Analyses

The effects of task predictability and ward size on two measures of staff qualifications are shown by the first two regressions in table 2.2 (first two columns). These regressions indicate that the greater the predictability of tasks on the ward, the lower the qualifications of the staff, both in terms of the RN ratio in the subunit and in terms of the extent to which members of the nursing staff engage in professional activities. While task predictability affected both aspects of staff qualifications negatively, greater size predicted a lower RN ratio but not fewer professional activities. This divergent effect suggests that these indicators are tapping different aspects of staff qualifications.

Table 2.2 also reports two regression equations predicting ward differentiation, the equations varying only in that the first used RN ratio as a measure

Table 2.2. Regressions on qualifications and differentiation of ward staff ($N = 99$ wards)

	Staff Qualifications		Staff Differentiation	
		Professional		
Predictor	RN Ratio	Activities	(1)	(2)
Task predictability	−.032**	−.467***	.014***	.015***
	(.015)	(.175)	(.005)	(.005)
Ward size	−.004**	.003	.001*	.001**
	(.002)	(.024)	(.001)	(.001)
Staff qualifications				
RN ratio			−.010	—
			(.033)	
Professional activities			—	.000
				(.003)
Constant	.729	2.13	.697	.670
R^2	.077	.069	.122	.122
F	4.017**	3.563**	4.414***	4.384***

Note: Entries are unstandardized regression coefficients; their standard errors are given in parentheses.

$*p \leq .10$ $\quad$ $**p \leq .05$ $\quad$ $***p \leq .01$

Table 2.3. Regressions on centralization of routine and policy decisions at the ward level ($N = 99$ wards)

Predictor	Centralization of Routine Decisions		Centralization of Policy Decisions	
	(1)	(2)	(1)	(2)
Task predictability	−.400*	−.464*	.044	.032
	(.231)	(.240)	(.038)	(.040)
Workflow predictability	.270*	.258	.042*	.040
	(.155)	(.161)	(.025)	(.027)
Ward size	.063**	.047	−.001	−.004
	(.030)	(.030)	(.005)	(.005)
Staff qualifications				
RN ratio	3.94***	—	.790***	—
	(1.44)		(.237)	
Professional activities	—	.116		.027
		(.129)		(.021)
Constant	−2.56	.082	.151	.673
R^2	.136	.075	.144	.059
F	3.696***	1.911	3.963***	1.464

Note: Entries are unstandardized regression coefficients; their standard errors are given in parentheses.

*$p \le .10$ **$p \le .05$ ***$p \le .01$

of staff qualifications, while the second used professional activities. In both regressions only task predictability and ward size were significant predictors of staff differentiation. The direction of these relationships was positive, as predicted, but contrary to our expectation, staff qualifications were not directly related to the level of differentiation.

The analysis for centralization of decision making is reported in table 2.3. Task predictability was included in all of these equations. We had expected no relation between task predictability and our measures of centralization, but preliminary analysis of the Simon-Blalock prediction equations revealed significant correlations between these variables after controlling for the effects of staff qualifications and workflow predictability. Task predictability was therefore added to each regression.

The first two columns of regressions report the analysis for centralization of routine decisions, and the last two, the analysis for centralization of policy decisions. The RN ratio was used as a measure of staff qualifications in the first regression of each pair, and professional activity was used in the second of each pair. In the first regression for centralization of routine decisions, all terms—

task and workflow predictability, ward size, and RN ratio—were significant, and while workflow predictability was associated with increased centralization of routine decisions, as expected, task predictability was negatively related to such centralization. Furthermore, the RN ratio did not have the expected effect on centralization: staff qualifications were expected to decrease rather than increase centralization of decision making at the ward level. In the second regression predicting centralization of routine decisions (differing only in the indicator of staff qualifications used), all relationships were similar in their direction of effect, but only task predictability remained significant.

In the pair of regressions predicting centralization of policy decisions, only workflow predictability and the RN ratio were significant predictors. Workflow predictability increased centralization, as predicted, but as in the first regression, the effect of the RN ratio on centralization was the opposite of that expected. As before, professional activities were not related to centralization.

It is interesting to note that task predictability exhibited a positive, though

Table 2.4. Regressions on standardization of ward procedures and policies ($N = 99$ wards)

	Standardization			
Predictor	(1)	(2)	(3)	(4)
Workflow predictability	.673**	.614**	.601**	.513*
	(.288)	(.293)	(.303)	(.306)
Staff differentiation	18.87**	17.55**	16.79***	14.94*
	(8.51)	(8.49)	(8.77)	(8.67)
Staff qualifications				
RN ratio	7.51*	6.98**	—	—
	(2.91)	(2.96)		
Professional activities	—	—	.010	.001
			(.256)	(.253)
Centralization				
Routine decisions	.203	—	.334	—
	(.201)		(.202)	
Policy decisions	—	1.66	—	2.61**
		(1.25)		(1.23)
Constant	−20.37	−20.35	−14.88	−15.44
R^2	.170	.171	.111	.128
F	4.285***	5.041***	2.947**	3.447**

Notes: Entries are unstandardized regression coefficients; their standard errors are given in parentheses.
*$p \le .10$ **$p \le .05$ ***$p \le .01$

not significant, effect on the centralization of policy decisions but a negative and significant effect on the centralization of routine decisions. We predicted no relation, and it is not entirely clear why task routinization should be associated with decentralization of decision making on routine matters. Workflow predictability also tended to be more strongly related to centralization of routine decisions; as predicted, it was associated with increased centralization of both types.

Table 2.4 reports four regressions predicting ward standardization. Workflow predictability had its clearest effect in these equations. All four regressions demonstrated the strong and independent effect of a measure of the ward's workflow on standardization, a measure of the ward's control system. As expected, the more predictable the workflow at the subunit level, the more likely it was that work procedures would be standardized at that level. The regressions also showed that staff differentiation consistently increased standardization, as predicted. Contrary to our expectations, however, RN ratios were found to be associated with increased standardization of policies and procedures, as they were with increased centralization. Consistent with other reported results, professional activities did not have any effect on the level of standardization. Finally, our expectation that centralization of decisions would increase standardization was not supported in three of the four equations.

Further Analysis of the Effects of Task Predictability

It is important to acknowledge that our measure of task predictability, while fairly elaborate, suffered from the important defect that it applied to only a subset of the patients treated on each ward. Not all postsurgical patients were included in the seventy-one categories measured, and what is even more important, many who were not postsurgical patients, including presurgical, medical, and obstetrical cases, were present on these wards but not represented in this measure. Indeed, more often than not, our measure of task predictability was based on a minority of the patients present on each ward on any given day. The average for all wards combined was only 24 percent of all ward patients included in the seventy-one postsurgical categories. By reexamining the effects of task predictability on ward characteristics for the wards in which a larger proportion of patients were included in our task predictability measure, we hoped to obtain a better indication of the effects of this variable.

Table 2.5 shows the regression analysis for staff qualifications and differentiation for two subsets of wards: thirty-one wards in which at least 30 percent of the patients fell within categories measured by our index of task predictability and seventeen wards in which at least 40 percent of the patients were included in these categories. A comparison of these regressions with those reported in table 2.2 reveals a marked increase in the coefficients for task predictability and in the total variance explained by the two regressions for staff qualifications.

Table 2.5. Regressions on wards with at least 30 percent and wards with at least 40 percent of patients characterized by task predictability

Predictor	Wards with At Least 30% (N = 31)			Wards with At Least 40% (N = 17)		
	Staff Qualifications			Staff Qualifications		
	RN Ratio	Professional Activities	Differentiation	RN Ratio	Professional Activities	Differentiation
Task predictability	-.107***	-.939***	.022**	-.123***	-1.43***	-.034*
	(.034)	(.403)	(.010)	(.044)	(.542)	(.018)
Ward size	-.003	-.002	.003**	-.008	-.111*	.003
	(.034)	(.052)	(.001)	(.005)	(.065)	(.002)
RN ratio	—	—	.014	—	—	-.026
			(.050)			(.088)
Constant	.997	3.610	.594	1.22	8.85	.550
R^2	.262	.162	.270	.423	.413	.404
F	4.967**	2.715	3.324	5.135**	4.922**	3.404**

Note: Entries are unstandardized regression coefficients; their standard errors are given in parentheses.

$*p \leq .10$ $**p \leq .05$ $***p \leq .01$

For both the RN ratio and professional activities there was a two- to threefold gain in the effect of task predictability, while the relative effect of size in these equations declined. Task predictability was an excellent predictor of staff qualifications in those wards in which our measure was based on a higher proportion of the tasks performed; however, restricting the sample to those wards in which our measure of technology was stronger made little difference in its effect on staff differentiation.

A note of caution may be in order in interpreting these results. Taking smaller subsets of the original sample may have the effect of randomly inflating the coefficients. In order to test for such a sampling error, we used a technique suggested by Johnston (1972, 197ff.) for comparing the power of a subset to that of the entire sample.[4] The sample was partitioned into two sets, one containing all wards with at least 30 percent (or 40 percent) of the patient census in the seventy-one rated categories and a complementary set of those wards having less than 30 percent (or 40 percent). By computing separate regressions for each of the two complementary sets, we allowed the slope and intercept to vary independently in each. For each subset, this should yield a better fit with the data than we obtained in a single regression for the whole sample. We could then compare the total of the sums of squares obtained in the two subsets with that obtained from the regression fit to the whole sample. The difference indicates the gain in power obtained by partitioning the sample.

For both measures of staff qualifications in each subset of wards, the increase in the explained variance was significant at least at the .1 level. These results increase our confidence that our predictions about the effects of task predictability would have been more strongly supported had this measure been based on a larger proportion of the tasks being performed on these wards.

The Relative Effects of Technology and Size

With respect to the relative effects of technology and size, our analysis at the subunit level showed that both were important predictors of RN ratios, staff differentiation, and the centralization of routine decisions. In our presentation of results to this point we have relied on unstandardized regression coefficients. While these are useful for evaluating the significance of each coefficient, they are not appropriate for comparing the relative effects of these variables, since

---

4. The formula for the test of significance of this difference was

$$F(pk - p - k + 1, n - pk) = \frac{(SS_1 + SS_2) - SS_t/(pk - p - k + 1)}{(SS_{r1} + SS_{r2})/(n - pk)},$$

where SS_1, SS_2, and SS_t are the regression sums of squares for the two subsets and the total sample, respectively, SS_{r1} and SS_{r2} are the residual sums of squares for the subsets, p is the number of subsets, k is the number of variables in the equation, and n is the number of observations.

Table 2.6. Comparison of the relative predictabilities of ward technology and structure (N = 99 wards)

Predictor	Dependent Variable		
	RN Ratio	Staff Differentiation	Centralization of Routine Decisions
Ward size	−.189	.194	.212
Task predictability	−.205	.281	−.182
Workflow predictability	—	—	.184
RN ratio		−.030	.274

Note: Entries are standardized regression coefficients.

they reflect the different units of measurement for each variable. Table 2.6 presents, in standardized form, the three principal regressions in which size appeared as a significant predictor.

The first regression in table 2.6 indicates that size had an effect on RN ratio almost equal to that of the technology variable, task predictability. In the second regression, however, the effect of size on staff differentiation was considerably less than that of task predictability. And the effect of size on the centralization of routine decisions was slightly greater than the effect of either task or workflow predictability, but it was not greater than their combined effects. Finally, it must be recalled that size was not related to other measures of staff or ward characteristics, including professional activities, centralization of policy decisions, and standardization, while each of these variables was found to be strongly affected by either task or workflow predictability.

While this analysis does not bear at all on the issue of the relative effects of size and technology at the organizational level, it does indicate that for subunits the effects of size were not as pervasive as those of technology but were clearly an important determinant of some staff characteristics and at least one feature of the control system.

These results provide rather clear support for our principal argument that the technology of a subunit can be assessed at two very different levels—that of individuals each confronting their specific tasks and that of the subunit, which must assign and accomplish a set of tasks encompassing all members. What is more important, these two levels of technology have different organizational consequences for the subunit. Even though all variables were measured at the subunit level, as we move from measures that assess the modal characteristics of the tasks performed to measures of workflow for the entire unit, the effects of technology shift from the characteristics of workers to the subunit systems of coordination and control. Distinguishing the effects of aggregated measures of individual tasks and staff characteristics from measures of workflow and social structure at the subunit level was proved useful in this study and may be fruitful in further research.

Predictable tasks were associated with lower qualifications of staff members both in terms of their initial level of training and in terms of their continuing professional activities. At the same time, however, task predictability predicted greater differentiation, indicating greater staff specialization. We also found that size had a positive effect on differentiation but a small or negative effect on staff qualifications. Various measures of staff qualifications or expertise have often been combined with indicators of differentiation to form a general index of structural complexity. The divergent effects of task predictability and size suggest that staff qualifications and differentiation should not be combined in this way. They are alternative modes of complexity: predictable tasks give rise to greater staff differentiation but lower individual staff qualifications; unpredictable tasks reduce staff differentiation but raise staff qualifications.

While task predictability decreased both the level of nurses' training and the extent of professional activities, ward size reduced only training. Large wards were apparently assigned a smaller proportion of registered nurses. It is plausible to argue that these wards receive some scale benefits, with the more highly trained nurses assuming the more professional responsibilities, while other, less qualified staff members carry out the more routine tasks. This explanation is also supported by the finding that larger wards were more likely to be highly differentiated.

Quite consistently throughout the analysis, the extent of professional activities appeared to be a response by individual workers to the characteristics of the tasks they performed. The number of courses attended, journals read, and associations joined was affected only by the average predictability of the tasks performed, not by the predictability of workflow at the subunit level and not by subunit size. Professional activities, in turn, were not related to other subunit characteristics, such as ward differentiation, the centralization of routine or policy decisions, or standardization.

We have noted that task predictability, while not statistically significant, has a positive effect on the centralization of policy decisions but a negative effect on the centralization of routine decisions. This suggests that the more predictable the tasks, the greater the possibility of separating policy from routine decisions. This is consistent with the observation of Reeves and Woodward (1970) that routine technology allows for the separation of policy making and execution.

While predictability of tasks primarily influenced attributes of individual staff members, more predictable workflows at the subunit level increased the bureaucratization and centralization of the control system. Both the centraliza-

Figure 2.2. Determinants of staff qualifications and differentiation (standardized regression coefficients with $N = 99$)

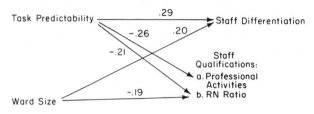

tion of decision making and the standardization of procedures were increased by workflow predictability. Our analysis suggests that it is the characteristics of the technology at the subunit level, rather than at the level of the tasks carried out by the individual workers, that best predicts the configuration of the control system.

The size of the subunit had clear effects on both the characteristics of the staff and the subunit structure. Larger wards had not only lower staff qualifications and greater differentiation but also greater centralization of routine administrative decisions. The independent effects of size cannot be ignored, even though in general they appear to be smaller than those of technological predictability. Also, we observed that the relative impact of size on staff qualifications declined as our sample was restricted to those wards to which our measure of task predictability was most applicable.

It should be emphasized when comparing the relative impact of technology and size on subunit structure that all of the subunits studied performed the same basic type of work, that is, patient care. We ignored the units not concerned with patient care, such as laboratories, administrative services, and hotel support departments, in which the individual tasks and workflows were likely to be much more predictable (Neuhauser 1971; Shortell, Becker and Neuhauser 1976). So if we have demonstrated effects of technological differences in our sample of wards, then we would expect to find even larger effects of technology in studies encompassing a more diverse set of organizational subunits. It is possible that with improved measures and increased variance of technological predictability, the effects of workgroup size might be relatively insignificant.

Results reporting the determinants of staff qualifications and of the subunit control system are summarized in figure 2.2. We use standardized regression coefficients in this diagram in order to facilitate comparison of the effects of different independent variables. Since standardized coefficients are affected by the variances in a sample, such comparisons as these within a single sample are valid, but they should not be extended to other samples.

Figure 2.3. Summary of relationships observed and hypotheses supported

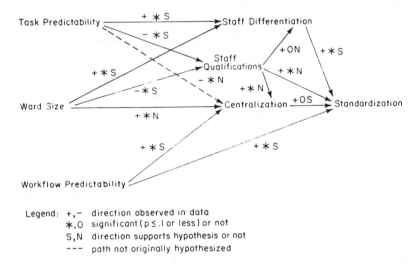

Legend: +,− direction observed in data
        ✱,0 significant (p ≤ .1 or less) or not
        S,N direction supports hypothesis or not
        --- path not originally hypothesized

Figure 2.3 summarizes the direction, significance, and support for the hypotheses discussed in this chapter. An unexpected result warrants some discussion. Although we had expected staff qualifications to reduce both standardization and the centralization of decision making, we found that the RN ratio increased both of these aspects of the control system of the ward. It appears that nurses in these wards were not behaving as autonomous professionals demanding the privilege of exercising individual discretion, as physicians are likely to do (Freidson 1970), but as persons lacking an extraorganizational base of power and working within the administrative framework of the hospital in a heteronomous professional arrangement (Scott 1965; Hall 1968; Etzioni 1969). The absence of any association between the measured individual behavior, professional activities, and these ward characteristics supports the view that individual professional orientation is of little consequence in predicting structural characteristics in the absence of professional power. While RNs are the most qualified members of the ward staff, their power is based more on organizational position than on individual expertise. They are responsible for the work of the ward and occupy the supervisory positions, exercising authority over practical nurses, nurses' aides, and orderlies. To maintain control, they centralize decision making within the ward and establish strict rules and procedures to govern ward routines. Thus, these semiprofessionals, instead of resisting bureaucratic constraints, use them and extend them to enhance their own ability to control the behavior of subordinate workers (Heydebrand 1973).

SUMMARY

This study demonstrates that task and workflow predictability have differential effects on the characteristics of the staff and the structure of organizational subunits in acute-care, general hospitals. It supports the general proposition that the effects of technology are strong close to the primary work locations within organizations. Since we have shown that technology is composed of at least two levels, with distinguishable effects, we are led to suggest that the variety of subgoals and the coordination requirements presented by varying subunits may account for the characteristics of overall organizational control systems. This expectation would help to resolve the ambiguity in some arguments about the relative effects of technology and environment on organizational structure. It suggests that technology measures should be the more powerful predictors of structural characteristics at the lower levels of organizational structure.

We have also attempted to interpret the absence of relationships. Our results show that investigators should not be surprised by the absence of relations between the characteristics of individual tasks and organizational structure. Indeed, we found little effect of task characteristics on subunit structure. More care in formulating predictions that relate variables at the same levels of analysis should improve our grasp of organizational behavior.

PART II

Defining and Measuring Hospital Performance

3 · Costs and the Quality of Care in Hospitals: A Review of the Literature

W. Richard Scott and Ann Barry Flood

In the early 1970s, when our study began, the most professionally and politically salient questions regarding hospital performance revolved around the quality of care provided for all patients and access to it for underserved populations such as the aged and the poor. This concern, soon after spawning a number of regulatory and professional quality-assurance programs, was nearly eclipsed by a change toward trying to contain the costs of hospitalization. These attempts were led by representatives of the federal and state governments, charged with paying for improved access to care for special populations, and by businesses, which saw payments for employee health benefits as an unfillable black hole. The focus of our study during this period widened from a nearly exclusive concern for the quality of care as a measure of hospital performance to a focus that included the intensity of services and lengths of stay in hospitals as indicators of the resources consumed in the delivery of care. In this chapter we discuss the primary factors contributing to the increasing costs of hospitalization, particularly during the ten years preceding and following our study (including the situation in the mid-1980s), and review the theory and evidence linking hospital structure to hospital performance as defined by the costs and quality of care.

Over the past three decades, the cost of care in hospitals has continued to rise, regularly outstripping the general cost-of-living indices. But factors contributing to the increase have changed: factors prominent in the 1960s are less significant in the 1980s, and new factors have been introduced. Moreover, because of the increased salience of the topic, many more studies of hospital costs have been conducted recently than earlier in the period under review, and the later studies have employed larger samples and more sophisticated methods—although they have not always produced better data.

Most observers would agree that the quality of hospital care has also increased over the same three decades, but by no means at a rate commensurate with increases in costs. While quality itself may not have improved dramatically, there has been considerable progress in its conceptualization and measurement. A number of studies assessing hospital factors related to the quality of care have been carried out, but much more research attention has been devoted to costs, and only a handful of studies have attempted to examine both cost and quality issues simultaneously.

Taken as a whole, the literature on hospital costs and quality of care is large and growing rapidly. It is not possible to include all of even the major studies in a single review, but we have attempted to include a fairly representative sample. Our primary focus is on studies that examine the influence of hospital characteristics—intraorganizational variables—as independent factors influencing cost and quality. Particularly in the area of cost, however, we also review the effect of other more general factors.

INCREASING HOSPITAL COSTS: CORRELATES AND CAUSES

There is widespread agreement that hospital costs have risen at an extraordinary rate in this country during the past three decades. Fuchs (1974, 93–94) summarizes the major trends in hospital costs up to 1971:

> From 1959 until 1965 per capita expenditures of community hospitals grew fairly steadily at a rate of about 8 percent annually, while the figure for all services in the U.S. economy for the same period was only 5 percent annually. . . .
>
> After 1965 hospital expenditures started to explode. Between 1965 and 1971 per capita expenditures grew at approximately 14 percent annually—a rate that amounts to a doubling every five years! Service expenditures in the economy as a whole during this period grew at only 7 percent annually.

During the 1970s and up to the present, the annual rate of increase has continued at the same or even a slightly higher level, averaging 14.5 percent between 1970 and 1978 (Gibson 1979) and increasing to 15.4 percent per year for 1980 and 1981 (Gibson and Waldo 1982).

While there is general agreement about the facts of increased hospital costs, there is not a complete consensus as to its cause. Many factors appear to contribute to increased costs, but each is of variable importance depending on time and place. This overview begins by briefly reviewing several general factors that have led to increased costs for all types of hospitals. Following this review, we attempt to identify those hospital characteristics that cause some hospitals to experience higher costs than others. Unless otherwise indicated, our focus is on nonfederal, short-term, acute-care, general hospitals—the so-called community hospitals that in 1981 accounted for 84 percent of all hospital expenditures (Gibson and Waldo 1982).

General Factors Affecting Hospital Costs over Time

There are numerous ways to usefully categorize the many factors related to increased costs of hospitals. This review identifies five types of factors: (1) increased utilization; (2) increased prices for inputs; (3) increased intensity of services provided; (4) increased reliance on indirect and passive payment schemes; and (5) increased costs associated with regulation.

Utilization

Utilization of hospital services increases as a function of population growth, changes in the age composition of the population, and changes in individual demand for services. From 1960 to 1978 the population of the United States increased by about 10 percent. However, utilization of hospitals increased at a much faster rate: the number of inpatient days increased by approximately 21 percent, while outpatient visits during this period almost doubled, increasing by 86 percent (Gibson 1979). Virtually all of this additional volume was accommodated by an increase in the capacity of existing hospitals rather than by the addition of new hospitals. Thus, between 1965 and 1980 the number of nonfederal, short-term "community hospitals" increased by only 1.6 percent, while the average size of these hospitals increased by 31.8 percent, from 129 beds to 170 beds (Feldstein 1983).

The population not only grew but also aged during this period. Between 1965 and 1978 the number of persons in the United States aged sixty-five or over increased by about 30 percent, from 18.5 million to 24.1 million. Analyzing average expenditures for health by different age categories, Enthoven (1980, 31) estimated that the pattern of aging contributed about 7 percent to the doubling in real per capita spending for health services that occurred from 1965 to 1978.

Demand for health services is a complex function of many individual and contextual variables that have been the subject of much research. Social psychologists such as Mechanic (1962), Kasl and Cobb (1966), and Rosenstock (1966) have focused on variations among individuals in their perception and evaluation of symptoms, expectations regarding treatment benefits, and knowledge and beliefs concerning health and illness. Sociologists such as Suchman (1965) have emphasized the more contextual elements effecting utilization, such as social group affiliations and referral systems among lay persons as well as professionals. Later investigators have developed more comprehensive models that include both classes of variables. Aday and Andersen (1974), focusing on family patterns of utilization, identified three groups of variables: (1) predisposing conditions, such as demographic variables (age, sex, marital status), social-structure variables (education, occupation, ethnicity), and health beliefs; (2) enabling conditions affecting the ability to secure services, such as family resources, health insurance coverage, community resources (e.g., medical care facilities and transportation), and a regular source of care; and (3) perceived need for services as affected by the subjective perception of illness, clinical evaluation of illness, and reaction to illness. Cummings, Becker, and Maile (1980) developed an even more comprehensive system of variables building on earlier research and using the authors of these models as judges to select and group variables for inclusion. Six categories of variables emerged from this synthesis, including (1) accessibility of health services, including availability and the individual's ability to pay; (2) attitudes toward health care, including beliefs about benefits and the quality of available care; (3) perceived threat of illness; (4) knowledge about disease; (5) social interactions, norms, and social structure such as friendship and family systems; and (6) demographic characteristics. (These and other individual utilization models are reviewed in Becker and Maiman 1983.)

Because of improvements in private hospital insurance coverage and especially because of government programs such as Medicare and Medicaid, national survey results reveal that utilization patterns now are much more clearly a reflection of demographic (sex and age) and morbidity differences and less determined by socioeconomic status. Data from the National Health Interview Survey collected from 1964 through 1979 reveal that by 1973 the poor were being hospitalized at higher rates than the nonpoor, reflecting their generally poorer health status. Despite these improvements, racial differences have persisted: "Low-income whites continued to be hospitalized more often than low-income nonwhites" (President's Commission for the Study of Ethical Problems in Medicine and Biomedical and Behavioral Research 1983, 69). Other factors continuing to influence utilization of inpatient hospital services are identified in a national household survey conducted in 1975–76 by Aday, Andersen, and Fleming (1980). They found hospital use to be higher for those over sixty-five, women, those not living in rural farm areas, and those who reported having a regular source of medical care. Aday, Andersen, and Fleming (1980, 236, 120) concluded that "the distribution of hospital services in the United States appears reasonably equitable," noting that "some of the inequities that exist for ambulatory physician services do not necessarily obtain for hospital service use."

Numerous studies have shown that utilization patterns are influenced by the availability of medical services, but there is a controversy over whether this is the result simply of accessibility or whether physicians tend to induce demand for their services and act thereby to fill empty hospital beds. Roemer (1961) was among the first to propose that hospitalization rates more closely reflected the number of available beds in an area than they did differences in the morbidity of the populations being served. And a series of studies conducted by Wennberg comparing similar populations in small areas in New England reported a positive association between the number of surgeons serving an area and the surgery rate in that area (Wennberg and Gittelsohn 1973). However, this association was not confirmed in an analysis of data from the National Medical Care Expenditures Study conducted in 1977. Employing multivariate techniques to take into account the effect of a patient's physical condition, age, sex, and nature of illness, Wilensky and Rossiter (1983) concluded that while the density of physicians did tend to increase the number of physician-initiated visits in ambulatory-care settings, it did not increase the likelihood of surgery for patients.

Finally, it is important to point out that during the period under review, utilization patterns have shifted, so that, on average, today's hospitalized patient population is more severely ill—presenting a more complex and difficult set of medical demands—than hospitalized patients thirty or more years ago. This change is itself a result of two trends: (1) increases in the complexity or severity of illnesses among patients being admitted to hospitals, with less ill patients being cared for in an ambulatory or outpatient surgical setting; and (2) reduced lengths of stay for all types of patients, so that patients with improved health status are being discharged earlier (Goldfarb et al. 1980). However, a portion of the reduction in lengths of stay may be attributable to increases in multiple short stays, in which the same patient is discharged but then readmitted (Luft 1981b).

Inflation

Economists attempt to distinguish between an inflation effect, referring to increases in the prices of the input factors used to produce medical care services, and a service-intensity effect, referring to changes in the quantity, quality, and/or mix of medical care inputs. Most analysts appear to agree that the inflation of medical care prices has been substantially higher than the general rate of inflation. Moreover, there is general agreement that inflation accounted for a growing proportion of the increase in costs in the 1970s compared with in the 1960s, with its strongest effects occurring in the period 1974–79. For example, Andersen and May (1972) estimated that while only about 7 percent of the increase in hospital costs was due to inflation during the period 1960–65, inflation was responsible for 23 percent of increased costs in 1965–70. Gibson (1979) estimated that the inflation rate was much higher during the 1970s, accounting for about 50 percent of the increase in health care costs from 1969 to 1973 and for over 70 percent of the increase from 1974 to 1979. Since 1980 the rate of inflation has subsided somewhat.

The extent of inflation is difficult to estimate in the medical care sector because its definition is tied to the concept of productivity which in turn is tied to the concept of output. Increases in the price of input factors are, by definition, noninflationary if they are tied to increases in productivity. And productivity increases, by definition, when more or better output is achieved for a given level of input. The difficulty, as we discuss below, is that there is little consensus among health services providers or researchers about how to define or measure health outputs. Hence, there can be little agreement about the extent to which increases in an input factor, such as wages of medical technicians, are inflationary in their effect on health care prices (National Academy of Sciences, Panel to Review Productivity Statistics 1979). In spite of these problems, it is useful to attempt to distinguish between increases in the quantity or quality of medical inputs and increases in the costs of a given input.

Service Intensity

Medical care inputs are usually subdivided into labor and nonlabor inputs, the latter including equipment and supplies. Most studies index changes in the quantity, quality, or mix of labor inputs by measuring labor costs. Among the factors causing higher labor costs in hospitals are higher average pay, shorter work weeks, increases in the average skill level of personnel, and increases in the number of staff members per patient (Lave 1966). In addition, collective bargaining has played a role in wage increases since 1974, when the National Labor Relations Act was extended to employees of nonprofit hospitals.

During the 1950s and early 1960s, increases in the number of workers per patient and in their wages were a significant factor in increased hospital costs. A study examining the cost of care in thirty-nine acute-care hospitals in Maryland between 1953 and 1962 reported that two-thirds of the increased total costs were due to increases in hospital wage rates (State of Maryland Commission 1964). Fuchs (1974, 93) argued that a good part of the differential between increases in hospital expenditures and those for all services in the U.S. economy for the period 1950–65 was attributable "to sharp increases in the number of personnel per patient and to wage increases that exceeded those in the general economy. This may have been a true 'catching up' period for hospital employees, who prior to World War II typically worked very long hours at very low wages. The period of most rapid growth in both personnel per patient and earnings per employee was from 1950 to 1955." However, Feldstein (1971, 1981) showed that wage rates in hospitals have continued to rise more rapidly than those for comparable occupations, so that hospital workers did not simply "catch up" but rapidly exceeded the earnings of their counterparts in other sectors. Feldstein (1971, 67) attributed this situation in part to a tendency on the part of hospital administrators to engage in "philanthropic wage setting": concern with the well-being of their staff as well as their patients expressed by the payment of higher than market wages to personnel. Administrators were able to act on their philanthropic impulses because the rapid rise in demand for health services, stimulated by public and private insurance, had given them greater budgetary freedom.

Other analysts have rejected this interpretation or have argued that it is but one among several possible explanations of wage increases. Thus, Salkever (1979) suggested that Feldstein's demand thesis should be supplemented by a recognition of the operation of several supply-side factors, including a decline in unemployment rates during the 1960s, a decline in racial discrimination, and increased availability of welfare payments. The first two factors operate to reduce the discrepancy in wages across industries for low-skill jobs; the last, to reduce the size of the available labor force by providing an alternative means of support for marginal workers. Sloan and Steinwald (1980a) conducted analyses using 1 percent samples of the 1960 and 1970 U.S. population censuses to compare wage rates in hospitals with selected reference-group industries and concluded that the evidence did not support the contention that hospital workers were overpaid. "Rather, a substantial part of the wage gains of the 1960s resulted from an upgrading of the hospital work force" (7). Thus, Sloan and Steinwald argued that wage increases for hospital workers had not been inflationary but resulted from improvements in the quality of labor inputs to hospitals—assuming, of course, that improved inputs lead to improved outputs.

Increases in the number of staff members per patient appear to have become a more important factor during the period under review. A study by the State of Maryland Commission (1964) estimated that during the 1950s only about one-sixth of the increased cost of hospital care could be attributed to the hiring of additional staff members. The data reported by Andersen and May (1972, 68) show that while an increase in staff personnel accounted for only about 13 percent of the total increases in hospital costs during the 1960–65 period, it accounted for approximately 25 percent of the increase during the 1965–70 period. Fuchs (1974, 94) reached a similar conclusion: "The number of personnel per patient after 1965 jumped by 3.4 percent annually, compared with a 1.7 percent annual rate from 1960 to 1965." For the extended period 1955–75, Feldstein (1981) calculated a 2.6 percent average annual increase in the number of employees, noting that the number of employees per patient-day rose from 2.03 in 1955 to 3.39 in 1975.

Nevertheless, most observers agree that although labor costs increased during the period of review and did so more rapidly than labor costs in comparable sectors—whether because of philanthropic managers or better-qualified workers—labor costs account for only a small proportion of the increases in hospital costs. According to Feldstein (1981, 3), "From 1955 to 1975 labor cost per patient-day rose at a rate of 9 percent a year. But as a fraction of the total hospital bill, labor costs actually decreased from 62 percent in 1955 to 53 percent in 1975. In other words, nonlabor costs rose faster than labor costs."

Nonlabor costs include both medical "technology"—medical supplies and specialized equipment—and nonmedical facilities and consumables such as hotel, food, and linen. The equipment used is increasingly costly, specialized, and elaborate, and the supplies and materials prepared, prepackaged, and disposable. Feldstein (1981) estimated that during the period 1955–75 there was an overall increase of 11 percent in the cost of nonlabor inputs (compared with 9 percent for labor inputs), of which two-thirds (7.2 percent) was attributable to increases in the volume of nonlabor inputs, and one-third (3.6 percent) to increases in their price. McMahon and Drake (1978), however, insisted that there had been a dramatic shift between the earlier and the more recent period. They utilized data collected by the American Hospital Association (AHA) to argue that while increases in nonlabor costs in 1969 were due primarily to increases in the quantity of goods and services purchased, by 1975 the same level of increases in nonlabor costs was due primarily to increases in the prices paid for these purchases. Sloan and Steinwald (1980b) pointed out that McMahon, an executive officer of the AHA, was not an entirely disinterested observer but concluded that their own independent observations were consistent with McMahon and Drake's.

Changes in the technology of medical care have in general been associated with increases in costs. Thus, studies by Scitovsky and McCall (1976) reported that during the period 1964–71, for a broad range of illnesses costs rose more than they would have if only the price of inputs had changed. Particularly costly were those technical changes that resulted in shifting care settings to more specialized facilities, such as intensive-care units. Support services such as laboratory tests increased dramatically over the period under review. A study of changes that occurred between 1951 and 1971 in a large, multispecialty group-practice setting reported that the average number of laboratory tests for perforated appendicitis increased from 5.3 to 31, and for breast cancer from 5.9 to 27.4. Comparable increases in service intensity were found for x-rays, intravenous solutions, and electrocardiograms (National Center for Health Services Research 1977).

Some types of technical changes had a direct lowering effect on costs but an indirect perverse effect. For example, the introduction of new equipment such as multichanneled blood-test analyses and the computerized tomography (CT) radiographic scanner reduced the cost of providing these services to individual patients, but their availability at lower cost in turn led to more patients being provided with these services, contributing to increased costs of medical care (Knaus, Schroeder, and Davis 1977). While some of the increased usage of these services represents an improvement in the quality of care to patients, much of the increased use did not result in better outcomes, so that the overall effect on costs was inflationary, despite the reduction in cost per service.

Several analysts have attempted to estimate the relative contribution of changes in utilization, inflation, and service intensity to increases in hospital costs. Recognizing that these effects have shifted somewhat over time, we report two estimates for only the more recent period. Gibson (1979) estimated that during the period 1970–78 only 6 percent of the increase in costs was due to

Table 3.1. Percentage of personnel expenditures
for hospital care, by source of funds
for selected years

Source of Funds	1950	1965	1980
Direct patient payment	30	17	11
Private health insurance	18	42	34
Total public	49	39	54
Federal		(18)	(41)
State and local		(21)	(13)

Source: Data from Gibson and Waldo 1982 (24, table 5).

population growth; 29 percent was due to increased intensity of services provided; and 65 percent was due to increased costs of the inputs purchased, that is,
to inflation. Joskow (1981) arrived at a very similar set of estimates: for the
period 1970–79 he attributed 10 percent of the increases to utilization, 30
percent to service intensity, and 60 percent to inflation. Part of the discrepancy
in these estimates is due to Gibson's decision to restrict the first factor to
population growth and to treat changes in the level of demand for hospital
services as part of his service-intensity measure. Joskow combined both of
these variables in his utilization factor.

Payment Schemes

Over the past thirty years, dramatic changes have occurred in the arrangements by which hospital care is financed in this country. Based on statistics
compiled by Gibson and Waldo (1982), the major trends are quickly summarized in table 3.1. As is clear, direct patient payments for hospital care fell from
30 percent to 11 percent by 1980, with third-party payers covering almost 90
percent of hospital costs in 1980. Private insurance companies accounted for
nearly 40 percent of the third-party payments, while public agencies accounted
for over 60 percent. Since the introduction of Medicare and Medicaid in 1965,
the federal share has more than doubled, while state and local governments
carry a reduced proportionate burden. However, the relative role of the federal
and state governments has begun to shift again under President Reagan's New
Federalism: states are being asked to pick up a larger share of hospital costs,
primarily under Medicaid (Lee and Estes 1983).

A major federal role in financing health care was a long time coming in the
United States, and when the political breakthrough finally came in the
mid-1960s with the backing of a strong Democratic coalition of Congress and
the executive branch, it was possible only through what Starr (1982, 374)

termed the "politics of accommodation." Physicians agreed to participate only at the price of preserving intact their autonomy to make decisions about patient services and retaining a reimbursement method based on the fee-for-service system; hospitals' cooperation was purchased by the lawmakers' agreeing to reimburse them according to their costs rather than according to some prearranged schedule of rates.

In an early analysis, Klarman (1969) began to discern the effects that these new federally funded reimbursement programs were having on costs. His analysis suggested that while the program did not appear to result in "abnormal" or excessive increases in the number of persons seeking care, it did have substantial effects on service intensity (see also Somers and Somers 1967). Klarman (1977) later examined the types of expenditures most heavily affected by Medicare and Medicaid—expenditures for short-term hospitalization, physicians' services, and nursing homes—and found that these expenditures rose at an average annual rate of 9 percent during the period 1960–65, before the advent of these two major health care financing programs, and increased by 16 percent during the period 1966–74, following their passage.

Most informed observers of the health care scene point to these changes in payment schemes as the major cause of cost increases. Enthoven (1980, xvii) asserted that "the *main cause* of the unnecessary and unjustified increase in costs is the complex of perverse incentives inherent in our predominant system for financing health care." He noted that the fee-for-service system strongly preferred by physicians "rewards the doctor with more revenue for providing more, and more costly, services." And the third-party payment system removes from both provider and patient incentives to conserve on services or to contain costs.

Feldstein (1981, 153) arrived at a very similar conclusion: "Hospital costs have risen rapidly because insurance has increased the demand for hospital care. Hospitals have responded to this increased demand by raising prices and providing a more expensive style of care. This change in the apparent quality has further increased demand, setting off another round of price and quality increases." Under insurance, Feldstein included both private health insurance and public reimbursement programs, that is, programs that reduce or eliminate the connection between patient and payment.

Feldstein tends to treat patients as the source of the increasing demand for medical care, and, of course, they are the ultimate consumers. But numerous observers have noted that physicians are the major decision makers, determining who is admitted to a hospital, how long they stay, and what services they receive. In the role of the patient's purchasing agent, physicians will naturally want to ensure that their patient receives the best care available, resulting in more and higher-quality services at increasing cost. Redisch (1978) pointed out that while physicians have a direct role in ordering more and more costly services, it is in their economic interest to reduce their own inputs to patients by transferring functions and costs to the hospital. By allowing house staff and nurses to take on more responsibility for the care of patients, physicians can increase their own productivity, seeing more patients and thus enjoying higher earnings without increasing prices. The possible cost savings entailed in substituting lower- for higher-priced labor (e.g., nurses for physicians) are not realized, because two bills are submitted: one for hospital services and one for the physician's supervisory oversight.

By 1970 it was apparent to all that medical care costs in general and hospital costs in particular were seriously out of control. Having acted in the 1940s with Hill-Burton to increase the capacity and improve the distribution of hospital facilities and in the 1960s to improve equity of access to hospital services with Medicare and Medicaid, the federal government was then forced to seek ways to curtail costs and to ration services. The new emphasis became regulation.

Regulation

Sloan and Steinwald (1980b) identified three useful categories of regulatory programs: (1) investment controls, which attempt to contain hospital capital and service expansion; (2) reimbursement controls, which attempt to regulate hospital service rates and revenues; and (3) utilization-quality controls, which attempt to set and enforce criteria governing admissions to hospitals and length of stay. Here we select only major examples of each type and comment on the evidence regarding their impact on costs.

Investment controls developed out of the health planning movement and have been described as "planning with teeth" programs. Prime examples include Section 1122 of the Social Security Act Amendments of 1972, authorizing state-designated planning agencies to review hospital plans for facility or service expansion, and the National Health Planning Act of 1974, which created the system of Health Systems Agencies (HSAs) to oversee the allocation of resources to medical care facilities. Both acts placed primary reliance on a certificate-of-need (CON) mechanism, by which designated agencies review proposed expansion or technology improvement projects in order to determine eligibility for federal funding or reimbursement for interest and depreciation costs.

Numerous empirical studies have attempted to examine the efficacy of CON reviews as mechanisms of cost control. In general, the evidence suggests that the pattern of expenditures is altered under CON controls but that overall costs are not much affected. Thus, an early study by Hellinger (1976) employing a cross-sectional analysis of state data for the period 1971–73 found no differences in total plant assets between states having a CON agency and states lacking one as of January 1973. Moreover, states having CON agencies in place less than half a year were observed to have higher plant investments, suggesting that hospitals anticipated CON legislation by increasing their investments prior to the activation of the program. In a much-cited study, Salkever and Bice (1976) also investigated the effect of CON controls using state data for the period 1969–72. Distinguishing between total assets, bed supply, and assets per bed, they reported positive but insignificant effects of CON controls on total assets, negative effects on bed supply, but positive effects on assets per bed. Salkever and Bice (1978, 452–53) concluded that "contrary to expectations of the public interest theory, our findings suggest that CON controls contributed to cost increases during the 1968–1972 period. CON regulation did not deter total investment in the hospital sector; instead, it altered its composition by discouraging expansion of beds and thereby encouraging (or at least facilitating) expansionist urges of hospitals to find expression in investment in new equipment and facilities."

Using data at the hospital level rather than the state level, Sloan and Steinwald (1980b) examined data from 1,228 hospitals for the period 1969–75. Employing more detailed measures of both CON controls and hospital expenditures, they reported findings consistent with those of Salkever and Bice, namely, the CON effects on total investments were generally positive but insignificant and that effects on bed supply were negative and significant. Also like Salkever and Bice, they found compensatory responses by hospitals, but the increases were in labor rather than nonlabor inputs. Sloan and Steinwald (1980b, 170) also replicated Hellinger's finding of "an anticipatory response by hospitals to impending implementation of CON controls." Joskow (1981) questioned the conclusions from these studies on the grounds that the studies may have been premature in the sense that the CON programs being evaluated had been operational for too short a period. He therefore replicated the study for all fifty states for the years 1973–79 to determine the effect of the presence of CON programs on expenditure growth. He concluded: "There has been no apparent effect of CON regulation on the growth of hospital expenditures, other things held constant" (154).

Reimbursement controls are a collection of supply-side constraints that attempt to alter the incentives of hospitals to provide various types and quantities of services by regulating hospital charges, reimbursement rates, and budgets. With the exception of a short period in the early 1970s when hospitals were subject to generally imposed federal cost controls under the Economic Stabilization Program (ESP), reimbursement controls operated primarily at the state level up until 1982.

The ESP under President Nixon existed in varying phases from 1971 to 1974. In some phases wage levels were frozen; in others ceilings were placed on wage and nonwage price increases. Ginsburg (1978, 319) compared increases for the period 1971–73 with those for the period 1969–71 and concluded that the ESP had been "very effective in reducing rates of increase of hospital employees' wages, but not with regard to hospital costs." Feldstein's (1981) analysis of the effects of ESP supported Ginsburg's conclusion regarding its effect on wage increases and reported that nonlabor inputs per patient-day also fell sharply under these controls. From their analysis based on data from 1,228 hospitals previously cited, Sloan and Steinwald (1980b, 171) concluded: "Of all the regulation variables considered, ESP has the most definite negative effects on input use." However, their data suggest that contrary to Ginsburg's conclusion, real wages of hospital personnel increased during this period, although total expenses declined.

Largely in response to rapidly escalating Medicaid costs, in the early 1970s states began to devise programs for regulating reimbursements to hospitals. The state programs vary greatly in scope and stringency: some are mandatory, while others are advisory; some set reimbursement rates prospectively, and others retrospectively; some set rates for all payers, and others are restricted to selected programs; some base reimbursements on budget review, while others employ a formula that includes variables pertaining to individual hospital characteristics; and some base payment on patient-day, some on case, and some on specific services rendered. Joskow (1981, chap. 6) provided a good description of the variety of state regulatory programs developed between 1970 and 1980. Hellinger (1978) and Salkever (1979, chap. 4) reviewed and assessed a number of empirical studies designed to evaluate the effectiveness of one or another of these state systems. Reviewing the experience in western Pennsylvania, Rhode Island, New Jersey, and New York, Hellinger (1978, 398) cautiously concluded that "overall, . . . firm conclusions concerning the dampening effect of prospective reimbursement on hospital inflation in the four experiments reviewed are not easily drawn." And Salkever (1979, 154), having reviewed studies of rate-setting programs in Indiana, New Jersey, New York, and Rhode Island, was no more sanguine: "Evidence of a negative rate-setting effect on average unit cost is generally meager, being weakest in the New Jersey and upstate New York studies and somewhat stronger in the Indiana study."

Meanwhile, back at the federal level, Medicare expenditures from 1973 to 1981 increased by 20 percent per year, leading Congress in 1982 and 1983 to exact "the two most significant changes in the history of Medicare" (Enthoven and Noll 1984, 1). The first was the Tax Equity and Fiscal Responsibility Act (TEFRA), by which Congress placed a ceiling on rates of increase in hospital revenues and, at the same time, extended Medicare coverage to all federal employees who previously had not been eligible. Another provision established a cost-per-case basis for reimbursement; however, these specifications were in effect overridden by the enactment the following year of the Prospective Payment System, based on fixed payments per case classified by Diagnosis Related Group (PPS/DRG). Under this system, reimbursement for inpatient services covered by Medicare shifted from a retrospective approach based on actual expenditures to a prospective budget determined by prices set in advance based on DRGs. The DRG system classifies all patients into one of 470 groups based on primary diagnosis, secondary diagnoses, surgical procedures, age, and sex

(Fetter et al. 1980). Prices for each category are determined by a complex formula based on average costs for treating this type of patient. In addition, adjustments are made for urban/rural location of hospitals and teaching status. Lohr and Marquis (1984) provide a detailed review of the major provisions of both TEFRA and PPS/DRG.

The PPS/DRG approach is modeled on the cost-containment system implemented in New Jersey. It is based on the assumption that limiting hospitals to a predetermined amount per case will create incentives for hospitals to restrict services to the minimum necessary consistent with quality care. According to Enthoven and Noll (1984, 8), "Essentially, what the new system does is to take the TEFRA cap on expenditure growth and apply it separately to each DRG." Since the new approach first went into effect for hospitals on or after 1 October 1983 (depending on their fiscal year) and is to be phased in over a three-year period, data available on its effectiveness in controlling cost increases are only preliminary (Wallace 1984; Wood 1984) but suggest that there has been a significant reduction in lengths of stay.

Utilization and quality controls were primarily a matter of individual hospital initiative until the enactment in 1965 of Medicare and Medicaid which required all participating hospitals to put in place utilization-review (UR) committees to review the appropriateness of admissions, lengths of stay, and services delivered (Gertman et al. 1979). Similarly, the meeting of accreditation standards to ensure minimum quality was professionally encouraged but not required of hospitals until the passage of Medicare.

These arrangements, in turn, led to the creation of a nationwide system of utilization review and quality control with the establishment in 1972 of the Professional Standards Review Organization (PSRO) program. This program put into place a national system of 195 area-based review organizations of elected physicians backed by an administrative and technical support staff to monitor utilization and quality of federally funded hospital care within each area (Goran et al. 1975).

Although the program was originally designed to include a strong quality-assurance component, by the time PSROs had become operational in 1977–78, the name of the game was cost containment. Carefully conducted evaluations by a research team in the Health Care Financing Administration, the responsible federal agency, based on studies comparing active with not-yet-active PSRO areas and newer with older programs discerned no consistent or statistically significant differences in hospital utilization related to PSRO functioning (Health Care Financing Administration 1980).

Under the recently adopted PPS/DRG approach, a new system of private contract organizations, termed Professional Review Organizations, will replace the PSRO system. This new review mechanism is charged with monitoring the costs and quality of services dispensed to Medicare patients and reviewing all hospital requests for exceptions to DRG-based payments.

This brief review of regulatory efforts by public agencies at the federal and state levels only hints at the variety and complexity of the programs developed to contain hospital costs. It also suggests that with the possible exception of the use of direct cost controls under the ESP, these efforts have been largely ineffective. Not only have most studies failed to find that regulatory programs reduce costs but a few studies have suggested that they actually increase costs. In an analysis of PSRO performance, Ginsburg and Koretz (1979) reported that although the program was associated with a slight reduction in hospital use, the savings realized were less than 30 percent of the costs of operating the program. Analysts have long noted that in addition to the costs associated with the operation of regulatory programs, there also tends to be an economic burden on the systems being regulated. A study by Drake (1980) of hospitals in the Carolinas and in Michigan attempted to determine the costs imposed on hospitals complying with five types of regulations—CON, utilization reviews by PSROs, personnel-management requirements, fire codes, and safety codes. He estimated that for the year 1977 the costs of compliance added 1.5–2.0 percent to total hospital costs. Kinzer (1977), in a less systematic study of a more highly regulated state (Massachusetts) suggested that the costs of regulation may have been twice as high as Drake indicated.

Feldstein raises a more crucial issue: in the absence of any clear standards on health care quality, it is dangerous to allow external parties to control the medical encounter. As Feldstein (1981, 7) argued, "Direct regulation of hospital costs is inappropriate because there is no 'technically correct' way for the regulators to set an appropriate maximum quality of hospital care . . . the direct regulation of hospital costs would in the long run make the nature and quality of hospital services completely unresponsive to the preferences of patients and their physicians."

Hospital Factors Affecting Hospital Costs

The general types of factors contributing to the rise in hospital costs during the past three decades, just reviewed, affect all hospitals in roughly comparable ways. They focus attention primarily on changes over time in costs for the hospital industry as a whole rather than on differences in costs among hospitals at a given point in time. We turn now to factors influencing the costs of hospital care that relate more clearly to differences among hospitals.

Hospitals are highly variable in their organizational characteristics. Even if psychiatric, long-term-care, and other specialized facilities are excluded and attention is focused on general, acute-care facilities, a wide range of types is apparent. In this section, we examine those differences among hospitals that have been reported to affect the cost of care. These include (1) services and/or case mix, (2) size, (3) teaching status, (4) characteristics of the medical staff, (5) type of ownership, (6) system membership, and (7) management practices.

Services and Case Mix

Hospitals are multiproduct firms. While their primary outputs are those associated with inpatient care, most hospitals also produce varying quantities of education, research, outpatient care, and community services. Each of these types of outputs is intrinsically difficult to measure, and to attempt to combine them raises serious issues of commensurability and relative importance or value. In this section we focus only on the problem of measuring quantity and costs of outputs; difficulties associated with assessment of quality differences are considered in the following section.

Even when attention is restricted to inpatient care, there are great differences among hospitals in the types of patients treated and, hence, in the types of services provided and outputs produced. As Lave (1966, 58) pointed out, "The average patient day of a 30-bed rural hospital is vasty different from that of a 600-bed teaching hospital. In comparing the cost per patient day in the two hospitals, the difference in product must be taken into account. (Not taking account of the difference is analogous to ignoring the difference between a Volkswagen and a Rolls Royce.)" In order to take into account differences among hospitals in the types of work performed, early studies such as that by Berry (1967) grouped hospitals according to their types of facilities, although Berry acknowledged that this approach represented a "second-best approximation to grouping by product homogeneity." In another early study, Feldstein (1967) used the percentage of cases in each of eight medical-surgical departments as a proxy for case mix. Most later approaches have focused attention directly on patient characteristics, in particular the distribution of patients across variously defined diagnostic categories. Thus, an early influential study by Lave and Lave (1971) developed a measure of "role differentiation" among hospitals based on diagnosis and surgical procedures as recorded in patient data obtained from the Hospital Cost and Utilization Project (HCUP). Employing diagnostic categories based on seventeen broad International Classification of Diseases Adapted (ICDA) groups, as well as a more detailed set of forty-eight categories, and applying them to assess the case mix of sixty-five hospitals in western Pennsylvania, they were able to show evidence of considerable variation among "similar" hospitals in the types of patients treated and in the relative stability over time in the case mix for a given hospital.

In the present context, differences among facilities or patients in hospitals are of little interest unless they can be shown to affect differences in costs among hospitals. These studies were able to do so. For example, Feldstein (1967) estimated that even his crude index of case mix explained 27 percent of the variation in total costs per case among his sample of British hospitals (see also Berry 1970). And as hospital costs became an increasingly salient issue, investigators began to construct measures of case mix specificially designed to maximize explained variance in hospital costs. (Of course, when the issue is quality of care rather than costs, different approaches are used to assess differences in case mix. Examples of these are given in the following section and in chap. 4.)

Thompson, Fetter, and Mross (1975) developed their AUTOGRP system in an attempt to group patients into diagnostic categories and, by taking into account such additional factors as age, sex, use of surgery, and complications, to predict differences in the use of hospital resources (see also Fetter et al. 1980). This system eventually became the basis for the DRG classification now being used to determine reimbursement formulae for Medicare patients. It is significant that the DRG system is currently under attack on the grounds that it accounts for too little of the variance in costs per case (Horn and Sharkey 1983; Enthoven and Noll 1984). Although we can expect further refinements to be made in techniques for measuring case-mix differences among hospitals, it has now been firmly established that hospitals vary significantly in the types of patients treated and that these differences account for a substantial amount of the variation among hospitals in the costs of treating patients.

Size

Due to economies of scale (Stigler 1958), the costs associated with producing a given unit of output are often observed to decline as the scale of the production organization increases. There is continuing disagreement, however, as to whether economies of scale apply to human service organizations such as hospitals (Brown 1972).

Although as of 1975 over half (53 percent) of the short-term acute-care hospitals had less than a 100-bed capacity, the average bed capacity of hospitals in the United States had steadily increased during the past fifty years. Thus, voluntary nonprofit hospitals grew from an average bed capacity of 104 in 1928 to an average of 196 by 1975; and during the same period, for-profit hospitals, which are much smaller on the average, increased from 31 to 94 beds (White 1982, 154). Nevertheless, the range in bed capacity among hospitals is very large and continues to be a very significant characteristic of this industry.

As already noted, hospitals that vary in size are also likely to vary in case mix, types of facilities, and, hence, types of outputs, so that it is important to take these factors into account in assessing the effects of size on costs. In his early study already noted, Berry (1967) examined data for 15 percent of the hospitals in the United States grouped into forty categories, so that each contained hospitals with "identical" facilities, and then regressed costs per patient-day on the total number of patient-days for each type of hospital. He concluded that the pattern of results was consistent with an economies-of-scale argument, with larger hospitals exhibiting somewhat lower costs per patient-day. In a similar approach, Carr and P. Feldstein (1967) examined data from 3,147 hospitals, relating average costs per patient-day to the average daily census within each of five "service-capability" groups, as measured by number of facilities, services, and programs. They concluded that "economies of scale in the provision of care appear to exist over a wide range of sizes in each of the service-capability groups" (61). These early studies were challenged, however, on the grounds that the number of hospital facilities or measures of service capability were not adequate proxies for differences in case mix or services. As Jeffers and Siebert (1974, 295) noted, "The mere availability of services and facilities reflects neither rates of utilization nor the intensity with which services are rendered." Using the distribution of patients across eight hospital departments as his index of case mix, M. Feldstein (1967) concluded in his study of 177 nonteaching hospitals in England that when case mix was taken into account, size had little effect on costs per case.

One reason why it is difficult to draw firm conclusions from these and similar studies is that different cost measures were employed. While Berry and Carr and P. Feldstein used average cost per patient-day as their indicator of costs, M. Feldstein emphasized cost per case. Indeed, M. Feldstein's study found that while costs per patient-day tended to decrease as size increased, which is consistent with the other studies and with economies-of-scale predictions, these savings were offset by what Feldstein referred to as the "case flow" effect, the number of cases per bed per year. Case flow tended to decrease as size increased because length of stay was greater in larger hospitals, presumably reflecting case mixes of greater complexity and severity.

These early results have been replicated in more recent studies. Thus, Sloan and Steinwald (1980b), in their study employing pooled, cross-sectional data from 1,228 hospitals over the period 1969–75, reported that scale economies were observed when costs were computed on adjusted patient-days but that the reverse was true when costs were based on adjusted patient admissions.

Generally speaking, there seems to be diminished interest in the question of hospital size as a factor in determining costs. In part, this is because there is now widespread consensus that in comparing costs among hospitals, costs per case rather than costs per patient-day is the appropriate measure; and size does not appear to have the expected effects on costs per case. It is also widely acknowledged that larger hospitals are different kinds of organizations than smaller hospitals, with different structures, processes, and outputs (Neuhauser and Andersen 1972), so that size cannot be treated as an isolated variable. Finally, as an increasing number of hospitals share services or move into some kind of cooperative association with other hospitals and medical care units, the size of a particular establishment becomes a less meaningful attribute.

Teaching Status

Some hospitals not only provide patient care but engage in a variety of professional teaching programs. The term *teaching hospital* refers to hospitals engaged in the training of physicians, although many hospitals conduct teaching activities for other types of health care personnel. But even the meaning of the term is somewhat ambiguous, and it is used in several ways. The most restrictive definition limits the label to those major teaching hospitals that are members of the Council of Teaching Hospitals of the Association of American Medical Colleges. In 1982, 411, or about 7 percent, of all nonfederal, short-term hospitals were members of the council. A more inclusive definition appends the label to hospitals affiliated with a medical school. In 1982, 1,059, or 18 percent, of nonfederal, short-term hospitals met this criterion. Most broadly defined, a teaching hospital is a hospital that has been approved to participate in one or more residency training programs by the Accreditation Council for Graduate Medical Education. As of 1982, 1,237, or 21 percent, of the nonfederal, short-term hospitals were in this category (AHA 1983, table 10A).

Most analysts agree that teaching programs tend to raise the average cost of patient care. Thus, in their early study employing data from 3,175 acute-care hospitals, Carr and P. Feldstein (1967) reported that within each of their five "service-capability" groups, total costs were higher for hospitals operating internship and residency programs. Affiliation with a medical school did not have an additional significant effect on costs after the presence of training programs for house staff was taken into account. And in a study of a random sample of 982 hospitals combining data from 1964 to 1973 in a cross-sectional time series, Lave and Lave (1978) reported that controlling for complexity of facilities, size, occupancy rate, and length of stay, the average cost per case was highest in major teaching hospitals, intermediate in nonmajor teaching hospitals, and lowest in nonteaching hospitals. They also identified four basic reasons for higher costs in teaching hospitals: "(1) the cases treated are likely to be more complex; (2) for a given case, more tests and so forth may be ordered; (3) the salaries of interns and residents are included in total costs; and (4) in teaching hospitals physicians are more likely to be salaried and thus physician costs are sometimes incorporated in the hospital costs" (564).

Costs of treatment are known to be higher in teaching hospitals, but how much higher? Sloan, Feldman, and Steinwald (1983) employed data from several sources for the years 1974 and 1977 for a national sample of 367 short-term, general hospitals to compare the costs per adjusted patient-day and per adjusted admission of nonteaching hospitals and the three types of teaching hospitals (hospitals with residency training programs, hospitals with medical school affiliations, and major teaching hospitals that were members of the Council of Teaching Hospitals). Sloan and colleagues estimated that compared with nonphysician costs in nonteaching hospitals, those in teaching hospitals were higher by the percentages shown in table 3.2. This study suggests that the type of definition of teaching hospital employed does make a difference and that when case mix is taken into account, major teaching hospitals are at most 15 percent more costly per case (i.e., admission) than nonteaching hospitals.

Table 3.2. Percentage increase in expenses for teaching hospitals and nonteaching hospitals, 1974 to 1977

Types of Teaching Hospitals	Expenses per Adjusted Patient-Day	Expenses per Adjusted Admission
Hospitals with residency training	5.2	2.0
Hospitals with medical school affiliations	9.7	5.2
Hospitals belonging to Council of Teaching Hospitals	19.7	13.9

Source: Sloan, Feldman, and Steinwald 1983.

Characteristics of the Medical Staff

The size, nature, and degree of organization of the medical staff varies greatly among hospitals (Roemer and Friedman 1971), but relatively little research has attempted to link these characteristics to hospital costs. Probably the most direct and important connection that has been identified is the nature of the payment arrangements linking physicians, patients, and hospitals. Luft (1981a) reviewed a large number of studies comparing costs of care provided by physicians to patients in Health Maintenance Organizations (HMOs)— systems in which a group of physicians assumes a contractual responsibility to provide a specified range of medical services to a population of subscribers who have agreed to pay a fixed payment that is independent of the use of services— with costs of care for comparable patients using conventional fee-for-service providers. Luft reported that in spite of the great variation within these two categories of providers, costs in HMOs were 10–40 percent lower. Moreover, most of these savings can be attributed to differences in hospitalization rates: patients in HMO plans were hospitalized at rates 10–40 percent below those of conventionally insured populations (Luft 1978, 1981a).

The studies reviewed by Luft have been criticized on the grounds that the differences observed may have been the result of differences in the types of individuals selecting one or the other payment arrangement. This alternative explanation has recently been tested and rejected by an experiment conducted by Rand in which 1,580 individuals were randomly assigned to receive care free of charge from either a fee-for-service physician of their choice or an HMO-type organization, the Group Health Cooperative of Puget Sound in Seattle. While there were no differences between the two groups in outpatient visits, the rate of hospital admissions for the HMO patients was about 40 percent less than that of the fee-for-service group, and the overall calculated expenditures for all services were about 25 percent less for the HMO patients (Manning et al. 1984).

Whether or not physician payment arrangements also influence costs for patients who have been hospitalized is less clear. Some evidence that they may do so is provided by a study by Luke and Thompson (1980) comparing the behavior of physicians in a prepaid group practice with those in a fee-for-service group practice using the same hospital facility. They examined cases treated by physicans from these two groups over a three-month period during 1977, adjusting for differences in case severity and diagnosis. They noted no significant differences between types of physicians in the use of technical services—laboratory and radiology charges—but did observe a significant difference in their use of physician consultations: fee-for-service physicians both requested and rendered more consultations than did physicians in the prepaid group practice. Luke and Thompson speculated that this difference may have reflected the importance of consultations and referrals as sources of physician revenue under fee-for-service arrangements. But these authors also acknowledged that within-hospital use of services was probably less affected by differences in payment arrangements than were admissions patterns.

These studies of the medical staff were based on examinations of the characteristics of individual physicians, for example, whether the doctor was a member of a prepaid group practice. It is also possible to examine the characteristics of the medical staff as a corporate body and to determine whether or not the characteristics of the staff itself influence costs. Sometimes the same or similar variables can be measured at the level of either the individual physician or the medical staff, and it is possible to observe different, and sometimes conflicting, findings. The following studies illustrate both the use of varying levels of analysis and contrasting results.

Two studies attempted to determine the effect of physician specialization on hospital costs. Pauly (1978), working at the level of the medical staff, examined data collected in 1975 from fifty nonmajor teaching, short-term hospitals in California. After adjusting for case-mix differences using a method based on average charges for diagnosis groups, he found total costs and costs per case to be higher in hospitals with a higher proportion of specialists. Rhee, Luke, and Culverwell (1980), however, in their study of physicians in Hawaii conducted at the level of the individual physician, found specialists to be engaged in behaviors likely to reduce hospitalization costs. Data based on a sample of 3,316 patients in sixteen major diagnostic categories treated in twenty-two hospitals by 506 physicians were scored using Payne's (1966) process categories to assess conformity with "established medical practice." The more highly specialized physicians had higher scores on the appropriateness of their admissions decisions; a higher proportion of their patients scored as exhibiting a shorter-than-expected length of stay; and a lower proportion of their patients scored as exhibiting a longer-than-expected length of stay. Although cost data were not collected, these are the types of decisions that would be expected to lead to reduced hospital costs.

Another study relating length of stay to the characteristics of the medical staff was conducted by Becker, Shortell, and Neuhauser (1980). These analysts measured the degree of autonomy—the extent to which physicians are free to determine what, when, where, and how they perform their clinical work—of the medical staff both as a group and as individual physicians in forty-two short-term, nonteaching hospitals in Massachusetts in 1971–72. Controlling for case-mix severity, the quality of care using a medical-surgical death rate and an index of complications, and extended-stay beds in the hospital's service area, these investigators found that a medical staff with greater autonomy was associated with a hospital having shorter preoperative lengths of stay for Medicare patients. In contrast, they found that greater autonomy for individual physicians was associated with longer overall lengths of stay for Medicare patients. Again, we note that the same variable (autonomy) apparently has different effects at the level of the medical staff than at the level of the individual physician.

One final characteristic of the medical staff that appears to have important effects on hospital costs can be noted. In the study described above, Pauly (1978) measured a second attribute of the medical staff: output concentration. Similar to the industrial-organization measure of concentration, this variable assesses the extent to which outputs (patients) are tightly concentrated around a few attending physicians or widely distributed across many. He reports that the more highly concentrated the medical staff, the lower the total and the per-case costs.

Type of Ownership

As of 1982, there were 6,915 hospitals of all types in the United States. Of this number, approximately 350 were federal hospitals, primarily Veterans Administration and specialized facilities (tuberculosis); another 700 or so were primarily psychiatric hospitals or hospitals specializing in long-term care. The remaining 5,863 facilities made up the population of general, acute-care, short-term hospitals. It was on this group of hospitals that we focused attention. Table 3.3 gives the number of hospitals, beds, and adjusted expenses per patient-day for three subtypes of these nonfederal, general hospitals in 1982.

The largest subtype of general hospital is the nongovernmental, not-for-profit category often termed *voluntary*. It includes church-owned hospitals; community hospitals owned by independent, nonprofit corporations; and a number of other types, such as industrial hospitals and Kaiser Plan hospitals. The state- and local-government category consists primarily of county and community hospitals. The investor-owned or proprietary hospitals are those owned by individuals, partnerships, or corporations and operated for a profit.

It is improtant to point out that data supplied by the Federation of American Hospitals (FAH), which represents the investor-owned hospitals, vary considerably from those reported by the AHA. Thus, in its 1982 directory, the FAH (1982) reported a total of 1,016 investor-owned hospitals rather than 748.

Table 3.3. Distribution of hospitals, beds, and adjusted expenses per patient-day, by hospital type, 1982

Type of Hospital	Number of Hospitals	Number of Beds (thousands)	Total Adjusted Expenses per Patient-Day
Federal	346	114	—
Nonfederal, short-term	5,863	1,015	$2,493
Nongovernmental, not-for-profit	3,354	712	2,570
State and local government	1,761	212	2,337
Investor-owned (for-profit)	748	91	2,224
Total, all types	6,915	1,360	—

Source: Selected data from AHA 1983, table 1.

It may be that this accounting included a substantial number of nongeneral or long-term-care hospitals. According to the FAH data, the total number of proprietary hospitals changed very little since 1975, but the percentage of independently owned versus system hospitals decreased from 64 percent in 1975 to 38 percent in 1982. This movement of independent hospitals into systems, characteristic of the not-for-profit as well as the for-profit group, is discussed below.

Note that the AHA expenses data suggest that after adjustments to take into account differences in case mix among hospitals, total expenses per patient-day were highest in not-for-profit hospitals, intermediate in state- and local-government hospitals, and lowest in investor-owned hospitals. This may reflect true cost differences or imperfect adjustments for case mix.

There are studies to suggest that the for-profit hospitals are more responsive to incentives to curtail costs (Rushing 1974; Kushman and Nuckton 1977). But other studies report that the cost savings achieved are reflected in higher profits, not in lower prices (Lewin, Derzon, and Margulies 1981). Unfortunately, there have been relatively few systematic studies of performance, cost, and pricing differences between not-for-profit and for-profit hospitals, so that answers to important economic questions are scarce. Moreover, the apparent resurgence of the proprietary sector and, more generally, the movement to a more competitive environment for all hospitals raises not only economic but medical, legal, and ethical issues as well (Gray 1983; Meyer 1983).

System Membership

The descriptive statistics on the distribution of hospitals by ownership type mask the most important current change in hospital structure, namely, that hospitals today are less likely to be organized as independent, freestanding enterprises and are increasingly likely to be involved in some mode of interinstitutional collaboration. As of 1980, over 80 percent of U.S. hospitals participated in some form of sharing of services—from laundry and laboratory to clinical specialties and administrative management—and over 30 percent had entered into some kind of formal system (Goldsmith 1981). The variety of these new interinstitutional arrangements is great and defies easy categorization. Brown and McCool (1980) attempted to identify modes of collaboration ranging from program affiliation, shared services, and contract management to consortia, condominiums, holding companies, and total consolidation, but they acknowledged that there are important organizational variations within as well as between categories (see also Zuckerman 1979).

Collaborative arrangements are as likely to involve not-for-profit hospitals as they are for-profit hospitals. Statistics compiled by Ermann and Gabel (1984) reported that the number of not-for-profit hospitals moving into systems increased from 727 in 1978 to 967 in 1982, an annual average growth rate of 11.4 percent, compared with the increase in for-profit hospitals from 628 in 1978 to 773 in 1982, an annual average growth rate of 5.3 percent. The for-profit and not-for-profit systems also differ in several important respects: the for-profit systems are much larger on the average, containing more hospitals and extending over a larger geographical area, usually several states, while the not-for-profit systems have fewer hospitals and are more regionally concentrated into one or two states. At the same time, not-for-profit systems occur throughout the country, while for-profit systems tend to concentrate in the Sunbelt states, where favorable regulatory and reimbursement practices exist.

Analysts have generally agreed that systems have advantages over independent hospitals in raising capital and that they may realize some important economies of scale with respect to a number of services. It is also alleged that systems use highly skilled personnel more efficiently than independent hospitals and that for-profit systems in particular use fewer staff members per unit of output. The evidence to support these assertions was assembled and reviewed by Ermann and Gabel (1984), but it should be noted that few systematic studies have been conducted in this rapidly changing area. Moreover, systems differ greatly in their structure and performance, and it is difficult to separate selection from structural explanations for any differences observed. Further, several studies have found evidence that the age of the system has an important impact on cost, with start-up costs making costs per case higher for the first few years. Whether age or natural selection to eliminate unsuccessful systems or components is responsible for this trend has not been studied.

Starr (1982) hypothesized that system hospitals, particularly those that have moved into a multidivisional form with a separate corporate headquarters overseeing the operation of a number of medical care organizations, may secure important cost savings by restricting physician autonomy in decisions regarding admissions, service intensity, and length of stay. Whether new corporate managers are able to acquire this kind of control over decisions historically reserved to the individual clinician and the medical staff remains to be seen.

Management Practices

Relatively few studies have focused on the effects of varying administrative arrangements or management practices on hospital costs. Among the few analysts who have investigated such managerial factors is Neuhauser. In an early study, Neuhauser (1971) employed data from thirty short-term-care community hospitals in the Chicago area to test a series of predictions relating management practices to several measures of efficiency. All thirty hospitals participated in the Hospital Administration Services (HAS) data-collection program, which provided them with a statistical analysis of monthly costs, manpower, and output data based on standardized definitions. Three varieties of management control practices were identified: (1) the specification of working procedures by hospital superiors for subordinates, as measured by questionnaire responses of department heads and the use of written job descriptions; (2) the visibility of organizational consequences to managers, measured by how accurately the administrator was able to compare his or her hospital with others in the area on a series of measures; and (3) the use of reports as a managerial tool. Efficiency was assessed by several indicators, including a unit-cost index based on cost data from seven nonmedical departments, a man-hour index based on data from the same departments, expert judgment of hospital efficiency, and occupancy rate. Results suggested that specification of procedures, visibility of consequences, and the existence of a number of administrative reports were all significantly associated with improved efficiency. Neuhauser (1971, 49–54) estimated that together with measures of hospital size and the complexity of facilities, these measures of managerial practices accounted for 28–60 percent of the variance in the efficiency of the nonmedical departments, depending on which indicator of efficiency was used.

A more recent investigation utilized many of these same variables in studying forty-two general, short-term-care, nonteaching hospitals in Massachusetts (Shortell, Becker, and Neuhauser 1976; Becker, Shortell, and Neuhauser 1980). Four types of efficiency measures were developed: (1) direct costs per patient-day in three nonmedical support departments; (2) direct costs per patient-day in four medical support departments; (3) overall costs per case; and (4) average length of stay for all patients. After taking into account case-mix severity and medical-surgical death rate, the investigators found that the visibility of consequences to administrators was related to greater efficiency for all four measures. Other measures of managerial awareness were also associated with lower costs or reduced lengths of stay but were not consistent across all efficiency indicators.

In the traditional hospital structure, a fairly clear demarcation has existed between the spheres of authority of the administrative group on the one hand

Table 3.4. Perceptions of hospital administrators

Factor	Cost Savings Potential	Administrators' Power	Physicians' Power
Length of stay	1	5	5
Admissions	2	6	2
Quality	3	7	6
Intensity	4	9	4
Teaching	5	4	7
Efficiency	6	3	8
Scope of services	7.5	8	3
Input prices	7.5	2	9
Case mix	9	10	1
Investments	10	1	10

Source: Allison 1976.

and the medical staff on the other. Each body has tended to exercise control over a somewhat separate set of decisions, and these decisions, in turn, have had varying degrees of influence over hospital costs. Allison (1976) attempted to obtain a relatively systematic description of this division of decisions between physicians and administrators. Surveying all hospital administrators in the state of Michigan, Allison asked them to rank their power relative to that of physicians for ten factors and to rank the cost-savings potential for each factor. The results are given in table 3.4. These rankings emphasize the administrators' perceptions of limitations on their power to influence hospital decisions that affect costs. They also suggest that serious attempts to curtail cost increases will need to involve physicians if they are to succeed.

Even this brief overview reminds us of the extent of the variations among hospitals—how much they differ with respect to such basic characteristics as size, ownership, internal organization, and external connections. Although no one would argue that the evidence is straightforward or always consistent, in combination the studies do strongly support the proposition that these differences among hospitals significantly influence the costs of delivering care to patients. We next ask whether such differences affect the quality of care provided.

THE QUALITY OF CARE IN HOSPITALS

Because of the concern over rising costs of hospital care, hospitals increasingly have become the targets not only for efforts to contain rising costs but also for regulatory, professional, and political demands to improve effectiveness. Effective performance encompasses more than controlling costs through efficient production of services; it also concerns the quality of services provided. Up to this point our review has concentrated almost exclusively on studies concerned with costs. We turn now to focus on issues and factors influencing the quality of care in hospitals.

How can one tell when a hospital is effective? There is general agreement that such a question is too simply put. It implies that there is a single, meaningful criterion by which to judge effectiveness in hospitals, when in fact hospitals are complex organizations, involving many subunits producing many types of outputs and attempting to achieve many diverse and often competing objectives. Even when we limit our concern to health outputs, there are many dimensions to the quality of care—accessibility, appropriateness, sufficiency, timeliness, efficacy in producing the desired result. The quality of care can be described as a portmanteau concept: "it carries a great many things, keeps them in no particular order, and does so in a way that conceals them from view" (Kahn 1977, 237).

Elsewhere we review the many conceptual and methodological issues involved in defining and assessing the quality of care in hospitals (see below, chap. 4. See also Luft 1981a; and Scott and Shortell 1983). Here we briefly consider only one of these issues: what the primary indicators are that may be employed in assessing quality.

Indicators of the Quality of Care

Donabedian (1966, 1980) usefully categorized the various indicators to measure the quality of care into three groups: structure, process, and outcome. Of course, such measures may be evaluated at the level of the individual patient or aggregated in various ways so as to categorize the quality of care provided by specific providers, groups of providers, hospitals, and so forth.

Structure refers to "the relatively stable characteristics of the providers of care, of the tools and resources they have at their disposal, and the physical and organizational setting in which they work" (Donabedian 1980, 81). These characteristics include the qualifications of the provider (experience, training, licensure, and certification) or average staff qualifications, type and quality of facilities, and accreditation and program approvals at the hospital level. *Process* indicators refer to the set of activities that go on between the providers and the patient, including the management of both the technical and the interpersonal processes involved. Examples include preparing a patient history, conducting a physical examination and adhering to norms of good practice. *Outcomes* are the changes in a patient's health status that can be attributed to receiving health care and are broadly enough defined to refer to physiological, social, and psychological function and attitudes, including satisfaction with any aspect of the care provided. Examples include postsurgical infections, death, and satisfaction with the outcome or process of care at an individual level, or the rate of each at a physician or hospital level. The implied interrelationships among these three types of measures can be diagrammed as

$$structure \longrightarrow process \longrightarrow outcomes$$

because structural characteristics of the settings can influence the process of care, which in turn can influence the outcomes obtained.

Most authors embrace these distinctions but disagree about which indicators have the most face validity in measuring the quality of care. One group argues that the primary object of study in medical care is the process of providing it, and outcomes and structures are both indirect measures of the process (McAuliffe 1978, 1979; Donabedian 1980). Others argue that outcomes are the primary objective of medical care, and thus process measures are once removed from the actual phenomena to be evaluated, and structural measures twice removed, since they reflect only the capacity for the provider or organization to perform well (Scott, Forrest, and Brown 1976; Scott 1977; Luft 1981a). Part of the disagreement about the validity of the indicators is based on conceptual differences regarding which aspects of care are to be evaluated, and part occurs because of the weak causal linkages among the three types of indicators and the low association among indicators of the same type (Brook 1973). For example, a structural indicator of good quality based on the excellence of the facilities does not necessarily mean that good process will result. In turn, well-performed interpersonal management of a patient may not produce good health but may lead to patient satisfaction.

It is important to recognize that there are biases, strengths, and weaknesses for each type of measure. For example, structural measures offer the advantage of being relatively easy to measure and compare across institutions but may be biased in favor of large or teaching hospitals, since these institutions may be able to attract well-trained physicians and modern and sophisticated technology. Studies that examine causal relationships between hospital structural arrangements and hospital performance, using *structural* measures of performance are particularly likely to observe tautological or spurious relationships.

Process measures also have problems and biases. A process measure based on a doctor's orders can be relatively easy to collect and reliably recorded in a patient chart. However, an assessment of the quality of the orders—their necessity and adequacy—requires comparison with a standard that, if implicit, can take into account changes in medical knowledge and particular information about the patient's case but may vary from rater to rater. On the other hand, explicit standards can be applied more reliably but may be based on outdated or incorrect standards (see Donabedian 1981 for a more extensive discussion). Process measures can be biased toward finding high quality in hospitals having a major affiliation with a medical school if the measures are based on the application of the most recent medical knowledge and technology or on providing the most extensive diagnostic workup.

Outcome measures also have their drawbacks. Outcome measures focus on the actual changes produced and so avoid making a judgment on the medical knowledge or technology used but may be so infrequently observed (such as deaths) as to require very large data bases or may be difficult to measure reliably (such as postoperative morbidity, which is not regularly or uniformly recorded in patient records and can vary from rater to rater). Measures of patient satisfaction have the advantage of including the patient's perspective, but such data are not readily available. Moreover, patients are not expected to be able to evaluate either the technical quality of care received or the aspects of care they do not observe. Outcome measures can also introduce biases of a different sort. For example, some hospitals, such as major teaching institutions, function as referral centers for very difficult cases. An outcome measure of quality that does not adequately control for case-mix differences will be biased against these types of hospitals.

Finally, all three categories of indicators are subject to numerous common problems that beset attempts to accurately measure complex, changing variables (see chap. 4 for a more detailed review). These include problems of remoteness, of sampling procedures, and of timing of assessment. Briefly, while some measures of quality are based on direct observations of processes or outcomes, others are based on more remote information sources such as charts and patient abstracts. Perhaps the most remote type of evidence employed involves assessments based on physician or hospital reputation as assessed by "expert" observers. Sampling issues involve how activities of patients or providers are selected for study and the extent to which the units sampled are representative of the larger population of concern. Different conclusions about the quality of care may result depending on the timing of data collection. For example, the number and types of procedures performed on patients vary greatly depending on whether the patient is in the early or later stages of hospitalization; and the point at which outcomes are assessed has a critical effect on judgment of quality. Patients are often less well following medical intervention than before because of the invasive effects of the procedures themselves on health status.

With these brief comments and caveats, we turn now to review evidence relating the quality of care to the characteristics of the hospitals providing medical care.

Hospital Factors Affecting the Quality of Care

There is substantial evidence that hospitals differ not only in the types of patients they treat and the costs of this treatment but also in the quality of care they deliver. Regardless of whether measures of structure, process, or outcome have been used, researchers have found consistent evidence that care in hospitals does differ significantly, even when case mix is carefully controlled (see Moses and Mosteller 1968; Brook 1973; SCHCR 1974; National Academy of Sciences Institute of Medicine 1976; and chap. 5 in this volume). There is also evidence that hospitals differ substantially in the way they are organized, in the characteristics of their staff and facilities, and in their relation to their environment. The obvious next question, and the primary concern in this section of our review is, Which differences in the organizational aspects of hospitals relate to the quality of care delivered, and why?

Firm conclusions about the hospital factors that explain the quality of care based on the few quantitative studies available would be both premature and oversimplified. The few studies differ in the number and types of hospitals studied (ranging from case studies of one hospital or one multihospital system to the universe of voluntary hospitals), the organizational features examined, and the methods for assessing the quality of care. Nonetheless, there is some convergence in research findings which we will emphasize in this brief review. (See also Goss 1970; Palmer and Reilly 1979; Rhee 1983; and Scott and Shortell 1983 for reviews of hospital organization and the quality of care.)

Teaching Status

As already noted, the definition of a hospital's teaching status can vary from having a residency program to having a major teaching responsibility. Goss (1970) summarized the early evidence in support of the generalization that teaching hospitals provide better care. The majority of these early studies compared outcomes or audits of process in a limited number of both teaching and nonteaching hospitals and employed relatively crude adjustments to take into account patient variation by type of hospital, usually by restricting the examination to only a few types of cases. Among these studies was Kohl's (1955), which reported lower percentages of "preventable" perinatal deaths among patients in two teaching hospitals than in two nonteaching hospitals in New York City. Lee and colleagues (Lee, Morrison, and Morris 1957; Lipworth, Lee, and Morris 1963) contrasted case fatalities, adjusted for age and sex, for three types of common surgical procedures and found that in Great Britain teaching hospitals had lower mortality rates than nonteaching hospitals. Two studies based on process measures of quality for a sample of Teamster families treated in approximately 100 hospitals found that care was better in teaching hospitals in general and especially so in hospitals with a major affiliation with a medical school (Morehead and Donaldson 1964; Trussell, Morehead, and Ehrlich 1962). The Commission on Professional and Hospital Activities (CPHA 1970) studied the mortality, adjusted for age, sex, and extent of surgery, of 96,317 cholecystectomy patients treated in 938 U.S. hospitals and found evidence that both larger size and the teaching status of the hospital were associated with lower mortality.

In contrast, our studies reported in this volume found no or mixed evidence that teaching status was associated with lower mortality. In the seventeen hospitals of the IS, no association of adjusted mortality and morbidity rates with teaching status was found (Flood and Scott 1978 [see also chap. 9 in this volume]). In the 1,224 ES hospitals, the effects of teaching appeared to vary by type of disease-surgical category (chap. 11) and by the type of indicator of teaching intensity (chap. 12), after controlling for patient-level variation in health status and hospital-level measures associated with teaching status such as size and expenditures.

Fleming (1981) used a national household survey of 490 patients to examine the relation between teaching status and patient satisfaction. Contrary to her predictions, even after adjusting for patient demographic characteristics, she found that patients were likely to view teaching hospitals, which tended also to be large hospitals, unfavorably. In interpreting her results, she argued that low satisfaction with the care in teaching hospitals is a valid indication of poor quality because there is evidence that stress may compromise whatever advantages teaching hospitals offer in superior technical care (although the causal relationship suggested is tenuous at best).

In a recent study, Garber, Fuchs, and Silverman (1984) examined differences in mortality adjusted for age, sex, race, urgency of admission, area of residence, previous discharge, and one of twelve DRGs. Comparisons were made between patients treated by full-time teaching faculty (and residents) and patients treated by community physicians, with both groups practicing in the same major teaching hospital. They found evidence to support lower adjusted inhospital mortality among patients on the faculty service, although a follow-up study to compare survival at nine months after discharge found no differences between patients treated by the faculty and those treated by community physicians. Two other significant differences in treatment between the two groups were noted: the patients treated on the faculty service had greater expenditures per patient (after adjusting for illness) and a lower rate of orders not to resuscitate. The authors speculate that the greater use of diagnostic services by trainees may reflect the educational utility of the tests, an "unwillingness or inability to rely as heavily as the more seasoned private physicians on the clinical examination . . . (and) an unwillingness to allow patients to die . . . even when it led to little or no improvement in patient outcome" (Garber, Fuchs, and Silverman 1984, 1235).

Patient Case Mix and Volume

Both conceptual and methodological issues are involved in measuring case mix and using it to adjust quality-of-care indicators. Because hospitals can exercise control over their patient case mix and volume, at least to some extent, these measures are also of interest as indicators of the ability of the hospital to manipulate its environment successfully and as descriptors of the complexity of the cases they must be prepared to treat. Organizational theory based on an open-systems approach would argue that there is no one best way to organize to achieve quality care; instead the organizational features of hospitals should depend in part on the difficulty of producing the services and outcomes required for the set of patients treated (Neuhauser 1971; Scott, Forrest, and Brown 1976; Shortell and Kaluzny 1983).

While there is some evidence that certain structural features of hospitals are associated with more difficult case mixes (e.g., teaching hospitals tend to treat more difficult patient diseases; large urban hospitals, sicker patients; proprietary hospitals, younger patients of a higher socioeconomic level), the effect of structure on the quality of care that is contingent upon the difficulty of the case mix remains essentially unexplored.

The SCHCR study addressed this issue but found little evidence to support a series of contingency hypotheses (Scott, Forrest, and Brown 1976; Forrest et al. 1978). Using data from the seventeen-hospital study, we examined the relations between structural indicators of coordination and control and outcomes to see whether systematic differences by case mix could be observed. The small number of (hospital) cases and surprisingly similar indicators of overall case mix render these results tentative at best. Flood (1976) did find some evidence to support a contingent relation between physician qualifications and training and better adjusted postsurgical outcomes; individual physician qualifications were important predictors of quality only for those surgical procedures judged to be more complex by a national panel of practicing surgeons. (See Schoonhoven et al. 1980 for a description of the complexity ratings and procedures for collecting them.)

The evidence relating volume of cases treated at a hospital to the quality of care is more consistent and persuasive. Luft and colleagues (Luft, Bunker, and Enthoven 1979; Luft 1980) studied twelve procedures treated in 1,498 hospitals subscribing to the Professional Activity Study (PAS) of CPHA. They reported generally strong and consistent evidence of a relation between a greater volume of cases of a given type treated at a hospital and lower mortality. Mortality was adjusted at a hospital level for patient differences based on diagnosis, sex, age, comorbidity, and operative procedures. Shortell and LoGerfo (1981) studied two types of patients treated in ninety-six hospitals obtained from a stratified random sample of East North Central Region hospitals subscribing to PAS. Using a patient-level adjustment for case mix, they found mixed results for the two study procedures. Greater volume was associated with reduced adjusted mortality for patients treated for myocardial infarction but was not related to adjusted morbidity rates following appendectomy.

Flood, Scott, and Ewy (1984a, 1984b [see also chap. 11 in this volume]) also reported a strong relation between the volume of cases treated and lower mortality. Our results, based on a patient-level adjustment for case mix in the

ES hospitals, showed strong and consistent support for the relation between volume and adjusted outcomes for a variety of selected types of surgical and medical patients. We also examined the contingency hypothesis that volume is more important in predicting outcomes when the patient's case is more difficult. First we looked at the relation between volume and outcome for patients grouped by the overall difficulty of their diagnostic-procedure category. Second, we ranked patients within a given category by the severity of their disease, based on an estimate of their probability of dying. No support was found for the prediction that the importance of volume was contingent on the difficulty of the case. The relation between volume and outcome was also tested, adjusting for structural characteristics associated with high-volume hospitals, such as larger size and teaching status. The results were, if anything, strengthened. Luft (1980) reported similar results for his study.

As we discuss in chapter 11, below, one important question yet unresolved is whether the association between volume and outcome occurs because experience is beneficial or because referral and patient selection patterns operate to encourage more patients to go to hospitals with good outcomes (Donabedian 1984; Dranove 1984; Luft, Hunt, and Mearki 1985). We present some evidence that experience is one important factor in this process in chapter 11. Two other studies also attempted to address these issues. Sloan, Perrin, and Valvona (1985) studied seven surgical procedures in a national cohort of hospitals over the period 1972–81. After adjusting for patient characteristics, they found consistent evidence that a greater procedure-specific volume was associated with lower mortality but cautioned against concluding that an optimal volume for a hospital could be defined at this time. They also found that hospitals did not necessarily do equally well or equally poorly over all seven procedures, concluding that hospital factors such as the quality of the nursing staff or medical staff overall must not be the major determinant. In general, hospital mortality rates tended to decrease over time, apparently as a result of two factors: hospitals tended to improve over time as they gained in experience, and hospitals with the poorest initial records tended to cease performing the procedure. They interpreted these results as supportive of an effective mechanism for patient selection of appropriate hospitals at work already.

Kelly and Hellinger (1985), in a study of four surgical procedures based on patients discharged in 1977 from the 373 nonfederal hospitals in the HCUP data base, again found evidence to support the relation between procedure-specific volume and outcome. They were able to test directly whether individual surgeon volume or hospital volume was more closely associated with better outcomes. They concluded that there was no evidence to support a relation between volume and mortality at the surgeon level; instead, the relationship holds only at the hospital level, lending support to the argument that more general organizational factors are operating.

Staff Qualifications

The evidence relating physician qualifications was summarized by Palmer and Reilly (1979), who grouped the findings into nine categories: (1) medical school performance, (2) type of medical school, (3) postlicensure training, (4) specialty certification, (5) site of medical practice, (6) graduation from a foreign medical school, (7) age and experience, (8) continuing education, and (9) specialization. Overall, the evidence is somewhat mixed, with older studies tending to find more support for the association of individual qualifications with better-quality care. There is little or only indirect evidence to support the importance of medical school performance, continuing education, certification, or foreign training for predicting differences in the quality of care. Training, age, and experience show some relationship to quality but often exhibit complex or mixed results; for example, Rhee (1976) found evidence of a curvilinear relationship with age, while Brook and Williams (1976) found no relationship. Flood (1976) and, more recently, Kelly and Hellinger (1985) found evidence that board certification was associated with better outcomes, especially for more difficult surgical procedures. There is some evidence that physician specialization, and the limitation of treatment to patients whose disease is related to that specialization, predicts better care. Payne and Lyons (1972), Rhee (1976), and their colleagues (Rhee et al. 1981) reported that physicians who treated patients within their "domain of practice" provided better care as measured by the Physician Performance Index (PPI), an indicator of the quality of process. These results were replicated in a more recent study of 1,136 physicians in five sites in the Midwest (Payne, Lyons, and Neuhaus 1984).

Two studies reported no significant association between physician qualifications and the quality of hospital care but instead found that the site of practice predicts the quality of the physician's care. Starting with the Teamster studies, there is evidence that site of practice has a strong impact on practice; for example, Health Insurance Plan of Greater New York (HIP) centers were better than less structured group practices. Rhee (1977) analyzed the Hawaii data comparing 454 physicians treating 2,500 patients in twenty-two short-term general hospitals, using the PPI to measure the quality of the physician's process. He found that hospitals, varying in the extent of structured control over practice, were more predictive of quality than were the physician's qualifications. Rhee, Luke, and Culverwell (1980) analyzed the same data base and included appropriateness of hospitalization as an indication of quality. They found evidence again that site was more important than were an individual physician's qualifications. Flood et al. (1982 [see also chap. 8 in this volume]) analyzed the IS data on 500 surgeons treating 8,000 patients in fifteen hospitals and used adjusted measures of morbidity at seven days following surgery and mortality at forty days following surgery to indicate the quality of care. Using two models, we examined the relative importance of the physician's qualifications and the site of practice for explaining differences in the quality of surgical care. First, we used a nested analysis technique to examine at the patient level whether surgeon qualifications or hospital variables were more predictive of differences in the quality of care, adjusted for case mix. Second, we used hospital-level measures of the average qualifications of the surgical staff to discover whether better-quality hospitals tended to have surgeons who were on the average better qualified, thereby explaining why the site of practice might appear to explain quality that was really due to a better-qualified staff as a whole. In both types of analyses, we found that the physician's qualifications, either for each patient's surgeon or for the hospital's average level of qualifications of the surgical staff, did not predict quality differences, while the hospital site did.

Organization of the Medical Staff

Although few would challenge the assertion that individual physicians must be allowed to exercise discretion in caring for an individual patient, several recent studies have suggested that a strong medical staff organization is not inconsistent with either the appropriate exercise of autonomy or the assurance of high-quality care. Early evidence can be found in the Teamster studies, where physicians who worked full-time and were associated with the more highly structured HIP programs provided better-quality care based on process indicators. The first to propose and test the importance of a tightly structured medical staff, Roemer and Friedman (1971) conducted two studies of quality that lent further support to this hypothesis. The first study was based on a large number of hospitals and measured the quality of care based on structural indicators such as the qualifications of the staff and the extensiveness of the facilities. They found evidence that the more tightly structured the medical staff, based on seven dimensions of structure, the better the care as measured by structural indicators of quality. In the second study, based on nine hospitals, although the quality of care involved a more sophisticated and direct measure using a severity-adjusted index of mortality, the hypothesis was less well supported.

In a study by Neuhauser (1971) of thirty hospitals in the Chicago area, quality of care measured by expert evaluation, accreditation, and a severity-adjusted mortality was associated with measures of medical staff control, such as the use of reports from tissue committees, the autopsy rate, and some types of specifications of procedures. Also, contrary to what they had predicted, Shortell, Becker, and Neuhauser (1976) found in their study of Massachusetts hospitals that the higher the autonomy of the medical staff, the lower the quality of care.

The Hawaii study and our studies previously cited offer not only evidence of the importance of site over physician qualifications for predicting better-quality care but also some mixed support for the hypothesis that the more highly structured the medical staff organization at the site, the better the care. Flood and Scott (1978 [see also chap. 9 in this volume]) found in the IS that lower adjusted surgical outcomes (better quality) were positively associated with the power of the surgical staff to regulate its own members, as reflected by the strictness of admission requirements for new staff members and the power exercised over tenured surgeons. However, using the SIS data base, including virtually all medical and surgical patients treated during a five-year period in the same hospitals, we found that the tightness of control measures for the surgical staff was associated with higher adjusted mortality at the hospitals (Scott, Flood, and Ewy 1979 [see also chap. 10 in this volume]).

Shortell and LoGerfo (1981) found an association of medical staff organization with morbidity following appendectomy but not with mortality following myocardial infarction. For appendectomy, the frequency of medical staff committee meetings, the proportion of contract physicians, the presence of a medical staff director, and a greater concentration of physicians' practices at the study hospital were all associated with lower adjusted morbidity. Even these results were somewhat mixed, since medical staff participation in decision making was not associated with better quality.

Management Practices

Three aspects of the management of the nonphysician hospital staff have been found to influence the quality of care provided: coordination systems, the managerial efficiency of the nonmedical services, and power and control mechanisms.

Coordination systems. Several studies have documented a positive relation between the extent of coordination systems and the quality of medical care in hospitals. Georgopoulos and Mann (1962) concluded from their study of ten hospitals that coordination activities in the hospital are the single most important factor accounting for differences in the quality of care. They developed a large number of indicators of coordination that they found to be strongly linked to higher-quality nursing care and overall care, as assessed by the staff members at each hospital. Their measures tended to stress the more formalized methods for coordinating work. Noting that there was little evidence of such coordination mechanisms among the medical staff, they concluded that medical staff organization had little impact on the quality of care. By contrast, Roemer and Friedman (1971) focused on control over medical work and concluded that nurses had little independent impact on the quality of care.

Longest (1974) used the index of severity from Roemer, Moustafa, and Hopkins (1968) to adjust death rates in ten acute-care hospitals and found evidence that preventive, promotive, and regulatory forms of coordination were related positively to the quality of care, while corrective forms were not. Shortell, Becker, and Neuhauser (1976), in their study of forty-two Massachusetts hospitals, found that more coordination among ancillary units and nursing was associated with better care, measured on the basis of adjusted complication rates. Studies of turnover rates and job satisfaction for nurses have also been associated with better coordination (Price and Mueller 1981; Weisman, Alexander, and Chase 1981). Moseley and Grimes (1976) found evidence that better-quality care occurred in hospitals that organized their nursing and technical staff to perform specific roles and tasks.

While coordination generally is regarded as being beneficial to the quality of care, or at least not harmful to it, there is one mechanism of coordination that several authors have posited as being associated with poorer-quality care. Programming, or formal specification of procedures for job performance and sequencing, is hypothesized to be detrimental to producing quality medical services. Two theoretical models lead to this conclusion. One, the entrepreneurial model or technological contingency approach, argues that greater specification of procedures is an appropriate coordinating mechanism only if the task is of low complexity and has relatively predictable outcomes. In a hospital setting, the provision of "hotel services" fits this description; medical care does not. The other model, the professional model, using similar reasoning, argues that professional work is complex and uncertain and therefore demands specialized training and autonomy to apply expert judgments to specific patient needs.

Becker and Neuhauser (1975) found some evidence to support this argument that greater specification of procedures is associated with poorer medical care. They found that poor-quality care was associated with restrictions on the types of drugs available, suspension of privileges for poor medical record keeping, and highly specified medical procedures. Moseley and Grimes (1976) found no relation between standardization of personnel activities and differences in the quality of care.

In contrast, several authors found evidence contrary to the predicted direction of effect. Shortell, Becker, and Neuhauser (1976) had expected to find that less formalized methods for communicating among medical services departments would be associated with better clinical decision making, arguing that informality permits more flexibility to respond to specific patient needs and would therefore result in better care. They found the opposite to be true but noted that the extent of specification was not extreme. Scott, Forrest, and Brown, in their report of preliminary findings of the IS (1976), found evidence that more explicit nursing policies were associated with a better-qualified nursing staff and better-quality care.

In trying to explain the unexpected finding that more formalized procedures are associated with better care, most authors have concluded that the theory and tests of the relation between types of coordination and quality of care have been too simplistic. Flexible decision making in a complex, unpredictable task environment is not necessarily incompatible with all uses of formalized coordination.

Managerial efficiency in nonmedical tasks. As already noted, the entrepreneurial model suggests that nonmedical services provided in hospitals are more predictable and less complex and thus amenable to coordination via formalized methods. Shortell, Becker, and Neuhauser (1976) found support for the belief that greater specification of procedures for nonmedical services was related to their more efficient production, which in turn was related to better-quality medical care.

Control systems and the visibility of consequences. Several studies have reported somewhat mixed evidence concerning the effects of control systems in hospitals on the quality of care. We have already reviewed the evidence that medical staff organizational control over physicians can influence the quality of care. In Neuhauser's study (1971), the degree of influence of physicians in hospital affairs generally was related to worse outcomes, measured using severity-adjusted mortality; weak but positive associations were found for physicians' participation on hospital boards and on joint conference committees and experts' ratings of better care. In the Shortell, Becker, and Neuhauser study (1976), the quality of care as measured by adjusted mortality was associated with greater participation of department heads in hospital decision making but was adversely affected by greater physician autonomy in clinical work. Neither was related to adjusted postsurgical complication rates. In our IS, administrators' influence over decisions within their own domain was found to be associated with better outcomes for surgical patients, but it was associated with worse care when the measure was based on adjusted mortality of all surgical and medical patients during a five-year period. Examining the influence of administrators, physicians, and nurses, we found little consistent support for the importance of restricting influence to one's own professional domain in contrast to encroaching on the task domain of the other groups (Flood and Scott 1978 [see also chap. 9 in this volume]). Shortell and LoGerfo (1981) found some evidence to support the importance of physician participation in decision making to predict better outcomes, but the indicators for appendectomy patients differed from those for myocardial infarction patients.

In a study of seventeen acute-care hospitals, Morlock et al. (1979), using a case-mix-adjusted mortality measure, found a significant relation between the influence of the governing board in hospital decision making and better outcomes. Although influential boards were more likely to include medical staff, there was no direct correlation between physician membership on boards and hospital performance.

Another method for controlling performance in organizations is the use of incentives and evaluation based on feedback of performance. In entrepreneurial theory, greater specification of evaluation procedures is related to better performance, since if there is "visibility of consequences," the higher-level management can reward good performance. Becker and Neuhauser (1975) found that greater visibility of consequences by hospital administrators and hospital boards was associated with better care. Morse, Gordon, and Moch (1974) found that visibility, in conjunction with decentralized decision making, was associated with higher adoption of technology, which was their structural measure of the quality of care. Shortell, Becker, and Neuhauser (1976) reported that administrative visibility of consequences was associated with more efficient nonmedical services as well as with lower costs per medical case. They noted that the relation between visibility and effective performance depended, not on the volume of reports prepared, but on the volume forwarded to the board of trustees; however, they did not find visibility of consequences related to care quality per se.

Membership in a Multihospital System

As we noted in our discussion on costs of hospital care, there is widespread use of shared services and contractual relationships among hospitals, and a substantial and increasing number of hospitals belong to hospital systems with formal ties to the system-level corporation. Despite this trend, there are very few studies of the impact of these multihospital systems on the quality of care provided in the member hospitals. And these studies have used fairly crude and indirect measures of quality—either structural measures, such as accreditation, quality of medical staff, and the extensiveness of available medical services, or reputational measures based on opinions of the staff in the system hospitals. The paucity of studies on the quality of care in multihospital systems can be explained by the difficulties in assessing these systems (which can vary considerably in the number of services or programs affected and the power of the corporate board), the diverse types of hospitals included in systems (both within a system and especially across different systems), and the difficulty in conceptualizing and measuring the quality of care at the system level. As Studnicki (1979, 317) commented, "All the imperfections in our knowledge about the predictors and correlates of the cost, quality, and efficacy of health services will not be eliminated by changing the focus of inquiry to a higher level of abstraction, namely, multihospital systems." Ermann and Gabel (1984, 59) also pointed out that all of the empirical studies of the performance of multihospital systems "suffer from one serious methodological flaw. Systems do not randomly choose where to locate, but self-select into favorable market areas."

A few studies have suggested that the quality of care is improved in hospitals that join a system and/or that system hospitals tend to provide care equivalent in quality to similar nonsystem hospitals. There is also evidence that friction and job dissatisfaction may be higher in multihospital systems and that they are less likely to offer professional teaching or research opportunities. (See Zuckerman 1979; Starkweather 1981; and Ermann and Gabel 1984 for more extensive reviews.)

Treat (1976) studied thirty-two urban and rural hospitals before and after merger and matched them to thirty-two independent hospitals on the basis of size, facilities, and geographic location. He found that the availability of patient services tended to improve after merger in both urban and rural hospitals but that increased costs in the urban hospitals appeared to offset the benefits from improved services. He also found that rural hospitals increased their ability to attract qualified personnel. Cooney and Alexander (1975), however, in a matched study of not-for-profit hospitals, found continuing problems for rural hospitals in the recruitment and retention of physicians. Edwards (1972) and Neumann (1974) studied the eight hospitals in the Samaritan Health System of Phoenix and found that the hospitals improved in their ability to meet accreditation and licensure requirements following merger; staff reported that hospitals, particularly in rural areas, benefited from improved patient-care services. Biggs and colleagues (Biggs 1977; Biggs, Kralewski, and Brown 1980) studied thirty-two matched contract and traditionally managed hospitals. Overall they found little evidence of differences in any hospital performance measures, including patient-care services, programs, and facilities.

Money, Gilfillan, and Duncan (1976) studied sixteen hospital systems and reported that larger systems tended to be less effective in accomplishing their goals as reported by their employees and that corporate managers and managers directly connected to patient care tended to experience low job satisfaction. In a study of forty multihospital systems, Dagnone (1967) found more general problems with absentee administration and friction among staff members, who saw merger as a threat to their status and professional opportunities. McGrath, Rothman, and Schwartzbaum (1970) found strong opposition among physicians up to three years following a three-hospital merger. Finally, "system hospitals performed no research activities and participated in fewer teaching and residency programs" (Ermann and Gabel 1984, 60); both teaching and research have been used by some authors as structural indicators of the quality of care.

STUDIES EXAMINING BOTH COST AND QUALITY

The majority of studies reviewed have treated cost and quality of care as independent or twin measures of the effectiveness of hospital care. We argue that cost and quality of care are more analogous to Siamese twins: a change in one has the potential to alter significantly the other. Only a very few studies have attempted to examine simultaneously the cost and the quality of hospital care, the relationship between them, and the factors affecting this relationship.

While the titles of many studies imply that these issues are addressed, readers of this literature are often frustrated in their search for relevant materials. For example, we have already referred to Trussell, Morehead, and Ehrlich's (1962) well-known study *The Quantity, Quality, and Costs of Medical and Hospital Care Secured by a Sample of Teamster Families in the New York*

Area. The research does indeed deal with these topics, but not in such a fashion that we can determine the nature of the relation between the cost of care and its quality. Information was gathered concerning 283 Teamster families who had recently undergone hospitalization for one of a number of selected diagnoses. Data included gross charges for hospital care during the sampled hospital stay and the amount covered by Blue Cross and other insurance carriers and by out-of-pocket costs to subscribers. An evaluation of the quality of care for 406 hospital admissions reported by the sampled families was made by specialists expert in the disease for which the patient was hospitalized. As already noted, quality ratings of care were related to the teaching status of the hospital, ownership, and physician qualifications, but no attempt was made to relate the quality of hospital care to its cost.

Other studies have addressed the relation between the quality and the cost of hospital care but have used such questionable indicators of one or the other concept as to cast serious doubt on the validity of their results. For example, in a study entitled "Hospital Costs and Quality of Care: An Organizational Perspective," Morse, Gordon, and Moch (1974) employed data from 388 hospitals to examine the effect of such organizational factors as centralization of decision making on hospital costs and quality. In order to measure hospital quality, they decided to assess those factors affecting the "ability of the hospital to deliver high-quality patient care" (317). Their specific indicator of quality was the hospital's ranking on a scale of institutional adoption of a set of specific innovations in modern medical technology. In short, hospital quality was assessed by an index of the organization's technical capability. Rather than use process or outcome measures of care quality, Morse and his colleagues employed a structural measure of quality, which "has the major limitation that the relationship between structure and process or structure and outcome, is often not well established" (Donabedian 1966, 170).

The indicators of efficiency by these researchers were more conventional and acceptable and included occupancy rate, length of stay, and expenditures per patient. However, a serious limitation affecting the validity of these data as indicators of efficiency was the absence of any controls for case mix. The questionable measure of quality and the failure to take into account differences in case mix call into question the conclusions relating cost and quality to organizational factors.

Other studies are characterized by similar defects. For example, Cohen (1970) employed data from twenty-five of the forty-six short-term, general hospitals of the United Hospital Fund of New York to estimate the effect of differences in hospital size and quality on the average cost of care. However, using his index of quality involved dividing hospitals into three groups based on accreditation and medical school affiliation, that is, on other structural indicators presumed to be related to quality. Feldstein (1970, 295) commented that not only did the measure of quality used in Cohen's study suffer from an inability to discriminate well among hospitals but, "what is more important, in the equations used . . . , the measure may be indicating merely the higher costs per unit of output that are associated with medical school affiliation. These would not be costs of increased quality."

Neuhauser (1971), who studied administrative activities and performance—both cost and quality measures—in thirty Chicago-area hospitals, was able to develop more acceptable measures of both cost and quality. Further, he had the good sense to develop several indicators for each. His cost measures included indices of costs and man-hours per patient based on cost data from seven nonmedical departments. Differences in the volume of services between hospitals were controlled by multiplying each department's cost per unit by the average number of units supplied by that type of department for all study hospitals. However, because differences in patient mix were not controlled, some of the cost differentials may have been associated with variations in services provided rather than with inefficiency in producing a given type of service, as intended. Quality measures included quality ratings by expert evaluators, an index based on data compiled by the Joint Commission on Accreditation of Hospitals, and Roemer's index of severity-adjusted death rates, which provides, at best, a crude adjustment for differences in patient mix.

Neuhauser reported that the cost and man-hour indices were not related to care quality for his sample. Only one of the six correlations among the various indicators of cost and quality was significant; however, five of the six correlations were negative, suggesting that, if anything, the more efficient hospitals—those with lower costs per patient—exhibited higher care quality (Neuhauser 1971, 91).

A follow-up study by Shortell, Becker, and Neuhauser represents a noteworthy attempt to accurately assess both cost and quality in hospitals. This study was based on forty-two of the fifty-eight short-term, voluntary, nonteaching hospitals of 100 or more beds in Massachusetts (Shortell, Becker, and Neuhauser 1976; Becker, Shortell, and Neuhauser 1980). Hospital-level costs were assessed using three indices: direct costs in three nonmedical support departments, in four medical support departments, and overall. Hospital costs were standardized for department measures by dividing by the number of inpatient days of hospitalization; for overall costs, by dividing by the number of patients treated during the study period. The quality of care at each hospital was measured by the medical-surgical death rate and the postoperative complication rate following clean surgery. Adjustment for case mix was made at the hospital level by assessing the severity of the non-Medicare patients treated. Efficiency in clinical care was measured by the average length of stay (ALOS) of Medicare patients, the preoperative ALOS for Medicare patients, and the overall ALOS for all patients. Adjustment for differences in case mix and care quality was again made at the hospital level, using aggregate measures of the severity of illness for non-Medicare patients and death and complication rates for Medicare patients.

As with many studies of care quality employing outcomes such as mortality and complications, this study was hampered by the low rates of adverse outcomes. Fewer than 1 percent of the cases included in the study were reported to have postsurgical complications, and only 3.4 percent resulted in death. Such low rates resulted in weak statistical power for the study and did not provide very sensitive indicators of care quality. What is more important, the approach used in adjusting for differences in case mix, while representing an advance over previous investigators, utilized very broad diagnostic categories, was based on subjective judgments of unknown validity, and was applied at the hospital level.

The relation between hospital costs and the quality of care was examined by dividing the hospitals into those with low and those with high costs and into those with low and those with high death rates. Hospitals with lower death rates were found also to exhibit lower combined costs for nonmedical and medical support department per patient-day (Shortell, Becker, and Neuhauser 1976). The relation between clinical efficiency and care quality was examined at the hospital level by regression (Becker, Shortell, and Neuhauser 1980). First, the authors examined the relation between preoperative ALOS and death rate, arguing that preoperative ALOS is more subject to control by the hospital. Controlling for hospital case-mix severity, they found that higher death rates were associated with longer preoperative ALOS. "This seems to suggest that poorer quality of care and less efficient resource utilization go together. The relationship may not be as simple as it appears, however, when other data are taken into account" (Becker, Shortell, and Neuhauser 1980, 323).

In a zero-order correlation, longer ALOS for Medicare patients was strongly associated with a longer preoperative ALOS and a higher death rate but was not related to the case-mix severity. In regression analyses with ALOS of Medicare patients as the dependent variable, death rate was no longer significantly related to ALOS; preoperative ALOS was the most important predictor, and along with case mix and quality, it explained 41 percent of the variance at the hospital level. The results for all patients were similar but explained less of the variance in the overall ALOS.

The authors acknowledged the difficulty in interpretation caused by measuring these relationships for different groups of patients within the hospital: quality was based on all patients; case mix, on non-Medicare patients; and preoperative ALOS, on Medicare patients. They also speculated that longer preoperative stay may be more appropriate for patients needing treatment prior to surgery and could therefore signify better care rather than inefficient use of resources. In addition, the results from these studies are compromised in their interpretation by a lack of effective techniques for taking into account differences among patients that affect both the cost and the quality of care observed and/or by a failure to model at the appropriate level the relationships between cost of production of services, clinical efficiency, and outcomes obtained.

In our SIS, data from five years of patients treated in the seventeen IS hospitals were used to deal with both of these issues. Using inhospital death as an indicator of outcome and the set of medical care services received and the length of stay for each patient as indicators of service intensity and duration of care, we analyzed the set of approximately 670,000 patients first at the patient level, to make adjustments for individual health characteristics. After adjusting each measure for patient-level differences in initial health status, we found better-quality care to be related to a greater intensity of services received but unrelated to duration as indicated by length of stay (Flood et al. 1979 [see also chap. 7 in this volume]). In a related analysis, we examined the relation of quality and intensity of services to hospital costs per patient and to managerial practices (Scott, Flood, and Ewy 1979 [see also chap. 10 in this volume]).

It is not easy to summarize these results relating hospital characteristics to measures of services, outcomes, and costs. Briefly, after adjustment for case mix we found that hospitals with a greater capacity as measured by size and facilities tended to provide a greater intensity of services. We found that staff qualifications were for the most part unrelated to service intensity, duration, or quality. Costs per patient were unrelated to quality or intensity and duration of services at the hospital level when other hospital characteristics were considered. Coordination and control measures appeared to be important predictors of better quality and greater intensity of services, adjusted for case mix. Though the relation between quality, costs, services, and managerial practices were more carefully tested and modeled in the latter study, the findings do not present a clear or consistent picture of their association at either the hospital or the patient level.

4 · Conceptual and Methodological Issues in Measuring the Quality of Care in Hospitals

Ann Barry Flood and W. Richard Scott

CONCEPTUAL ISSUES IN MEASURING THE QUALITY OF CARE IN HOSPITALS

Conceptualizing quality of care for hospitals requires understanding what quality care is and what it is not, both for any given patient and for the hospital. There are many conceptual and methodological problems in defining and measuring the quality of care for the patient; these are compounded by the need to have aggregate measures for the quality of care delivered in a hospital. For what should the hospital be held accountable in the delivery of care quality: for the quality of services provided or for the quality of decisions leading to their provision? for providing the best care possible or for meeting minimal standards? Should the hospital be held accountable for the decision to hospitalize or to discharge the patient when many factors outside of the hospital's control affect such a decision? Such questions are implicitly or explicitly addressed when the quality of care in hospitals is assessed.

Assessing the quality of care in hospitals involves the evaluation of two interrelated dimensions in producing health outputs: the effectiveness of the care and the efficiency of its production. *Effectiveness* refers to the extent to which the desired health output is obtained. *Efficiency* refers to the ratio of inputs to outputs and measures the extent to which resources are minimized in producing a given output. Sometimes only one dimension is considered in defining or measuring the quality of care, but increasing emphasis has been placed on the direct or indirect consideration of both the costs and the effectiveness of care. Cost-effective studies are examples of the explicit consideration of both dimensions. Implicit use occurs in attempts to designate a standard for necessary and sufficient quality beyond which any additional "Cadillac care" should be paid for by the patient instead of by society through pooled insurance risks. (See President's Commission for the Study of Ethical Problems in Medicine and Biomedical and Behavioral Research 1982 for an illustration of implicit use in defining adequate care.)

These concepts are defined at the patient level. Applying them to organizational performance is neither simple nor straightforward. For example, Donabedian and colleagues (Donabedian, Wheeler, and Wyszewianski 1982; Wyszewianski, Wheeler, and Donabedian 1982) noted that efficiency in producing care in hospitals is determined by both *clinical* efficiency (the selection, timing, and sequencing of services necessary for each patient to produce the greatest increment in health for the use of resources) and *production* efficiency (the timeliness and quality in producing clinical services ordered for patients and the amount of resources consumed in their production). They concluded that clinical efficiency implicitly involves the quality of care, because the decisions involved, such as those regarding the appropriate timing of treatment or appropriate usage of services, are the responsibility of the physician, and inefficient ordering of services is an indication of poor clinical decision making. By contrast, they argued that production efficiency does not involve the quality of care, because the decisions involved, such as those regarding the hiring of sufficient personnel with the appropriate level of training or the purchasing of equipment, are the responsibility of hospital management and are not under the control of the physician. Shortell and colleagues (Shortell, Becker, and Neuhauser 1976; Becker, Shortell, and Neuhauser 1980; Shortell and Kaluzny 1983) have argued that production efficiencies in a hospital involve proper decision-making processes on the part of management and therefore should be achieved by (and studied by looking at) traditional management techniques and models of production.

We argue that production efficiencies, to the extent that they affect the outcomes of patients and the mix and timing of clinical services received, also involve the quality of care for the patient. In our own work we have focused on outcomes of patients and examined care quality in terms of the effects on outcomes rather than on whether standards of good clinical decisions have been met. In examining the amounts of each clinical service received by patients (and the mix of services, weighting each service according to its relative cost), we have attempted to measure efficiencies that include both the appropriateness of (clinical) decisions made by individual physicians and also the effects of (production) decisions made by the hospital and the medical staff on the clinical services and outcomes of patients in the hospital. Thus, while our primary focus in on the quality of care, we also include clinical and production efficiency as measures of hospital performance.

In this chapter, following Donabedian (1966, 1980), we organize our discussion around the three approaches to measuring the quality of care in hospitals—outcome, process, and structure—giving primary attention to approaches assessing outcomes and processes. These three approaches are defined and discussed in chapter 3. Here we briefly review their definitions.

Outcomes are the changes that occur in a patient's health status and are broadly defined to include the patient's physiological, social, and psychological function and attitudes, including satisfaction with any aspect of the care provided. Examples include postsurgical infections, death, and satisfaction with the outcome or process of care at the level of the individual or the rate of each at the level of the physician or hospital.

Process refers to the set of activities that go on between the providers and the patient, including the management of both the technical and the interpersonal processes involved. Examples include the diagnostic workup and the treatment of patients and adherence to norms of good practice. Illustrations at the hospital level are rates based on these activities and autopsy rates.

Structure refers to "the relatively stable characteristics of the providers of care, of the tools and resources they have at their disposal, and the physical and organizational setting in which they work" (Donabedian 1980, 81). These characteristics include the qualifications of the provider (experience, training, and licensure and certifications) or, at the hospital level, the average staff qualifications, the type and quality of facilities and services, and the accreditation status.

We first review each approach, commenting on the conceptual problems of measuring care quality both for individual patients and for patients aggregated to measure quality for a hospital.

Assessing the Quality of Care by Health Outcomes: The Patient Level

Luft wrote that the goal of medical care for a given patient is "the maintenance or improvement of one's health, rather than the mere consumption of medical services" (Luft 1980, 208). If we assume this goal, quality should be measured by the amount of health or the amount of improved health obtained—health outcomes—not by the services rendered. Of course, the amount of health a person has is affected by many factors besides the receipt of medical services, even assuming that the services are timely, appropriate, and well executed. Although some have stressed the importance of taking into account the positive aspects of health (e.g., the quality of life obtained or improvement of physiological performance measures) (see Poznanski et al. 1978; De-Nour 1982; Kaplan and Bush 1982; Grieco and Long 1984; and Bergner 1985), most measures of outcomes focus not on health but on morbidity (see Scott et al. 1976; Flood and Scott 1978 [see also chap. 9 in this volume]; and Shortell and LoGerfo 1981 for examples of hospital-level measures), physiological impairment (see Yates, Chalmer, and McKegney 1980; and Wagner and Draper 1984), or mortality (see Lipworth, Lee, and Morris 1963; Roemer, Moustafa, and Hopkins 1968; Goss and Reed 1974; Flood et al. 1979 [see also chap. 7 in this volume]; and Flood, Scott, and Ewy 1984a [see also chaps. 11 and 12 in this volume]).

Health outcomes or illness outcomes? This distinction is not merely semantic; the maximization of health is not simply the polar opposite of the minimization of major morbidity and death. There are several practical differences between these two approaches, each with important conceptual implications.

Skewed Distribution of Outcomes

One difficulty arises because only a very small percentage of patients, especially after controlling for diagnosis and physical status, is likely to experience death or major morbidity after receiving care in a hospital. For example, the overall mortality rate for patients in nonfederal, acute-care hospitals is approximately 3 percent (CPHA 1977); about 5 percent of all hospitalized patients have hospital-based (nosocomial) infections (Haley et al. 1985). To focus on minimization of major morbidity and death is to concentrate on the most important health risks but to describe the outcomes of only a minority of patients.

Short-term versus Long-term Outcomes

Another difference between these two approaches is their focus on short-term and long-term health. In the short run, most medical care provided in hospitals produces morbidity from which the patient must recover (independently from any need to recover from the disease); that is, although most patients leave the hospital "discharged, full recovery," they are rarely without some morbidity. A short-term focus on health at discharge that defines quality in terms of maintenance or improvement of health can lead to the undesirable conclusion that care that produces no morbidity (e.g., admission for observation) is superior to care that increases morbidity (e.g., surgical procedures), given patients with the same medical problem. There are two ways out of this dilemma: one can try to take into account the probability of short-term morbidity associated with different treatment modalities for the same medical problem, or one can look at long-term health benefits (thereby potentially including factors outside the control of the hospital, such as medical care services received after hospitalization).

Beneficial versus Unharmful Outcomes

A third difference is the focus on the positive versus the negative aspects of care. This distinction is built into the Hippocratic oath: the physician is enjoined to actively apply his or her knowledge and skills for the benefit of the patient and to do no harm. Health outcomes for hospitalized patients that are based on morbidity and mortality help to emphasize the second aspect: what harm to the patient, if any, occurred? For the majority of patients, major morbidity or death is not an expected outcome except under unusual conditions, including gross misconduct in the delivery of medical care. A positive outcome for these patients would tend to emphasize the health output benefits obtained: what good did the care do the patient? Nevertheless, health benefits are seldom measured in practice.

Because of the way outcomes are generally measured, the goal of medical care should be rephrased: it is to reduce morbidity and postpone death due to disease by application of effective clinical services. To this statement several authors would add the goal of prevention of morbidity or death.

Prevention of morbidity can refer to (*a*) screening tools for early detection and treatment of problems, such as mammography or fetal monitoring; (*b*) preventive therapy, such as a hysterectomy for carcinoma *in situ* or adjuvant chemotherapy with the goal of avoiding metastasized cancer; or (*c*) avoidance of iatrogenic morbidity accompanying treatment, such as reducing exposure to hospital-based infection, accidents from unintended puncturing of a vital organ during surgery, and adverse effects from avoidable use of interacting combinations of drugs (see Schimmel 1964; Melmon 1971; and Mason et al. 1980) or using prophylactic methods to prevent postoperative complications (Colditz, Tuden, and Oster 1985).

To assess the appropriateness of preventive measures, we need to return to the ultimate goal of medical services, namely, to reduce morbidity or postpone death due to disease. Thus, in order to examine whether preventive measures do more good than harm, the costs and risks associated with the preventive measures for the entire population served must be less than the costs and risks of (*a*) equally effective alternative preventive measures and (*b*) the therapy for the proportion of patients whose disease was prevented. A sophisticated examination of "prevented disease" requires taking into account the failure rates of the preventive measures and, for screening of early-stage disease, the number of patients found whose disease would have been detected early without the screening measure (Eddy 1980). In practice, persons responsible for applying preventive measures rarely attend to such evaluations, resulting in some questionable practices such as incidental appendectomies for populations at low risk of appendicitis (Sugimoto 1985). Colditz, Tuden, and Oster (1985) argued that one way to encourage adoption of cost-effective preventive measures in hospitals is through economic incentives. They suggested that systems like the prospective-payment system based on DRGs provide incentives for hospitals to apply cost-effective preventive measures. In particular they argued that hospitals could save money by preventing postoperative complications, which add to the lengths of stay and therapeutic regimens of patients experiencing the complications.

A related but separate issue is the extent to which appropriate, well-performed care can carry a risk of iatrogenic morbidity, which is not avoidable. For example, most aggressive drug therapy involves considerable risk of adverse side effects which may also need to be treated, and postsurgical fever and edema usually accompany major vascular surgical procedures. In other words, risks and choices are involved in both treatment and nontreatment.

Assessing the Quality of Care by Health Outcomes: The Hospital Level

The conceptual issues raised so far focus on the receipt of services and outcomes obtained by an individual patient. However, the measures of care quality most of concern in our research are those at the hospital level. Problems at the hospital level are of two types: (*a*) issues in measuring health outputs at the individual level that remain when measures are aggregated to the hospital level and (*b*) additional problems that arise because the unit of analysis is the hospital.

Conceptual Problems Related to Problems at the Individual Level

If patients were randomly distributed across hospitals with respect to those factors that affect outcome, such as their diagnoses and treatments, we could assume that individual-level differences would not affect hospital differences observed. However, this assumption is invalid. As argued in chapter 3, there is considerable evidence that hopsitals do differ in the types of patients treated; that is, case mix does make a significant contribution to differences in the aggregate measures of type and mix of services provided and outcomes achieved.

Besides the methodological issues discussed later in this chapter and in chapter 5, there are important conceptual choices to be made regarding which case-mix variables to take into account. Choices are usually based on clinical criteria such as the primary diagnosis explaining admission as grouped into DRGs. Further refinements of these categories to include stage of disease or more general physical status may be necessary to correctly predict the effects of case mix on patient outcomes and costs. (See the debate in *Health Care Financing Review* involving the DRGs used by Medicare and the classification system proposed by Pennsylvania Blue Cross: Conklin et al. 1984; Gertman and Lowenstein 1984; Kominski et al. 1984; Smits, Fetter, and McMahon 1984; and Young 1984). These refinements still leave out nonmedical factors influencing clinical decision making such as the patient's preferences regarding alternative therapies and sociodemographic characteristics such as race, education level, marital status, religious preference, and occupation (Hornbrook 1982a). Factors external to the hospital and patient that use the categories to evaluate hospital performance on outcomes also can influence clinical decisions.

We illustrate how the rewarding of hospitals for care with inappropriate incentives based on miscategorization of patients can lead to undesirable effects. Suppose reimbursement of a hospital (such as the Medicare Prospective

Payment System) is based on the patient's major diagnosis explaining admission, receipt of a surgical procedure, age, and selected comorbidity. Suppose also that a significant number of patients with a given diagnosis need two independent surgical procedures that can be performed coincidentally or separately, such as replacement of the hip joint in both hips. From the point of view of the individual patient, one hospitalization and one visit to the operating room with double replacement would use less resources and produce less morbidity and fewer days off work than would two separate hospitalizations, one for each hip replacement. However, if we compare costs and outcomes for individual patients having one versus two hip replacements, the patient with one hip replacement has less morbidity and consumes fewer resources than the patient with two. From a societal perspective, the hospital that is "efficient" in its use of clinical resources should encourage combining the two surgical procedures into one hospitalization. However, if the financial reimbursements to the hospital for the single and the double operation are identical, the hospital can receive higher reimbursement for unbundling the two procedures. Similarly, if a hospital practice of unbundling results in an evaluation of its patients' outcome and lengths of stay that credits the hospital for having two "live" patients and two "short" lengths of stay for the single patient undergoing two separate procedures and hospitalizations, then the hospital is further encouraged to promote unbundling of services into different hospitalizations, even though the total costs and morbidity for the patient (and for society) would thereby increase.[1]

Additional Conceptual Problems at the Hospital Level

For all the complexity of problems in defining the quality of care for a patient in terms of health outcomes, new issues arise when the unit of analysis is the hospital, and new problems occur in defining the boundaries of accountability. As Scott and Shortell (1983, 422) wrote, "Of the many factors that affect one's conception of organizational performance, none is more important than the view adopted of the fundamental nature of organizations." They argued that if hospitals are considered to be instruments primarily for the attainment of specific goals, then performance measures are likely to focus on goal attainment. Other conceptions of hospitals would emphasize the importance of organizational survival and system maintenance in contrast to pursuing specific goals. Open systems theories of organizations emphasize the importance of maximizing the organization's bargaining position in obtaining resources from its environment. (See chap. 8 for an elaboration of these arguments.) These

1. Originally, the Prospective Payment System of Medicare did provide the same amount for single and double hip replacement, because both types of patients were placed in the same DRG. After organizational responses such as we describe, Medicare altered their reimbursement in spring 1985 to pay twice the amount for a double hip replacement, thereby encouraging combining the procedures for those patients needing two.

different perspectives can lead to very different ways to answer the question, For what should the hospital be held accountable in providing quality of care?

Briefly, the hospital can be expected to have an impact on the production of health outcomes in several respects. First, the hospital is held legally accountable for the quality of tasks and decisions relating to medical care made by hospital employees. Second, even though physicians often are not salaried employees of the organization, the medical staff organization of a hospital is also held accountable for monitoring and controlling the quality of clinical decisions and performances through quality-assurance committees and other mechanisms for peer review. Third, hospital employees and resources can also interact with the process of making clinical decisions. For example, many patient-care decisions, such as whether and how long to hospitalize and when to operate, are influenced both by clinical decisions made at the doctor-patient level and by hospital-level resources such as the availability of hospital beds, discharge-planning services, operating rooms, or laboratory results.

The multiple goals of the hospital and the complexity of the many subunits and multiple occupational groups can be in conflict with providing the highest-quality and most efficient care. For example, the hospital may intend to provide high-quality care but also needs to be concerned with its own survival, that is, with obtaining sufficient capital to operate. To accomplish this latter goal, the hospital is encouraged to maximize its reimbursement for medical services, which under a fee-for-service reimbursement system can lead to incentives to provide more or more expensive care than necessary. As a second example, the organizational goal to be a teaching institution can impact the costs and outcomes of care indirectly by influencing the amount spent on clinical technology and to attract well-qualified physicians and by encouraging the care of especially difficult patient health problems. Teaching can also have a direct effect due to students' involvement in producing services. Garber, Fuchs, and Silverman (1984) compared teaching and nonteaching units within the same hospital and found that patients who were treated on the faculty service tended to have better outcomes in the short term but not significantly different outcomes after six months. In chapter 12 we present evidence that not all teaching hospitals are alike in predicting whether patient outcomes are improved or harmed by the presence of residents, suggesting that a more refined examination of "teaching" as a hospital goal is necessary in order to understand its impact on care.

In summary, the difficulty of defining health outcomes, the many factors that affect it in addition to medical care, the uncertainties involved in determining the type and extent of disease, and the risks and values involved in choosing therapy—all complicate the interpretation of health outcomes as a measure of the quality of care at the individual level. Even more complications exist at the hospital level, including problems in identifying the nature of organizations and appropriate measures of hospital performance.

We turn next to a discussion of approaches that focus on the quality of the medical care process rather than health outcomes.

Assessing the Quality of Care by Process: The Patient Level

Many authors writing about professional work such as providing medical care have noted the complexity of the decision making involved and the many factors besides the quality of professional services rendered that affect the outcome. Professionals tend to prefer to be evaluated on the basis of what they have done—the *process* of their work—rather than on the final product—the *outcome* of their work—largely because of the number of factors affecting the outcome that are beyond their control. (See Freidson 1970; Scott 1972; McAuliffe 1979; Donabedian 1980; and Brown 1983 for more details of this argument applied to physicians.) Several authors have strongly supported the superiority of measures of process as indicators of quality when the purpose is to evaluate an individual physician's care, such as in most quality-assurance activities (McAuliffe 1979; Donabedian 1980). Our primary focus, however, is to evaluate medical care performance in order to understand how characteristics of the individual practitioner and the organization can affect it. With this focus in mind, we discuss four conceptual issues for measuring quality based on measures of process.

Patient Health and Social Factors

Using measures of process to assess the quality of care without reference to the actual outcomes obtained obviates the need to decide which factors affecting *outcome* to control for before comparing care among professionals. Nonetheless, the decisions about the type and quantity of services to be provided also depend in large part on patient factors. Many of the sociodemographic and health-related patient factors already discussed affect outcomes in part because they also affect the services rendered. For example, the age, sex, and educational level of the patient may affect the physician's type and extent of instructions and advice about the best alternative for therapy, which in turn could influence the patient's decision to cooperate with recommended therapies (DiMatteo and DiNicola 1982) and therefore to obtain the health outcomes expected.

The Necessity of the Service

Unlike outcome measures, which generally assume that the decision to hospitalize or operate was appropriate, the quality of process care can include assessing the necessity of the service, for example, the appropriateness of the hospitalization, the timeliness of the surgical procedure, or the risk-to-benefit ratio of the service (Rhee, Lyons, and Payne 1978; Rhee, Luke, and Culverwell

1980; Greenfield et al. 1981). However, as Hendley (1984) editorialized, the distinction between necessary and unnecessary treatment is seldom clear-cut, leading to a middle ground of treatment decisions that are "justified but not mandatory." The most difficult problems arise in attempts to prevent unnecessary care when genuinely ill patients and/or their physicians seek access to costly therapy that has a low probability of being effective (Bayer et al. 1983).

Quantity versus Quality

Too little care is poor-quality medicine. However, this does not necessarily imply that more care is always better. In medical care, too much care also represents poor quality both because it exposes the patient to unnecessary risks and iatrogenic consequences and because of inefficiencies in using resources that do not benefit the patient. The difficult task, like that of Goldilocks, is to find the amount that is "just right." As Luft (1980) reminded us, "More care is not necessarily better, nor is it necessarily worse." When quantity is indicated by the number of days of hospitalization, more care does not necessarily represent better care, since many factors influence length of stay, including local medical practices or poor care resulting in the need for further treatment. As Simpson (1977) concluded, "The range in length of stay for particular conditions . . . results as much from force of habit or perverse necessity as from considered judgment." At the extreme, several studies have found that much care can be provided effectively without hospitalization at all. Research conducted on patients in the Portland Kaiser Foundation Health Plan found that 35 percent of surgical procedures were performed on an outpatient basis, with no difference in outcomes achieved and greater satisfaction for both the patient and the surgeon involved (Marks et al. 1980).

In some cases more care does lead to a better outcome (Rhee, Lyons, and Payne 1978; Flood et al. 1979 [see also chap. 7 in this volume]). Even in these circumstances the argument that there is a necessary association between quality and quantity of services assumes that there is no waste in production and that each increment of service adds to the quality. Many economists apply the law of diminishing marginal returns to health care, arguing that eventually a point is reached in the production of health where very little or no discernible benefit is gained from the increased consumption of medical services. Any service provided beyond the point where there is benefit is called "flat-of-the-curve" medicine, based on a graph of this phenomenon (see Enthoven 1980; 45).

Medical services include both diagnostic and therapeutic services. Focusing on diagnostic services, Donabedian (1966) and Vuori (1980) argued that there is a tendency for physicians to believe that more information about the patient (such as from diagnostic test results) will necessarily lead to better clinical decision making, while in fact at some point additional information can result in overload, or "logical inefficiency." That is, not only can the information be of no practical benefit (such as additional or different types of laboratory tests whose results improve the diagnostic accuracy from 95 percent to 97 percent, with no practical import to clinical decision making) but it can potentially obscure valuable information. McDonald (1976) provides an example of errors in prescription writing due to information overload.

Another factor that can act to increase the quantity of services without adding quality is legal pressure to establish beyond any doubt that a reasonable course of action was pursued. Such "defensive medicine" can occur, not because there is any expectation of benefit from additional information or services for the patient, but because the provider wanted to establish a record of considering all possible diagnoses or monitoring for signs and symptoms as a defense against potential allegations of malpractice. (See Tancredi and Barondess 1978 for further discussion of defensive medicine.) The legal and moral axiom is that it is better to treat a well person (particularly assuming that there is no serious risk) than not to treat a sick person. This axiom, coupled with the greater difficulty in establishing that someone claiming to be sick is in fact healthy and does not need services, promotes dispensing a greater quantity of services regardless of anticipated and real benefits to health.

Problems with Setting Standards

A process measure based on the doctor's orders can be relatively easy to collect from a patient's chart and reliably recorded. However, an assessment of the quality of the orders—their necessity and adequacy—requires comparison with a standard that, if implicit, may vary from rater to rater. On the other hand, explicit standards can be applied more reliably but may be based on outdated or incorrect standards (see Donabedian 1981). Such standards can have biases, such as toward finding higher quality in hospitals affiliated with medical schools if measures are based on application of the most recent medical knowledge and technology or on providing the most extensive diagnostic workup.

Assessing the Quality of Care by Process: The Hospital Level

Parallel to problems encountered concerning quality as measured by health outcomes, the difficulties in defining the quality of process care at the level of the individual are complicated further by the need to aggregate the process-based measure of quality to the hospital level. As with outcomes, differences in case mix need to be considered before comparing hospitals (or subunits such as medical staff organizations) using process measures. Of greater interest are new issues raised by hospital-level measures of the quality of process care.

Multiple Actors

The production of services for a given hospitalized patient involves not only direct patient-care services provided by the attending physician, such as we have been discussing so far, but services from many other providers as well: consulting physicians; physicans involved in specialized functions such as emergency-room treatment and ancillary services such as radiology, pathology, anesthesiology, and rehabilitation; nurses (including three shifts per day) on the wards and specialized units such as intensive-care units or the operating room suite; the technicians involved in the collection, administration, or monitoring of medical services; social workers to plan discharge dispositions; pharmacists to dispense medications; and so on. In the modern hospital, not only are many people involved directly and indirectly in the production of medical services for patient care but these people are members of many different divisions within the hospital (e.g., nursing versus medicine); the divisions often involve further subunits (e.g., nurses on different wards and in different shifts within a ward or physicians in different subdivisions grouped by speciality); and people can be members of multiple units (e.g., primary care nursing can involve a nurse in the care of patients in several different wards or over several shifts). The boundaries to designate which providers and which units have contributed what to the provision of a given service are as a consequence often unclear and arbitrary.

Moreover, the performance of a hospital is determined by more than a simple sum of the various parts. As Scott and Shortell (1983, 423) wrote, "One of the principal features of any system [is that] its performance is determined as much (if not more) by the arrangement of its parts—their relations and interactions—as by the performance of the individual components. A number of highly qualified physicians do not necessarily add up to a high-quality medical staff."

Multiple Tasks and Multiple Influences

As previously discussed, Wyszewianski, Wheeler, and Donabedian (1982) argued that patient-level efficiency can be maximized without necessarily maximizing hospital-level efficiency. For example, the clinical decisions could be excellent, but the laboratory may be slow in returning results, the hospital half-empty, and consultation requests from other physicians delayed for several days. Hospital production efficiency can also be affected by the external environment of the organization; for example, patients may not be discharged in a timely manner because skilled nursing care may not be available outside the hospital.

Information overload also has a counterpart at the hospital level. Rosen and Feigin (1982), reviewing quality-assurance efforts in eleven hospitals in New York, found that peer review efforts usually involved multiple medical staff and hospital staff committees, with little or no communication and sharing of information among the different committees. Each group collected an overabundance of data, which led to an inability to interpret the information and thus to act, resulting in what the authors called "a dead end phenomenon."

Assessing the Quality of Care by Structure

Included within the category of structural measures of quality are all assessments based on organizational features or participant characteristics presumed to have an impact on the effectiveness of performance. Examples for hospitals include measures of the adequacy of facilities and equipment, as well as the qualifications of medical and nursing staff as reflected in training and certification. These are the types of measures that have formed the basis of accreditation reviews, and they have been used by analysts as indicators of care quality (see Goss 1970; Neuhauser 1971; Roemer and Friedman 1971; and Heydebrand 1973).

If process measures are once removed from outcomes, then structural indicators are twice removed, for structural measures index not the work performed by structures but their capacity to perform work, not the activities carried out by organizational participants but their qualifications to perform the work. As Donabedian (1966, 170) noted, "The assumption is made that given the proper settings and instrumentalities, good medical care will follow. This approach offers the advantage of dealing, at least in part, with fairly concrete and accessible information. It has the major limitation that the relationship between structure and process or structure and outcome is often not well established." Since our primary interest is the relation between hospital structure and performance, we also argue that using structural indicators for quality for such research can lead to spurious or tautological observations.

Evaluating Quality as a Political Process

Some conceptual issues in assessing care quality transcend the distinctions among outcome, process, and structure and relate more generally to the process of evaluation of performance in organizations. Scott (1977) argued that evaluation processes in an organization involve making political choices about what will be assessed, how it will be measured, and what criteria will be used to evaluate it. The interested parties—those performing the evaluation, those being evaluated, and any others with an interest in the outcome of the evaluation—have different goals and interests which affect the evaluation process and outcome. Whose goals will be served by the efforts of participants and whose criteria will prevail in the evaluation systems are partly determined by differences in power among the participants. In a hospital setting, too, it is important to recognize the political bases affecting performance evaluations.

Multiple Goals for Each Interested Party

In providing care for a specific patient, there are usually multiple goals, with a potential to involve conflicting objectives. All the interested parties, including the patient and the providers, can identify several goals of treatment, but they may disagree on their relative importance and appropriateness. For example, a patient who is exceptionally anxious to treat a disease that cannot be definitively diagnosed at a given point in time may be most satisfied by receiving treatment, even if the doctor believes that treatment is not indicated by the clinical signs and symptoms and the insurance company is unwilling to pay for such care.

Variation in Treatment Goals by the Stage of the Disease

The goals of treatment for a given patient can vary over time depending on the stage or type of disease or on the convenience, availability of, and risks involved in treatment. For example, the goals of treatment of a cancer patient who is considered terminally ill will differ from those of a patient with the same diagnosis but for whom aggressive treatment offers a chance for remission or cure. In the first case, avoidance and relief of pain and nausea may be the primary objectives; in the second, these symptoms may be seen as necessary side effects to be endured.

Short-term and Long-term Goals

Considerations of time can strongly influence choices among therapies. Patients and providers can differ in their willingness to take on short-term risks in order to obtain long-term benefits—to practice what economists call time discounting—leading to variations in the value placed on short-term and long-term goals.

Attempts to Obtain the Most Favorable Evaluation

The person or organization being evaluated will use whatever influence it has in order to attempt to obtain the most favorable basis of evaluation and, failing this, to justify its performance. For example, a physician whose patient is experiencing a poor outcome may call attention to the unusual or difficult circumstances involved and attempt to emphasize the process indicators of the quality of his or her care. A physician treating a less demanding case mix may be inclined to emphasize the high rate of successful outcome. At an organizational level, a hospital that believes itself to be disadvantaged in evaluations of its performance—for example, by receiving too little reimbursement under the prospective payment system—is likely to point to the extra services it performs, such as teaching or research, or the unusually difficult case mix that it serves. (This point is discussed in more detail in the section on methodological issues, below.)

Evaluation as Symbolism

The evaluation process can serve symbolic purposes for the organization as well as provide useful information to evaluate performance and trigger mechanisms to improve quality. Hetherington (1982) argued that evaluations carried out by quality-assurance committees for the medical staff can serve to demonstrate compliance with accreditation requirements regardless of any effect they may have on medical care. Quality assurance can serve both functions, of course, but there is some evidence that only the symbolic function will be served unless the medical staff is committed to the evaluation task and has been actively involved in setting the standards as well as monitoring the care (see review in Hetherington 1982). Levy, Covaleski, and Johnson (1982) offered an even more complex example of gamesmanship involving internal evaluations. Powerful medical staff members wanted a hospital to undertake building a major new facility, which was not justified by the clinical needs of the hospital or the community. The hospital administration, even though it did not support the plan, prepared an elaborate evaluation and plan of the proposed facility, knowing that it would be turned down by a certificate-of-need review board. The evaluation procedure served to show the proponents of the facility that their project was refused by an external agency and not by the hospital administration.

In sum, political processes contribute to the difficulty of conceptualizing and choosing measures of the quality of care in hospitals in two basic ways. First, because there are many interested parties with different perspectives and values, the selection of which criteria to use is influenced by the power of the interested parties to promote their preferred choices. Second, the interested parties are motivated to exercise their power to select the criteria, depending upon the importance to them of the consequences of the evaluation (which can vary from having no or few consequences for any of the interested parties in the hospital—such as when a hospital participates anonymously in national research on the quality of care—to having very important consequences for the professional reputation or economic well-being of members of the hospital). This latter point is addressed more fully below.

METHODOLOGICAL ISSUES IN MEASURING THE QUALITY OF CARE IN HOSPITALS

For all the complex and difficult decisions involved in conceptualizing what is meant by quality of care in hospitals and why it is to be evaluated, the problems for the would-be evaluator do not end there. Selecting measures of care quality involves deciding not only which indicators to use but also what qualifying information should be taken into account, how to obtain the information, and what statistical and/or normative standards will be used to rate the extent of quality observed.

In this section, we describe two sets of methodological problems. First, we briefly note seven problems shared by all approaches to measuring quality.

These include the quality of the data collected, the completeness of the information, the generalizability of the findings, the comparability of the units of analysis, the standards selected for comparison, the reactivity of the evaluation process, and the general indices of performance. Second, we discuss varying approaches for taking case mix and patient variation into account, adjustments that are necessary if valid inferences are to be made concerning process and outcome measures of the quality of care.

Measurement Problems

The Quality of the Data

Measuring the quality of the data can be a problem for all indicators either because the desired information is not included in the medical record or because it was not recorded uniformly or accurately. (See Corn 1980; and National Academy of Sciences Institute of Medicine 1980 for a discussion of problems in measuring the quality of the data in medical records.) Moreover, the availability of data and the ease of collection tend to bias measurement to emphasize those aspects of quality more readily counted as opposed to those judged most clinically important.

Some researchers have used poorly recorded data as an indicator of a poor care process, arguing that the inadequate recording of information reflects a sloppy process and may compromise future care, which could benefit from knowing what care has already been rendered. In a study of outpatient care, Sullivan et al. (1980) found problems in assessing quality due to missing information, but they were unable to establish that missing data indicated either poor information gathering in the initial visit or problems for subsequent visits. They found that missing data were associated with an initial assessment of poor quality but were explained upon investigation by a failure to record important information used to make an appropriate clinical decision. In a study of emergency-room admissions, Greenfield et al. (1981) also questioned the assumption that poor recording of data necessarily represents poor care. They also found that poorly recorded data were associated with an initial assessment that poor-quality care had been given to the patient. However, after more careful review of the clinical situation, they found that poor recording was not indicative of a poor process but instead predicted admissions that were more likely to be appropriate. For patients with missing data, the data usually unrecorded during the emergency-room visit—the standard entry history and physical information—were not needed for deciding to admit the patient for further workup and treatment.

The Completeness of the Information

When to begin and end the collection of data and what population of patients to use as a comparison base are important measurement issues that depend upon the objectives of those performing the assessment. For example, if a process measure is used to evaluate the appropriateness of decisions to hospitalize, then the examination should include not only patients who were hospitalized but also patients who were not. In order to assess outcomes at discharge, patients discharged whose recovery was incomplete should be taken into account and/or "followed" after discharge. To determine hospital costs for treating a given illness, multiple hospitalizations for the same illness should be aggregated for a given time period.

The Generalizability of the Findings

When only a few selected diagnoses (or other groupings of patients) are assessed, the applicability of the results for other groups within the same hospital may be questioned. Three kinds of evidence support the expectation that performance, even when based on comparable indicators, varies within a hospital. First, subunits within any organization have been found to differ greatly in their performance. Second, the observation that treating a higher volume of patients for a given diagnosis leads to better outcomes (Luft, Bunker, and Enthoven 1979; Luft 1980; Shortell and LoGerfo 1981; Flood, Scott, and Ewy 1984a, 1984b; Kelly and Hellinger 1985; Sloan, Perrin, and Valvona 1985; and chap. 11 in this volume) suggests that outcomes would not be expected to be either uniformly good or bad within a hospital but would depend in part on the frequency of treatment of similar cases. Third, individual physicians differ in the quality of care provided to their patients, depending upon the type of disease being treated (Lyons and Payne 1974; Rhee et al. 1981).

The Comparability of the Units of Analysis

The assumption that a unit of service represents a comparable set of activities and a given level of quality may not be well founded. For example, a patient-day is sometimes employed as a unit of measurement for comparing hospital costs and outcomes. But service intensity depends upon the day during the stay (care is more intensive earlier in the stay and immediately postoperation), the ward (ranging from intensive-care units to low-skilled-nursing units), and the hospital (the ratio of nursing staff to patients and staff qualifications can vary significantly by hospital).

The Standards Selected for Comparison

Three basic types of standards are used to judge the level of quality attained. First, the indicator of care provided can be compared with a normatively defined standard describing appropriate quality or "standard practice." This is most common in process measures, where the standard of good process can be explicit or implicit (see Rhee, Lyons, and Payne 1978; and Fernow, McColl, and Thurlaw 1981). Second, the indicator of care can be compared with an empirically derived norm representing the average quality obtained by a large pool of patients across many institutions. Examples include standardized mortality and morbidity ratios (see Scott et al. 1976; Flood and Scott 1978 [see also chap. 9 in this volume]; Shortell and LoGerfo 1981; and Flood, Ewy, and Forrest [see also chap. 8 in this volume]). Third, one population of patients can be compared with another, assuming (1) that one population is defined as receiving good-quality care and is used as a standard against which the second can be compared (see Marks et al. 1980) or (2) that two populations may be compared but it is not clear whether one, both, or neither is receiving high-quality care (see Wennberg and Gittelsohn 1982).

The Reactivity of the Evaluation Process

One of the key control mechanisms used by organizations is the evaluation and monitoring of the performance of its members. It is therefore no surprise to find that the evaluation process itself is likely to affect performance. The impact of evaluation can vary, depending on whether the evaluating group is internal or external to the organization.

Evaluations internal to the organization. In order to illustrate several ways in which the process of evaluating performance in an organization can influence the performance of its professional members (and hence the quality of care), we categorize the evidence based on the model of Dornbusch and Scott (1975). They subdivided the evaluation process into four components—setting standards, selecting indicators, sampling or monitoring performance, and appraising—comparing sampled observations on indicators with standards to arrive at a performance evaluation.

First, there is evidence that the standards set can influence care. Several authors have found a significant change in medical practice following the establishment of explicit criteria for evaluating care. For example, after the surgical staff were informed that the tissue review committee would examine selected surgical procedures for the frequency of normal tissue removal per surgeon, there was a significant reduction in the rate of normal tissue removal (see McCarthy and Widmer 1974; and Dyck et al. 1977). Other studies have found that confronted with information suggesting that they are providing care markedly different from that provided by colleagues in the same institution or region, physicians will alter their performance to bring it more into line with the "average" performance of their colleagues (Fetter et al. 1977; Wennberg et al. 1977).

Second, there is evidence that the methods used to set criteria have an important influence on performance. Behavior is more likely to be altered when the local medical staff has participated in the setting of the standards than when standards have been imposed by an external group (Hetherington 1982).

Third, the process of sampling or monitoring performance has been shown to affect medical care. Cohen et al. (1980) installed a computerized system in a major teaching hospital to monitor and warn physicians whenever a hospitalized patient was given concurrent prescriptions with the potential for adverse interactions. Although the system was intended to have an impact on interacting combinations only, the monitoring of drugs resulted in an overall reduction in prescriptions per patient.

Fourth, the most important effects occur when performance is both actively monitored and evaluated, with important potential consequences for the person or group being evaluated. Becker and Neuhauser (1975) and Shortell, Becker, and Neuhauser (1976) found that the "visibility of consequences" (the extent to which key members of the hospital were aware of the performance) was significantly associated with better-quality care, as measured by outcomes adjusted for case mix. Morlock et al. (1979) found that involvement of the hospital board in quality assurance was associated with better-quality care.

Of course the power of evaluation to alter behavior can be overemphasized. Many other factors influence the process of evaluation and minimize its effect on behavior. For example, there can be counterincentives to altering the behavior (such as professional pressures to provide the best care regardless of cost). The evaluation process can produce information overload and ambiguous or contradictory findings, so that no clear response is possible (Rosen and Feigin 1982). Members may view the evaluation process as largely symbolic and as having no real import for their performance (Hetherington 1982).

Evaluations external to the organization. The evaluation process performed by groups external to the hospital is also likely to affect measures of medical care. When the evaluation is performed by an external group, organizational members are more likely to view the process as counter to their best interests and to minimize responses to it. For example, a hospital may decide to meet only minimal acceptable levels in complying with some accreditation requirements. (See Anderson and Shields 1982 for a review of various reasons why PSROs had limited effectiveness.) A more drastic response to a negative evaluation involves reorganizing so as to no longer fall under the jurisdiction of the external evaluator (for example, responding to CON requirements by creating a new corporation not under the jurisdiction of CON which then purchases major equipment for the hospital's use). For these reasons, the potential sanctions controlled by a group external to that organization are critical for determining how an organization will react to evaluations coming from such a group.

Three examples of evaluations by external groups serve to illustrate the relation between the importance of the evaluation to the organization and its degree of reaction to it. First, accreditation and approvals, usually based on structural measures, can have important effects on the hospital's reputation for high-quality care and on its eligibility for reimbursement or securing loans. The potential impact of failure to meet accreditation standards results in conformity to those aspects of structure and performance that are measured. Second, the newly organized PROs to monitor the quality of care for Medicare patients in hospitals have the power to deny payment to hospitals if poor-quality data and/or poor-quality care are found. A study predating the establishment of the PROs found no effect from a concurrent utilization review similar to that used by PROs but having no consequences for patients or providers who were noncompliant (Clendenning et al. 1976). In contrast, early evidence from Medicare's PPS reimbursement system, which provides strong economic incentives to reduce ALOS, shows that hospitals have responded to such external utilization review by significantly lowering the ALOS of their patients (Wallace 1984; Wood 1984). Third, participation in a major research effort to evaluate the quality of medical care in hospitals that has only a weak connection with management decisions through health policy—such as our study—is not likely to alter organizational behavior.

When a hospital is a member of a multihospital system (implying at least some corporate-level influence for important policy decisions), another layer of evaluators is introduced. Starkweather (1981, 15) reviewed "the many pluses and minuses (in such mergers), each calculated differently by the numerous parties which have something at stake" and noted the rifts that can arise among three major groups with vested interests: external groups, the corporation, and organizational groups at the level of the individual hospital, such as the medical staffs, the boards of trustees, the local administration, nurses, and other employees.

General Indices of Performance

Despite all the difficulties in measuring and modeling the quality of care of patients based on a single type of indicator, or perhaps because of them, several authors have tried to build an index of hospital performance that weights the various indicators and combines them into one overall measure of performance, using what Hetherington (1982) optimistically called the "effectiveness approach." Moseley and Grimes (1976) used a Delphi technique to obtain consensus from a group of experts on measures of performance and their relative weights. They then created an index of hospital quality based on a set of structural, process, outcome, reputational, and satisfaction indicators. Most authors, noting the poor correlation among the various indicators, do not attempt to combine measures but treat them independently.

Taking into Account Case Mix and Patient Variation

In order to compare the quality of care provided to patients by different providers or institutions directly, it would be necessary to assume that all patients were identical prior to receiving care or that any differences among patients would be distributed randomly among the providers or institutions; clearly neither assumption is tenable. Taking into account the initial differences in patient health status requires, instead, establishing some sort of methodological control, either by limiting the comparisons to groups of patients for which the assumption of equivalency is tenable or by deriving some empirical or normative standards for estimating the process or outcomes that would be expected to occur if good-quality care were provided.

Limiting Comparisons to "Equivalent" Groups of Patients

Several authors have limited their comparisons to a few selected "target" or "tracer" conditions in order to minimize differences in patient diagnoses or type of treatment (see Howie 1966; Arnold 1970; Brook et al. 1977; Flood and Scott 1978 [see also chap. 9 in this volume]; Rhee, Lyons, and Payne 1978; Fernow, McColl, and Thurlaw 1981; and Chassin 1982). Some have combined this technique with random sampling of patients within the targeted group (Morse, Gordon, and Moch 1974; Marks et al. 1980). Griffith (1978) suggested using target morbidity or mortality in hospitals, such as rates of hospitalization for preventable diseases, iatrogenic problems, or potentially overutilized surgical procedures, instead.

Adjusting for Case Mix

Hornbrook (1982a, 1–2), in reviewing different strategies for adjusting for case mix, noted that "case types have been defined in terms of diagnosis, prognosis, utilization, organ system, hospital department, and patient demographic characteristics [and have] been discussed from the point of view of the patient, the hospital, the physician, and society with little cognizance of the implications of the shift in focus." He suggested a heuristic device whereby the various methods would be organized according to the different points in the process of providing care, in an attempt to create equivalent groups of patients. Based on an ideal model of the process, he identified six activities that occur in sequence: (1) the initial presentation of symptoms, (2) determination of the primary diagnosis, (3) consideration of comorbidities, (4) receipt of therapeutic services, (5) changes in outcomes, and finally (6) determination of the social values added by the care. Any particular case-mix method can be classified according to the point(s) in time during this process at which it adjusts for differences among patients.

Using Hornbrook's classification, most methods to adjust case mix for hospitals have concentrated on patients grouped initially by diagnoses and may also include comorbidities and/or type of treatment (especially surgical procedures). The classification scheme helps to clarify the extensiveness of a method adjusting for case mix and to compare and contrast similar methods. For example, while Arnold (1970) and CPHA (1970) both focused on a single type of surgical procedure for a single diagnosis (cholecystectomy for gall bladder disease), only CPHA adjusted for comorbidity, age, and sex. (See Hornbrook 1982b for a review of seven major diagnostic classifications used to adjust hospital case mix; and see Palmer and Reilly 1979 for a classification of different studies by type of measure and the existence of any adjustment for case mix.)

Although the commonly used method for adjusting for case mix is based on diagnoses, Hornbrook (1982a) noted that problems can occur in classifying patients whose care does not fit the underlying ideal model. Major exceptions would include patients (*a*) receiving preventive care (including care appropriate for an early working diagnosis that was later found to be wrong); (*b*) experiencing symptoms with no identified pathology; (*c*) receiving treatment as a living organ donor; or (*d*) having a chronic disease for which different treatments are appropriate for different stages.

Hospital-level Adjustment for Case Mix

As Hornbrook correctly pointed out, the model underlying adjustment for case mix is based on medical care provided at a patient-provider level. Nonetheless, some authors have implemented the "adjustment" at the hospital level (see Roemer, Moustafa, and Hopkins 1968; Shortell, Becker, and Neuhauser 1976; Duckett and Kristofferson 1978; and Luft, Bunker, and Enthoven 1979). For example, Shortell, Becker, and Neuhauser (1976) obtained, for each hospital, the percentage of cases of non-Medicare patients treated in each of thirty-eight diagnostic-treatment categories during the study year. They then created a hospital-level measure of case mix by summing the products of experts' weightings of the relative severity of outcomes associated with each category and the proportion of patients in each category. They then used this measure in a hospital-level model to explain the medical-surgical death rate for all patients at the hospital.

Several authors have described the biases in measurement and the incorrect inferences that can result from examining the relation between two variables at the wrong level of analysis (Alker 1969; Hannan 1971). Using a hypothetical example based on the quality of outcomes in hospitals, let us suppose that four hospitals are being compared (see fig. 4.1). They differ markedly in the complexity and difficulty of treating their patient case mix, from hospital A, a small community hospital in a rural area, having a case mix at the lowest level of difficulty, to hospital D, a major teaching hospital in a large community, having the highest level of difficulty. At the hospital level, death rates reflect an increasingly difficult case-mix treatment as we move from A to D, and we observe a linear relationship suggesting that the more difficult the case mix, the higher the death rate.

Within each hospital, however, the relation between the difficulty of a patient's treatment and the likelihood of dying varies. In hospitals A and B, patients whose treatment is truly difficult are referred to other hospitals, and within the range of cases they treat, there is no association between the difficulty of the case and dying. For hospital C, there is a strong association between

Figure 4.1. Hypothetical case showing aggregation bias

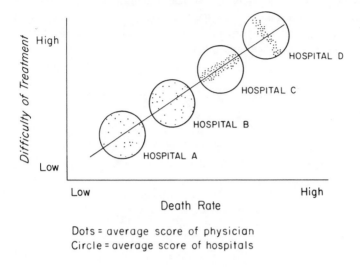

Dots = average score of physician
Circle = average score of hospitals

a more difficult treatment and a greater likelihood of death, paralleling the relationship at the hospital level. Hospital D specializes in treatment of cases at the highest level of difficulty and, through experience and preparation, has a superior record with this group and a moderate to poor record with patients under the care of new and less well supervised residents. Thus, if we measure the case mix and the death rate for these four cases at the hospital level and concluded that more difficult cases would have a greater likelihood of ending in death inhospital, we would be wrong for all hospitals except C. The quality of care measured by the overall death rate, adjusted for case mix, would not detect the variation in the death rate for patients within the hospital that is due to factors other than the difficulty of treatment. When the question to be addressed is the relationship between two variables for a given patient, the effects of patient variables on patient outcomes are most appropriately modeled and measured at the patient level rather than aggregated to the hospital level.

SUMMARY

In this chapter we have focused on the conceptual and methodological issues involved in assessing the quality of care in hospitals. Some of the problems arise from difficulties in assessing the quality of care provided to an individual patient. These problems are compounded by the need to aggregate them to a hospital level. New problems are added in evaluating performance at the organizational level. Political and value-based processes are at work at both levels, as are professional and organizational strategies. We have attempted to expose the assumptions and biases that necessarily accompany the choice of measurement of hospital performance. In the next chapter we detail our approach to this perplexing and important problem.

5 · A Methodology for Assessing Hospital Performance

Wayne Ewy and Ann Barry Flood, with
Byron W. Brown, Jr., and W. Richard Scott

In chapter 4 we describe some of the issues confronted in assessing the effectiveness of organizations. Here we propose to examine the quality and service intensity of surgical care as two important indicators of the effectiveness of hospitals viewed as organizations. Our approach was characterized by several important features.

1. *Our measures of quality focused on the outcomes of patient care rather than on process or structural indicators of effectiveness.* Having decided to use outcome measures as our primary indicators of care quality, we still had to select the specific measures. There exist an infinite number of possible measures, varying according to which phenomenon is to be emphasized (e.g., the extension of life or the quality of life) and when the phenomenon is to be assessed. Many researchers have attempted to define health-status indicators as reflecting the quality of life of the individual or measuring the improvement of health after care is provided. Many have struggled to define health such that it can be indexed and measured. There is little agreement among theorists as to how one measures the presence of good health (see WHO 1958; Sullivan 1966; Moore 1970; Donabedian 1980; and President's Commission for the Study of Ethical Problems in Medicine and Biomedical and Behavioral Research 1982). There is consensus, however, that death and morbidity are undesirable levels of health. We chose to measure outcomes by the assessment of the level of morbidity or the fact of mortality following surgery.

A secondary focus of our study was the examination of the process of care, based on the provision of selected clinical services and the length of hospitalization, measured both postoperatively and overall.

2. *It is well known that hospitals do not draw randomly from the entire pool of patients but vary as to the types of patients and conditions treated.* In

order to evaluate the quality of surgical care, we wished to adjust for any differences in patient outcomes that could be attributed to patient condition. It was important that the outcome we used as a measure of the quality of actual care delivered and the clinical services we used to indicate process take into account the differences deriving from these inherent risks. The physicians and organizational units should not be penalized for treating more difficult patients.

Early, relatively crude attempts to adjust outcomes for differences in patients were reported by Roemer, Moustafa, and Hopkins (1968) and Bunker et al. (1969). Roemer's approach was to use the length of stay weighted by the occupancy rate as an indicator of case severity. Goss and Reed (1974), attempting to apply this approach to different data, reported only mixed success due in part to regional variations among hospitals in the average length of stay. Moreover, the validity of the length of stay as a surrogate for severity is further questioned by the results of our own research, reported in chapter 7, below. The approach followed in the National Halothane Study (Bunker et al. 1969) foreshadowed our own effort by adjusting death rates for differences in the type of operation and other variables such as age, sex, and preoperative physical status. However, since this study was retrospective and utilized only data retrievable from charts, the amount and quality of data available were limited and characterized only a few hospitals.

3. *The state of medical knowledge about the disease, its diagnosis, and methods of intervention affect the outcomes possible for a given disease-operation.* While the members of the organization may be held culpable for not applying the techniques that are current medical knowledge, they should not be held responsible for failure to produce good outcomes for diseases that no one can treat better. Thus, it was important that the standards employed in the assessment of outcomes be made relative to the care provided by other members and in other organizations. And it was important that such assessments be made within a given disease-operation category. In this way, the comparisons of the levels of morbidity or occurrences of mortality were relative to the experience of patients having a similar disease and procedure.

4. *We must be careful not to overgeneralize on the basis of our conclusions.* Hospitals serve many goals, only one of which is patient care, and many types of care are provided in addition to surgical services. Our research design picked up patients only after a decision had been made to perform surgery. Since for many patient conditions the decision as to whether to operate is both controversial and critical, our design placed important limitations on any conclusions drawn about the quality of the surgical service. Moreover, only selected surgical categories were studied in detail.

In this chapter we first present an overview of the research design and methodology used to standardize outcomes and service—at a level common to all of the studies reported here. We then provide details about the design and methods specific to the Extensive Study, the Intensive Study, and the Service Intensity Study. To permit the reader to see the kinds of assumptions and choices we made, and why, we usually illustrate our choices with details from one study group of patients. For the reader interested in the full details of other groups, we provide a hitchhiker's guide through our reports, pinpointing where these fascinating worlds of detail reside. For the reader who wishes a briefer description of the relevant methods, they are reviewed in chapter 6, which also presents the results of our tests for differences among hospitals for outcomes and services. Results of linking hospital structure to performance are reported in chapters 8–12.

AN OVERVIEW OF THE OUTCOME METHODS USED

The specific techniques we employed in our studies of outcome and service intensity differed markedly, depending on the nature of the data used and practical considerations related to the number of hospitals, physicians, and patients and to the specific hypotheses under examination; however, they were quite similar in their underlying strategy.

The dependent variable (DV), whether it measured outcome or service intensity, was considered to depend on two classes of independent variables: patient characteristics and provider characteristics. Provider characteristics included those of the hospital, the physician, and other treatment personnel. The relationship can be formally written as

$$DV = F(\text{patient}) + G(\text{provider}) + \text{error}, \tag{1}$$

where F and G describe the functional relation between the independent effects (patient or provider) and the DV. The error term is the difference between the actual or observed DV and that predicted on the basis of the patient and provider effects. It reflects countless "random" influences, including unmeasured patient and provider effects.

Our primary aim was to examine the components of the provider function G. If we were to look at G by analysis of the DV data, the patient function F also had to be determined, so that its effects could be removed. One obvious approach was to estimate simultaneously both the F and G relationships, such as, for instance, by a multiple regression analysis. The alternative we chose, however, was a two-step process. We first estimated the effects of patient characteristics:

$$DV = F(\text{patient}) + \text{error}. \tag{2}$$

The function F in equation (2) is called the prediction function or the standardization function, depending on the context. In a subsequent analysis, we examined the effects of the provider characteristics, G, by relating the residuals from the first analysis (i.e., $DV - F[\text{patient}]$) to the provider effects. This relationship can be seen as a simple rearrangement of equation (1):

$$\text{Residual} = G(\text{provider}) + \text{error}, \tag{3}$$

where the residual for each patient is computed as

$$\text{Residual} = DV - F(\text{patient}).$$

This approach is analogous to an analysis of covariance proposed by Quade (1967), where the analysis of the main variables of interest (i.e., provider characteristics) is performed on the residuals from the covariate regression (i.e., patient characteristics).

There were two reasons for this methodological approach. First, we wanted our analyses to be "conservative" with regard to detecting provider effects. Suppose that some measures concerning providers correlate with measures of patient health; for example, teaching hospitals tend to treat patients with more serious diseases. In a nonrandomized study, to the extent that these measures about providers also correlate with the *DV,* interpretation or judgment must be used to decide to which factor this common effect should be ascribed. Continuing with our example, suppose that teaching hospitals tend to use more laboratory services for their patients. One reason for the higher use of services is the more serious diseases of the patients. Two alternative explanations for higher use relate to the process of teaching: use of laboratory tests for teaching purposes and use owing to the inexperience of residents. The two-step approach maximizes the predictive power attributed to the patient characteristics and thus minimizes the effects attributed to the provider characteristics. We preferred an approach that gave greater weight to using patient disease to explain higher use of laboratory tests in teaching hospitals, so that any relation we observed between teaching and the use of patient service could be argued to be "real effects," since they were likely to be an underestimate of the true importance of teaching hospitals.

The second reason for our methodological approach was one of practical computational considerations. We investigated different formulations of provider effects (i.e., sets of variables) based on various subsets of patient types each having a different F relationship. A single-step analysis to simultaneously estimate the necessarily complex F function covering all patient categories and the G function would have been prohibitively expensive, particularly for the logistic regression analyses, which we used for the dichotomous dependent variables such as mortality. In this case, the solution required iterative procedures using individual patient records. Summary correlation matrices could not be used as a starting point as in linear regression.

In describing our model so far, we have assumed the level of analysis to be at the patient level. That is, equations (1) through (3) all model the relation between patient characteristics and provider characteristics affecting the DV for a given patient. This provides the most sensitive model for estimating (and removing) the patient characteristics. Subsequent analyses directed at estimating provider characteristics were performed at a level appropriate for the specific hypotheses being investigated.

For some types of analyses, it was more appropriate to derive a DV modeled at the provider level. For example, if we wished to characterize the care of a given provider such as a surgeon or a hospital, we needed to aggregate the experience of the set of patients treated by that provider. A simple aggregation measure would have been to take the mean DV experienced by the set of patients for each provider. However, as we argue in chapter 4, standardization was necessary whenever individuals differed in their expected DV and the groups or populations being compared did not have the same mix of individuals (e.g., one group contains relatively more high-risk subjects).

The information about patient effects in equation (2) could be reassembled to describe the provider, for example, to get an overall index value for each hospital. For these calculations, the method we used can be viewed as a form of "indirect standardization" (see Mosteller and Tukey 1977; and Fleiss 1981). Indirect standardization is typically applied to a comparison of proportions of dichotomous events, such as deaths; but the ideas easily extend to DV measures that are not dichotomous, such as length of stay or the number of surgical procedures.

The fundamental calculation in indirect standardization is the expected value (E) of the DV, where the expectation is based only on the subject's relevant characteristics, not the *provider group* to which he or she belongs (in this case, the hospital in which the patient was treated). In our application, this expectation rule was derived from the combined experience of all study subjects. For example, suppose that the only patient factor affecting mortality was age; then $F(\text{age})$ for a patient would simply be the average mortality for all subjects of the same age as the patient. To compute an overall index for a hospital, the expected DV values are summed over all patients and compared (by either subtraction or ratio) with the sum of the actual observed DV values.

The form of the patient effect equation (F) is determined by the nature of the DV. For those DV that are multivalued (having more than two levels), a linear regression approach can provide a reasonable model:

$$Y = BX, \tag{4}$$

where Y is the DV, X is the set of patient characteristics, and B is the set of regression coefficients relating to X and Y. The regression coefficients, B, are estimated by analysis of all patients, disregarding any provider, or G, information.

When the DV is dichotomous (such as dead or alive), ordinary linear regression is not completely satisfactory, although it may work as a rough approximation. The principal problem in using linear regression as a prediction function for the dichotomous case is that the resulting predicted values are not constrained to the range (0, 1) as probabilities should be. For example, in the case where 0 corresponds to alive, and 1 to dead, an expected value of .5 can be interpreted as a 50 percent probability of dying. With linear regression, values such as 1.5 or 2, which cannot meaningfully be interpreted as "more dead" than other dead patients, can be obtained. The alternative we used to avoid these problems was logistic regression:

$$Y = 1/[1 + \exp(BX)], \tag{5}$$

where exp denotes exponentiation using the nature base, e.

Another form for the patient effect function, F, applies to both dichotomous and multivalued DV when there are only a few X variables and each has only a few distinct values, that is, where cross tabulation of the X variables results in only a small number of cells. In this case, one B coefficient is estimated for each cell, as in the age example above.

The predictive value, as well as the validity, of these models depends on the patient variables included in the standardization model F. Several factors limit the number and nature of variables that can be used. Practical considerations, such as whether the information is routinely recorded and abstracted, limit the availability of patient information. The use of available information is limited by the purpose of the standardization. In most analyses we focused on characterizing the patient's condition at the time of admission and on the surgical treatments received. Therefore, we used the patient's primary diagnosis (as it was eventually determined); indications of any comorbidity present at admission; the surgical treatments received; and demographic factors such as age, sex, and a height/weight index as surrogates for general health and comorbidity. With a few exceptions in our analysis of service intensity, we attempted to exclude from the standardization models any iatrogenic disease or complication occurring after admission. Surgical procedures were included because receipt of any surgical procedure has a major effect on the types of services received, the number of days stayed, and mortality and morbidity; however, whenever a procedure had a significant likelihood of being used to treat inhospital complications, it was not used for standardization. Because of the requirement to use only measures reflecting condition at admission and not complications of care provided, some rather powerful predictors were discarded. For example, abnormal laboratory values for nitrogen derivatives in the blood and the use of diuretics during hospitalization were both powerful predictors of death. However, such measures could reflect treatment of complications arising during hospitalization, such as kidney problems secondary to cardiovascular complications, and we did not wish to standardize for complications that may have been caused by poor-quality care.

The steps leading to the choice of predictor variables were complicated;

the specific choices differed in the various studies we carried out. The first step, and one of the most important, was the definition of rules for selection and categorization of patients. This step separated study patients from nonstudy patients and further divided study patients into more homogeneous subsets. Since separate models were developed for each category, this initial categorization is an integral part of the standardization model: it selects the appropriate intercept term for the model, as well as the category-specific regression coefficients. The details of variable selection and development of the standardization model are described below for each study.

METHODS USED TO MEASURE THE QUALITY OF CARE IN THE EXTENSIVE STUDY

The Extensive Study (ES) was based on the analysis of records of approximately 11 million patients, leading to computation of standardized death rates for each of 1,224 hospitals. It was designed to complement the Intensive Study (IS), as well as to be a freestanding project. This orientation, as well as practical considerations, heavily influenced the basic design decisions, such as selection of data sources, hospitals, types of patients, and overall analytic philosophy.

The principal objective of the ES was to measure the extent and sources of variation among hospitals in the quality of surgical care, as reflected by hospital death rates for selected types of patients, standardized or adjusted to remove the effect of differences in patient populations at each hospital.

The standardized death rates were computed from the Professional Activity Study (PAS) data submitted by the study hospitals. The Commission on Professional and Hospital Activities (CPHA) administers the PAS as a service to hospitals, a basic component of which is the collection of information on each patient upon discharge. The abstract is completed by the hospital and sent to CPHA for editing and error-checking before entering the PAS history file. The abstract's contents include information on admission tests, demographic characteristics, operations received, and final diagnoses. The accuracy of the PAS abstract information was of great concern in planning the ES. The items selected and the manner of use were designed to reduce the effect of any inaccuracies or omissions identified in the data (see Hendrickson and Myers 1973).

All U.S. hospitals participating in the PAS system for the full year of 1972 were included in the ES. These 1,224 hospitals represent approximately 20 percent of all nonfederal acute-care hospitals in the United States in 1972. Their 11 million discharges in 1972 represent about 33 percent of all discharges from this category in the United States that year. Compared with the 5,843 nonfederal short-term U.S. hospitals at the time of the study (AHA 1973), the ES hospitals were essentially identical in average bed size (151 beds for both) and teaching (26 percent in the ES and 27 percent nationally, based on the same definition of teaching). They tended to have lower average expenditures per day ($96 in the ES versus $105 nationally). They were less likely to controlled by the state or the local government (19 percent in the ES versus 30 percent nationally). The ES hospitals were located primarily in five of the nine major regions, although some hospitals were included from each region (30 percent were in the East North Central Region and 10–17 percent were in the West North Central, the Middle Atlantic, the South Atlantic, and the Pacific regions). About 40 percent were located in areas with a population size below 50,000; 16 percent were in Standard Metropolitan Statistical Areas (SMSAs) with a population of 2.5 million or more; and the remainder were spread evenly in the four SMSAs ranging from 100,000 to just below 2.5 million.

The types of patients selected for study were the same as in the IS portion of our study, described below. Briefly, study categories for both the IS and the ES were chosen to include a broad range of ages, both sexes, a variety of organ systems, a variety of surgical specialties among physicians, and surgical diseases amenable to staging by severity. An additional consideration for the ES was to select categories containing a large enough number of patients who experienced inhospital death to allow estimation of the quality of care based on this outcome, since it was found to be the only reliable measure available for this data base. The larger data base of the ES also permitted inclusion of trauma cases in some surgical categories, for example, hip fracture with and without trauma. Finally, the coverage in the ES was expanded somewhat to include patients in the nonsurgical counterparts of two surgical categories (i.e., ulcer and gall bladder) to test whether any differences in success rates in surgery were merely artifacts arising because of factors affecting the selection of patients to receive surgery.

The general methodological approach can be summarized briefly. Standardized death rates were computed by first estimating the probability of death for each patient—independent of any hospital effect—based on carefully selected standardizing variables reflecting the patient's preoperative status and the specific surgery performed and excluding any postoperative complications. In a sense, this probability approximates an average survival over all hospitals for the specific type of patient with a given disease (where the specific type is defined by the values of the patient's standardizing variables, such as age, sex, and comorbidity). Adding these probabilities together by hospital (over all patients or over some specified subset of patients) provided an expected number of deaths for each hospital under the null hypothesis that there are no true differences in mortality among hospitals. A standardized mortality ratio was then computed by dividing the actual number of deaths by this expected number. In this section we describe the basic analytic steps in computing the mortality ratios. Once such standardized mortality ratios were available, the basic investigation proceeded in two directions: determination of whether the standardized ratios differed more than expected by chance; and evaluation of hypotheses relating hospital characteristics to standardized mortality ratios. These methods are described in subsequent sections.

ES Measures of the Quality of Care

The only measure of the quality of care studied in the ES was whether the patient was dead or alive at discharge. Other measures— "inhospital complication" and death within forty days of admission—were considered but were not studied in depth. Inhospital complication was found to be unreliably recorded in the study hospitals. The measure of death within forty days of admission was originally created to parallel a measure of death used in the IS. It was later dropped because of differences in the definitions between the two studies (in the IS the forty days occurred after the surgery rather than after admission, and what is more important, in the IS patients were followed after discharge to obtain their status as dead or alive). The majority of ES patients (over 80 percent) who died inhospital died within forty days of admission.

Classifying Patients into Study Categories

The first task in deriving a standardized death rate was to select the qualifying patients in each hospital and assign them to relatively homogeneous categories. It is important to note that these categories represented only an intermediate step in computing the death rates (see fig. 5.1). The designation is, in effect, simply one of the standardization variables used in assessing the patient's prognosis and does not prevent aggregation of the categories or subsets of them in the final standardized ratios.

It was operationally convenient to perform the selection and classification into study categories in two steps. In the first step, patients were assigned to primary selection categories (PCs), on the basis of operation and diagnosis codes, using the Hospital Adaptation of the International Classification of Disease (HICDA) (see CPHA 1968). These selection categories are displayed in table 5.1. One primary category (PC 1) was defined in order to disqualify patients with evidence to secondary (metastatic) malignancies from the study. All fifteen PCs were ordered according to their seriousness, defined mostly in terms of decreasing probability of death. Any patient eligible for more than one PC was assigned to only one category, using the rule of assigning the patient to the PC with the lowest number (i.e., the most serious category). For example, any patient who underwent an incidental appendectomy along with his or her gastrointestinal procedure was classified according to the more serious PC: gastrointestinal. A patient tentatively assigned to a PC could still be rejected from the study for several reasons aimed at increasing the final homogeneity of the patients selected. For example, a patient with extensive surgery other than

Figure 5.1. Steps in the ES standardization process

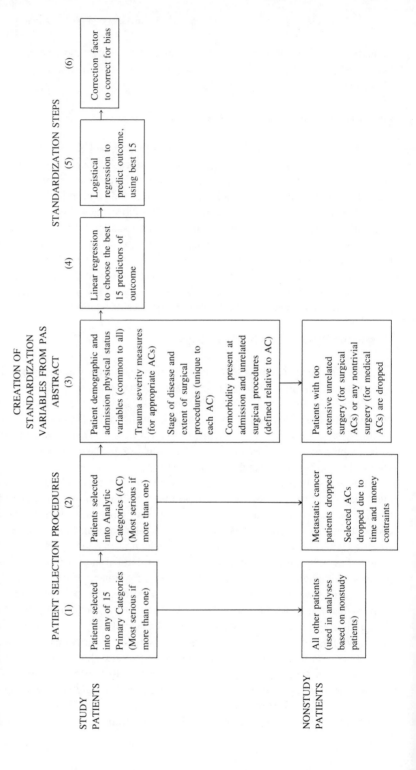

Table 5.1. The original patient categories of the ES and the subset selected for final analysis

---

I. Category used to disqualify patient from study
  PC 1. Secondary malignant neoplasms (dx: 196.0–199.0)[a]

II. Categories requiring surgical procedure and/or diagnoses[b]
  PC 2. Skull operations and/or diagnoses (op: 01.0, 01.2–01.6; dx: 800.0, 800.1, 801.0, 801.1)
  PC 3. Intraabdominal artery operations (op: 35.3, 35.5)
      AC 3.1. Intraabdominal artery operations
  PC 4. Lower limb operations and/or diagnoses (op: 87.6–87.8, 84.0–84.1; dx: 808.0–808.1, 820.0–820.5, 821.0–821.1)
      AC 4.1. Amputation of lower limb—current trauma diagnosis
      AC 4.2. Amputation of lower limb—no current trauma diagnosis
      AC 4.3. Hip fracture diagnosis with other trauma diagnosis
      AC 4.4. Hip fracture diagnosis with no other trauma diagnosis
      AC 4.5. Fracture of the shaft of the femur
      AC 4.6. Fracture of the pelvis
      AC 4.7. Arthroplasty of the hip
  PC 5. Lung operations (op: 25.1–25.4)
  PC 6. Gastrointestinal tract operations (op: 44.2–44.3, 44.6, 45.3, 45.5, 46.2, 47.0–47.3, 50.2)
      AC 6.1. Large bowel operations—cancer diagnosis
      AC 6.3. Large bowel operations—other specified diagnosis
      AC 6.4. Large bowel operations—other diagnoses
      AC 6.5. Stomach operations—cancer diagnosis
      AC 6.7. Stomach operations—ulcer diagnosis
      AC 6.8. Stomach operations—other diagnosis
  PC 7. Splenectomy (op: 38.2)
  PC 8. Biliary tract operations and diagnoses (op: 53.0–53.5, 53.9; dx: 574.0–575.9)[c]
      AC 8.1. Biliary tract operations
  PC 9. Prostatectomy operations and diagnoses (op: 65.1–65.5; dx: 185.0, 600.0)
  PC 10. Hysterectomy (op: 71.0–71.4)
  PC 11. Spinal operations (op: 83.4, 84.4)
  PC 12. Appendectomy (op: 49.0–49.1)

III. Categories requiring diagnoses and no surgical procedures
  PC 13. Biliary tract diagnoses—nonsurgical (dx: 574.0–575.9)[d]
      AC 13.1. Biliary tract diagnoses—nonsurgical
  PC 14. Ulcer diagnoses—nonsurgical[d] (dx: 531.0–531.3, 532.0–532.3, 533.0–533.3, 534.0–534.3)
      AC 14.1 Ulcer diagnoses—nonsurgical
  PC 15. Colon diagnoses—nonsurgical (dx: 211.3, 562.1, 563.0–563.1)

Note: Primary categories are designated PCs, and ACs are analytic categories. They are numbered to reflect the relative probability of dying, with the lowest number having the

Table 5.1. (*Continued*)

highest probability. The AC numbers are used for reference to the 17 final study categories throughout the original report (SCHCR 1974) and this chapter. In all, 18 additional AC categories in the remaining PCs were defined and staged in the original report, but only 6 PCs and all of their 17 AC categories were completed due to financial and time constraints. All 15 PCs and 33 ACs were used in the patient selection procedure. If a patient qualified for more than one AC or PC, he or she was assigned only to the category with the lowest number.

ᵃEntries in parentheses are the HICDA-1 codes for operations (op) and diagnoses (dx) included in each primary category (see CPHA 1968).

ᵇPatients in PCs 2–12 were disqualified if they had extensive unrelated procedures (rated 5 [see table 5.5]).

ᶜPatient with any primary malignant diagnoses (140.0–209.9) were disqualified.

ᵈPatients were disqualified for any primary malignant diagnoses (140.0–209.9) or any nontrivial surgical procedures (rated 2 or above [see table 5.5]).

those under study or with a primary (local) cancer diagnosis could be dropped from the study category.

In the second step, the final assignment to analytic categories (ACs) was made, and selected PAS abstract items were converted into variables for further standardization. The ACs within each PC also were ordered from the most serious classification to the least serious, on the basis of the probability of dying. Similar to the classification procedure for handling patients who qualified for more than one PC, whenever patients qualified for multiple ACs, the patient was assigned to the lowest AC—again, to ensure that the patient was assigned to the most serious category. In the original design, thirty-three ACs were defined within the fourteen broader PCs. Due to financial and time constraints, only seventeen ACs in six PCs were fully implemented. These seventeen study ACs, noted in table 5.1, form the basis of the remainder of our discussion of the methodology and results of the ES.

Standardizing Variables

Several rules were followed in choosing and defining the standardization variables. The first was that each variable must reflect the patient's presurgical condition, and not postsurgical complications or treatments other than surgery or other management activities. This rule led to the exclusion of all nonadmission tests and drugs given that could potentially reflect treatment and diagnosis of postsurgical complications. A second rule was to assume that a patient was normal in terms of a given attribute if the PAS item was not completed. This might result in an underestimation of a patient's risk, particularly if the unrecorded item actually was abnormal and abnormality carried a higher risk. In the extreme case, a hospital may show a poor standardized mortality ratio either because of poor performance or because it had a higher than average proportion of poor-risk patients with incomplete records. In order to take into account this possibility, the number of standardization items missing from the record was also recorded and used as a standardization variable.

The patient variables used for standardization can be classified into three major types: (1) those used to stage the extent of the study disease and operative procedures, (2) those measuring patient demographics such as age and sex and pretreatment physical status, and (3) those used to portray comorbidity and unrelated surgery. Variables in the first group were defined uniquely for each study category, while variables in the second group were common to all patients. Comorbidity and unrelated surgery were defined to be as uniform as possible across all patients, but their meaning was somewhat dependent upon the study category, as we illustrate below.

Standardizing for Stage of Disease and Operations

A separate procedure was necessary for each analytic category in order to use the information contained in the related diagnostic codes to stage the extent of disease present and to use the related operation codes to rate the severity of the related surgical procedures undergone. The definition of the variables to represent stage of disease and severity of operative procedures was reasonably straightforward once the diseases and operations were identified in terms of HICDA codes. The more frequent codes were usually included as simply binary indicator variables. An implicit ranking by severity of disease or operative procedure was created by having binary variables take on the value of 1 to indicate a patient with more severe codes. Less frequent codes were grouped into single variables, on the basis of being more or less severe, usually defined as the probability of dying. As an illustration, table 5.2 contains the definitions for staging disease and the extensiveness of operations for one of the categories (AC 8.1, operations on the biliary tract). (See SCHCR 1974, 374–37, for all categories.)

For some ACs (i.e., 4.1–4.4), the selection of patients and staging of disease required an additional set of standardization variables in order to rate the severity of trauma experienced. These ratings were based on the HICDA codes involving injury (800.0–959.9), which were first placed into eight anatomical groups plus a burns group. Within these groups, diagnoses were rated from 1 to 4 to reflect the increasing severity of the injury. No attempt was made to equalize these ratings across the nine groups. These ratings are illustrated in table 5.3, using selected injury diagnoses relating to the leg or the hip.

Standardizing for Demographics and Physical Status at Admission

The other standardizing variables were common to all study patients and are also based on the PAS abstract. The first basic type includes demographic variables, physical findings, and prescriptions. Table 5.4 describes these fifteen

Table 5.2. Staging disease and the extent of surgical procedures: Illustration using AC 8.1, biliary tract surgery

---

I. Selecting biliary tract study patients
Each patient must have one or more of the qualifying diagnoses and one or more of the qualifying surgical procedures.[a]

   A. Qualifying diagnoses
      1. Cholelithiasis, without acute cholecytitis or not specified (5749)
      2. Cholelithiasis, with acute cholecystitis (5740)
      3. Acute cholecystitis and cholangitis (5750)
      4. Cholecystitis and cholangitis, not otherwise specified (5759)
   B. Qualifying surgical procedures
      1. Cholecystectomy (535)
      2. Cholecystotomy (534)
      3. Incision of bile ducts (530)
      4. Excision of bile duct lesion (531)
      5. Anastomosis of bile duct (532)
      6. Plastic and repair of bile ducts (533)
      7. Biliary tract operations, other (539)

II. Staging biliary tract disease and the extent of related surgical procedures
   A. Diagnostic categories

1. Cholelithiasis[b]	1 = 5749 or 5740
2. Acute cholecystitis[b]	1 = 5740 or 5750
3. Cholelithiasis with acute cholecystitis[b]	1 = 5740
4. Obstruction, fistula, perforation[c]	1 = common bile duct obstruction (5760), gall bladder bile duct obstruction (5761), or spasm of Sphincter of Oddi (5765)
	2 = gall bladder or bile duct fistula (5762) or gall bladder or bile duct perforation (5766)
5. Other disease of gall bladder or bile duct	1 = gall bladder bile duct cholesterolosis (5363), gall bladder or bile duct hydrops (5764), or other gall bladder or bile duct diagnoses (5769)
6. Disease of the pancreas[c]	1 = chronic pancreatitis (5771) or other disease of the pancreas (5779)
	2 = acute pancreatitis (5770)

   B. Operation categories

7. Cholecystectomy	1 = 535
8. Incision of bile ducts for exploration	1 = 530

Table 5.2. (*Continued*)

9. Cholecystotomy	1 = 534
10. Minor biliary tract procedures	1 = excision of bile duct lesion (531) or biopsy of the biliary tract (538)
11. Other biliary tract procedures, rated only if no cholecystectomy	1 = anastomosis of bile duct (532), plastic and repair of bile duct (533), or other biliary tract operations (539)
	2 = anastomosis of gall bladder (536)
12. Cholecystography	1 = 934
13. Appendectomy	1 = 491
14. Liver biopsy, intra-abdominal approach	1 = 528

Note: Three- and four-digit codes are from HICDA (CPHA 1968), with decimals removed.

[a]The patient cannot have any metastatic cancer diagnoses (1400–2099) or be eligible for selection into PCs 2–7 (skull, abdominal, vessel, lower limb, lung, gastrointestinal, or spleen).

[b]If a patient has more than one of the biliary tract diagnoses for selection, only the primary reason for hospitalization (i.e., the first one listed) is coded.

[c]Two special rules apply: (1) a quadratic version of this variable minus one was also used; (2) if the patient's diagnoses qualify for both codes 1 and 2, use 2.

variables plus six quadratic versions of nondichotomous variables. Also displayed in table 5.4 are variables that were considered for standardizing but were rejected either because of significant missing data (e.g., race) or because the finding might reflect complications occurring during the hospitalization (e.g., a positive test for an unusual level of nitrogen derivatives).

Standardizing for Comorbidity and Unrelated Surgery

The second type of standardizing variables common to all study patients described the patient's comorbidity, that is, any diagnoses and surgical procedures other than those used to stage their particular AC. The PAS form allowed up to seven additional diagnoses and six additional surgical procedures to be recorded for each patient. For both unrelated diagnoses and surgical procedures, our procedure involved creating a severity rating for each HICDA code recorded on a patient's PAS abstract. We describe the ratings for unrelated diagnoses first.

The first step in evaluating comorbidity based on unrelated diagnoses was to rate each of the approximately 3,400 HICDA disease codes on a severity scale (0–9) based on their estimated effect on the probability of death. This

Table 5.3. Ratings of diagnoses involving trauma: Illustration of codes using selected diagnoses for the leg and the hip

Trauma Rating[a]	Diagnosis
1	Sprain or strain of hip or thigh (8430)
	Sprain or strain of knee or leg (8440)
	Sprain or strain of pelvis (8481)
	dislocated knee, simple (8360)
2	Fractured femur (neck), closed reduction (8200)
	Fractured femur (shaft), closed reduction (8210)
	Fractured ankle, open reduction (8241)
	Dislocated hip, simple (8350)
	Dislocated knee, compound (8361)
3	Fracture of pelvis, closed reduction (8080)
	Fractured femur (shaft), open reduction (8211)
	Fractured femur (lower end), closed reduction (8212)
	Injury to nerve in thigh, without open wound (9550)
4	Fracture of pelvis, open reduction (8081)
	Fracture femur (neck), open reduction (8201)
	Dislocated hip, compound (8351)
	Injury to nerve in thigh, with open wound (9551)

Note: These ratings were used for patient selection into categories and for staging of the severity of trauma for analytic categories indicating trauma or no trauma (e.g., AC 4.1–4.4).

[a]Trauma ratings, reflecting increasing severity from 1 to 4, were created for all diagnoses from 8000–9599 (HICDA with decimals removed); the diagnoses were first grouped into 9 categories: skull, spinal cord and nerves, thorax, abdomen, leg and hip, arm and shoulders, hands and feet, skin and superficial trauma, and burns (SCHCR 1974, 302–11). Rating levels are not comparable across these diagnostic groups. If a patient had multiple trauma ratings, the highest rating was used.

nontrivial task was complicated by the desire to have this scale as independent as possible of the other standardizing variables. The ratings were to reflect the differential effect of the condition on a patient of fixed age, sex, operation, and principal diagnosis. Diagnoses likely to reflect postsurgical complications were scored as 0 and were subsequently ignored in further analysis. The ratings of the codes were done by the SCHCR physicians in cooperation with the statisticians. These ratings are illustrated in table 5.5, which gives the ratings for seventy-seven codes pertaining to the cardiovascular system.

Using these ratings, we scored each of the patients' unrelated diagnoses (i.e., other than the diagnoses used for the category) from 0 to 9. For actual use as standardizing variables, only the ratings of the most severe and second most

Table 5.4. Standardization variables other than diagnoses or operation codes

Variable	Brief Description and Coding

I. Deomographic variables
  A. Used in standardization

1. Age[a]	In years; truncated to 100 on abstract; missing set to 35
2. Sex	0 = male; 1 = female or missing
3. Poverty indicator	1 = expected source of payment is Medicaid or charity; else = 0
4. Height/weight index[a]	Coded 1–9 for low to high; based on sex-adjusted norms for 20-year-olds

  B. Not used in standardization[b]

Race	White, Asian, black, "nonwhite"
Source of payment	Medicare, Workman's Compensation, Blue Cross, commercial insurers, self-pay

II. Physical findings specifically designated to occur at admission[c]
  A. Used in standardization

5. White blood cell count[a]	In thousands; 0 = 0–10 or missing, 1 = 11–20, 2 = 21–99
6. Systolic blood pressure[a]	0 = 220 mm Hg or more
	1 = 190–219
	2 = 160–189
	3 = 140–159
	4 = 120–139, or missing
	5 = 100–119
	6 = 90–99
	7 = 80–89
	8 = 50–79
	9 = 49 mm Hg or less
7. Diastolic Blood Pressure[a]	Coded same as systolic except missing coded as 7
8. Urine sugar	1 = test positive, else 0
9. Urine albumin	1 = test positive; else 0
10. Temperature	0 = 98°F or less or missing; scaled 1–7 for 99, . . . , 104, 105+
11. Hemoglobin	Hemoglobin or hematocrit (hospitals choose which to record uniformly for patients): 1 = hgb 10 or less; 1 = hct 35 or less; else 0

  B. Not used in standardization[b]

Emergency indicator	1 = surgery on day of admission or within six hours of admission (hospitals choose which time for patients); else 0

(continued)

Table 5.4. (*Continued*)

Variable	Brief Description and Coding
III. Other physical findings or drugs	
A. Used in standardization	
12. Pathology report of most important operation[a]	0 = no disease, no report, or no tissue; 1 = surgical removal not clearly indicated; 2 = tissue disease that generally requires removal
13. Oral antidiabetics	1 = given; else 0
14. Insulin	1 = given; else 0
15. Thyroid or antithyroid	1 = given; else 0
B. Not used in standardization[b]	
Blood sugar	1 = 150 mg % recorded (fasting or 2 hr PP); else 0
Blood chemistry: cholesterol	1 = abnormal high result for cholesterol test; else 0
Diuretics	1 = given; else 0
Antihypertensives	1 = given; else 0
Vasodilators	1 = given; else 0
Blood test for nitrogen	1 = abnormal high for nitrogen derivatives; else 0

Note: Variables were the same for all study categories.

[a]A quadratic version was also used $((x - 1)^2)$, resulting in 22 variables to be used for standardization.

[b]These variables were not used because they could not be assumed to reflect only pretreatment values or because significant data were missing.

[c]The admission period includes two days prior to hospitalization and one day after, unless surgery occurred on that day.

severe unrelated diagnoses for each patient were used. Based on preliminary work, these two variables had predictive power similar to or better than other measures considered (such as the sum of all ratings) and had the advantages of being simple to compute, of not being overly sensitive to the recording of many less serious diagnoses (as might occur with an extensive physical workup), and of preserving most of the information about each patient's unrelated diagnoses, since the average number of additional diagnoses was about 1. While the rating system can be faulted because different raters might well come up with different ratings of the 3,400 codes, we argue that the methods chosen were better than ignoring the diagnoses or simply counting the number recorded. And despite problems arising from potential variation in recording unrelated diagnoses, the

Table 5.5. Severity ratings used to score comorbidity for study patients (selected cardiovascular diagnoses)

Rating[a]	Code[b]	Diagnosis
0	4100–4109	Acute myocardial infarction
	4110, 4140	Acute or asymptomatic ischemic heart disease
	4130	Angina pectoris
	4210–9	Acute and subacute endocarditis
	4220	Acute and subacute myocarditis
	4270–79	Congestive heart failure and arrhythmias
	4300–4361	Acute cerebrovascular episodes
	4382	Cerebral edema
3	4381	Encephalomalacia and necrosis
	4389	Unspecified lesions, cerebrovascular disease
4	4380	Residual cerebral paralysis
	4384–85	Cerebral arteritis and nonpyogenic thrombosis
5	4370	Generalized ischemic cerebrovascular disease
	4402, 4409	Arteriosclerosis, generalized arteries of extremities
6	4010	Essential benign hypertension
	4260	Pulmonary heart disease
	4290–99	Cardiac enlargement
	4400–4401	Arteriosclerosis in aorta, renal artery
7	3940–80	Chronic rheumatic heart disease
	4020–50	Secondary hypertension
	4120, 4122–29	Chronic ischemic heart disease, except aneurysm of heart
	4240–49	Chronic disease of endocardium
	4250	Cardiomyopathy
8	4121	Aneurysm of heart
9	4000	Malignant hypertension

[a]Conditions presumed to be preexisting are coded from 1 to 9 for increasing severity. A rating of zero is assigned if the condition is considered to have some likelihood of being a postoperative complication.
[b]Codes are from HICDA (CPHA 1968), without decimals.

fact that a common set of rules was applied to data for all hospitals should result in a reduction of any bias in the death rate comparisons that do not use the diagnosis information.

Unrelated operations were rated in a manner parallel to that used for unrelated diagnoses. The approximately seven hundred HICDA operation codes were first divided into fifty-eight groups, primarily on the basis of anatomic region. The codes within each group were rated by the SCHCR physicians and statisticians using a scale of 1–5 to reflect the extent of surgery involved. This rating by definition reflected pure surgical trauma and ignored the seriousness of the disease for which the surgery is typically done, as well as other health-related factors such as age, sex, or physical status, since these variables were included directly. The goal was to have comparability of codes across the fifty-eight Surgical Extent Region (SER) variables—thus an unrelated procedure on the gall bladder that was rated 4 was supposed to be about as traumatizing as a level-4 unrelated procedure to the large bowel. Table 5.6 illustrates these ratings, using operations on the stomach.

Based on these ratings, each of the patient's unrelated operations was coded. Then two variables were created for standardizing unrelated procedures: the rating of the most extensive procedure and the number of anatomic areas receiving "nontrivial" surgery (ratings of 2 or more). In addition, these standardizing variables were used to identify patients to be excluded from the study. In all ACs, patients who had received extensive unrelated operations (i.e., a rating of 5) were dropped. In ACs 13.1 and 14.1 (the nonsurgical categories), any patient with a nontrivial surgical procedure (i.e., rated 2 or above) was dropped. This rule allowed patients who had received certain diagnostic procedures, such as simple biopsies and minor sutures, to remain classified as nonsurgical patients.

Predicting Death on the Basis of the Standardizing Variables

Altogether between forty and sixty-five potential standardization variables were implemented for patients in each study category. About thirty were identical or nearly identical across all categories. For variables that were not dichotomous (e.g., age or the highest rating of unrelated diagnoses), both linear and quadratic terms were included to provide an implicit scale transformation. Only the most powerful variables were used in the standardization model. While ten or fewer variables probably would have been adequate in most categories, we chose to use fifteen variables in the model for each category. We did not use all forty to sixty-five because very little predictive power would be gained, at a very great cost in terms of computational complexity and resources.

Although the final standardization model was based on logistic regression, the principal tool used for selecting the "best" set of fifteen standardization variables for each AC was stepwise linear regression of the outcome measure (i.e., dead/alive) on the full set of standardization variables. Our preliminary studies had indicated for this type of data that linear and logistic models were in close agreement in selecting the most important predictor variables from a larger set, but the linear model was considerably less expensive to analyze. The predictive power of both models, as measured by multiple correlation coefficient (R^2), plateaued very quickly after the first few variables were entered.

Table 5.6. Severity ratings used to score unrelated surgical procedures: Illustration using stomach operations (SER variable 25)

Rating[a]	Code	Operation
2	440	Gastrotomy
	442	Local excision of lesion of stomach
	448	Biopsy of stomach
	450	Gastrostomy temporary
	451	Gastrostomy permanent
3	441	Pyloromyotomy
	446	Vagotomy
	452	Closure of gastrostomy
4	443	Partial gastrectomy
	453	Anastomosis of stomach
	454	Revision of anastomosis
	455	Pyloroplasty
	456	Gastroorrhaphy and other plastic surgery
	459	Stomach operations, other
5[b]	444	Complete gastrectomy
	445	Radical gastrectomy

Note: For each study category, only those procedures not used to classify the study operation were coded. In addition, special exclusion rules or ratings were defined for each study category where appropriate. For example, the ratings 2–4 for the procedure in this table were reduced by one for gall bladder patients because the abdomen was already opened for the study procedure. See SCHCR 1974 (374–437) for details of special rules by category.

[a]Ratings are scaled from 1–5 for measuring the extent of the surgery (only levels 2–5 appear in this variable). There were 58 such variables defined, incorporating all HICDA operation codes. This system of variables and ratings identifies the number of anatomic areas receiving surgery (as opposed to the number of HICDA codes recorded, which may reflect the coding system more than the surgery) and measures the extent of the surgery in each area. See SCHCR 1974 (312–16) for details of all SER variables.

[b]Patients with any additional surgery rated 5 were dropped from the study. See SCHCR 1974 (285) for a complete list.

The final step in computing the predicted probability of death for each subject was to fit a multiple logistic function, using the fifteen selected standardization variables. A separate analysis was carried out for each of the seventeen final ACs. (For details of the variables chosen, their mean and standard deviation, and the coefficient and its standard error for each AC see SCHCR 1974, 342–58.)

In the follow-up to the original SCHCR study, an additional step was added at this point. Tabulations of death rate for patients classified by predicted probability of death (within each AC) led to the observation that the logistic models did not fit as well as they could: there was a small amount of systematic departure between observed and predicted in the center of the probability range and in the extremes. Based on these tabulations (actually the BX part of the logistic formula [see eq. (5), above]), we derived a "correction" formula to remove this bias. When computing the predicted probability for a patient, we computed the original BX from the standardization (X) variables. From this original BX value, using a low-order polynomial transformation (one for each AC), we obtained a modified BX and used it to compute the probability of death. The effect of this extra step on the accuracy of the death rate standardization turned out to be quite small (Forrest et al. 1978, 45–53).

Standardized Mortality Measures for Individual Providers

After we had computed the observed (dead/alive) and expected (logistic probability) outcomes for each patient, the computation of standardized mortality ratios, as well as other summarizations for provider analyses, was relatively simple. The designation of which sets of patients to use in computing these measures was, of course, a function of the specific hypotheses to be tested. There is no logical necessity for the entire set of ACs of patients to be used; various subsets, including the individual study categories, could also be defined. Our approach was to start with the all-study patient set and, following predefined rules, to split these into smaller subsets of interest, if sufficient statistical power remained. Two methods of grouping patients were used in the ES: first, patients were aggregated by subsets of AC; second, within each AC, they were aggregated by the probability of death. Three subsets of ACs were used: all surgical categories of patients (fifteen ACs), all nonsurgical categories (two ACs), and a set of surgical procedures (seven ACs) selected on the basis of being relatively more homogeneous in terms of their qualifying operation and diagnosis codes. For the latter aggregation method, patients in each AC were divided into three "risk-level" subsets (high, medium, and low probability of death), the cutoffs being set so that approximately a third of the deaths would fall in each subset. (These aggregations and their rationale are explained more fully in chap. 11, below.)

Tests for Differences in Hospital Performance

To test the null hypothesis that hospitals do not differ in terms of their true (i.e., expected or standardized) death rates, we used a ratio measure. For each hospital, for whatever set of patients was of interest, we computed the indirectly standardized mortality ratios (ISMRs) as the ratio of the total number ofobserved deaths divided by the total number expected. It should be noted that hospitals with poorer performance than expected have a ratio greater than 1.0, while hospitals performing better than expected have a ratio between 0.0 and 1.0.

To take into account random patient (binomial) variation, we calculated the variance for the ISMR for hospitals, i, as

$$V(\text{ISMR}_i) = \frac{\sum_{j=1}^{n_i} p_{ij}q_{ij}}{E_i^2},$$

where n_i = the number of patients in hospital i; p_{ij} = the probability of dying for patient j in hospital i, based on the logistic regression; $q_{ij} = 1 - p_{ij}$; and $E_i = \sum_{j=1}^{n_i} p_{ij}$, the total number of expected deaths. Note that when p_{ij} is small (as it is in predicting deaths), the variance is approximately the inverse of the sum of expected deaths in the hospital $(1/E_i)$, so that the variance depends upon the expected deaths, not the number of patients at the hospital per se.

The statistic used to test the null hypothesis was

$$\Phi = \sum_{i=1}^{H} \frac{(D_i - E_i)^2}{V(D_i)},$$

where H = the number of hospitals in the study; d_{ij} = the outcome observed for patient j in hospital i; $D_i = \sum_{i=1}^{n_i} d_{ij}$, the total number of observed deaths; and $V(D_i) = \sum_{j=1}^{n_i} p_{ij}q_{ij}$, assumed to be a known constant. Under the null hypothesis of no hospital differences, the expected value of the number of observed deaths in a hospital (D_i) is equal to the number of deaths predicted on the basis of patient characteristics (E_i); that is, $E(D_i) = E_i$.

With a large E_i, Φ will tend to follow a chi-square distribution. However, for a small E_i, as in our case, we developed an exact formula for the variance.

$$V(\Phi) = \sum_{i=1}^{H} \left\{ 2 + \frac{1}{V(D_i)} - \frac{6 \sum_{j=1}^{n_i} p_{ij}^2 q_{ij}^2}{[V(D_i)]^2} \right\}$$

The test statistic, $Z = (\Phi - H)/\sqrt{V(\Phi)}$, was assumed to have a standard normal distribution, since H is reasonably large.

In using the adjusted outcome ratios to investigate the relation between outcomes and hospital characteristics, the statistics and methods described up to this point were identical for the Extensive Study and the Intensive Study. For the Intensive Study, because of the smaller sample size, we made a further refinement based on an empirical Bayesian adjustment (Lindley 1965). Because a ratio with many expected adverse outcomes is a more precise estimate of the true underlying ratio than one based on fewer expected outcomes, larger hospitals by chance alone would tend to be more centrally ranked than smaller hospitals. The Bayesian adjusted score pulled each hospital's ratio toward the overall average (about 1.0) by an amount dependent on (1) the overall variation observed among hospitals and (2) the variability of the individual hospital's ratio, so that less reliable ratios were pulled more toward the center. (The results of these tests for true differences among hospitals are reported in chap. 6.)

Tests for the Magnitude of Differences in Hospital Performance

The more useful but difficult analysis was the estimation of the extent of differences among hospitals. Initially two methods were developed, but one proved to be more satisfactory and was used for our subsequent analyses. To estimate the variance of the true ISMR, we calculated two terms: (1) the mean ISMR squared plus the variance of the ISMR and (2) an independent estimate of the mean ISMR squared. By subtracting the second term from the first, we obtained an estimate of the variance (σ^2) of the ISMR:

$$\sigma^2 = \left[\frac{1}{H} \sum_i \frac{D_i^2 - D_i}{E_i^2 - \sum_j p_{ij}^2} \right] - \left[\frac{\sum_i D_i^2 - (\sum_i D_i)^2}{\sum_i E_i^2 - (\sum_i E_i)^2} \right],$$

where all summations over index i go from 1 to H, and over j from 1 to n_i. (The results of these analyses, based on hospitals with two or more cases each, are presented in chap. 6.)

Tests for Hospital Characteristics that Explain Differences in Performance

Having first established that hospitals do differ in their performance, with careful adjustment for case mix, we turn to the primary analyses presented in this book: tests of hypotheses about which provider characteristics explain the differences in performance. For these analyses we used both parametric (i.e., linear regression and correlations) and nonparametric techniques (i.e., cross tabulations). Aggregation levels, categories of patients, and the types of standardized measures differed as appropriate for specific hypotheses. In general our approach was to use a variety of related measures and statistical techniques to examine the consistency of our findings. Results reported in chapter 11 and 12 for the ES are those for which a number of tests provided significant and consistent patterns of support for the results presented, taking into account the potential for multicollinearity and the number of tests performed.

METHODS USED TO MEASURE THE QUALITY OF CARE IN THE INTENSIVE STUDY

The quality-of-care measures in the Intensive Study (IS) were based on 8,593 final-study patient records obtained prospectively from several different sources in seventeen hospitals during the period 15 May 1973 to 28 February 1974.

The principal objectives of the IS paralleled those of the ES: to measure the extent and explain the sources of variation in the quality of surgical care in nonfederal U.S. hospitals. Using our overlapping study design, the IS and ES permitted analyses of the quality of care that had different strengths and weaknesses and together could provide strong corroboration or refutation of the extent of differences in hospital performance and the factors explaining those differences. In the ES, the primary strengths of the study lay in the proportion of hospitals represented and in the size of the patient population included—permitting the study of disease categories where adverse outcomes are relatively rare. A secondary strength of the ES was that it used data that were relatively easily available and uniformly collected and could serve as a basis for additional studies of quality on a national scale. These same aspects of the data base provided the study's primary weaknesses: it was based on retrospectively collected data not specifically designed to be used in a study of the quality of care and had minimal control over the reliability and validity of the data for comparisons across hospitals.

The IS was developed to address the need to obtain an adequate data base in order to adjust outcomes for patient differences. Although it was based on a relatively small number of patients and hospitals, it used data specifically designed to study the quality of surgical care and uniformly collected in all hospitals for all study patients. It was not limited to a study of death as the only outcome following surgery but included several measures of morbidity. And it was not limited to a single inhospital episode; it could trace the patient outside of the hospital and examine for multiple related hospitalizations within set periods of time. (See Moses [1984] for a discussion of the limitations and strengths of studies using all patients receiving a given treatment in a given time period.)

One important set of methodological questions required using our overlapping patients in the seventeen hospitals to compare and contrast the IS and ES methods, primarily in order to determine whether medical abstract data could provide a reasonable data base for assessing hospital performance. (These tests and their results are described in chapter 6, under the Little Extensive Study.)

In addition, another study, called the Service Intensity Study (SIS), was conducted in the seventeen hospitals. The SIS, however, used the full set of surgical and nonsurgical patient records for a three and one-half-year period to study outcomes and clinical services, adjusted for patient mix. (There is a brief description of the SIS methods at the end of this chapter; the results are given in chapter 6.)

The Selection of the IS Hospitals

Several important theoretical, methodological, and practical considerations governed the choice of hospitals in the IS. The charge to the research team was to perform a study of national scope, so that representation of all nonfederal short-term hospitals was desired. However, funding for a prospective study was limited to at most twenty hospitals, so practical considerations suggested the need to define the available pool of hospitals more carefully. First, we wanted to ensure there being enough patients to provide a reliable study of outcomes in both the prospective study and in a validation study to compare the results for patients in each IS hospital using both the ES data sources and methods and the IS data sources and methods. To accomplish this, we required that the hospitals have PAS data available for a period of three years prior to the study, as well as the study year, and that they perform, during a six-month period, at least 125 surgical procedures of the types chosen for the prospective study. Second, in order to provide the most representative sample, we chose a stratified design based on three provider characteristics identified as potentially important for quality of surgical care: the size of the hospital, its teaching status, and the average expenditures per patient-day. We also chose to restrict the potential roster of CPHA hospitals to all nonfederal, nonprofit, general hospitals, since there were so few hospitals in any other categories. These restrictions altogether resulted in a potential pool of 742 hospitals—from the original roster of 1,224 hospitals—of which 300 were chosen by stratified sample and 270 agreed to be contacted regarding participation in the IS and released one year's worth of PAS data. The year's worth of data were examined for further evidence that the hospital treated a sufficient number of patients in the study categories, resulting in 160 qualifying hospitals. A second stratified sample of these hospitals was drawn and examined for representation of all major geographic areas. In all, thirty-two were contacted to participate in the IS portion of the study; sixteen agreed to participate, and a seventeenth, administratively linked to one of the study hospitals, asked to be included at its own expense.

These seventeen hospitals are not properly regarded as representative of all U.S. short-term, nonfederal, nonprofit hospitals or even the ES hospitals for two major reasons. First, these seventeen selected themselves from among the original thirty-two hospitals and can therefore be argued to be organizations that are more self-critical and interested in identifying sources of differences in hospital performance. Second, the conditions for qualifying as a potential hospital tended to bias the selection toward larger hospitals (their average census was 237, compared with a national average for these types of hospitals of 124). They were also slightly more likely to be involved in teaching residents (35 percent of the seventeen hospitals, compared with 27 percent on a national level). On the other hand, all major geographic areas were represented, and their average expenditures per day were similar to the national average for comparable hospitals. (See table 5.7 for a characterization of each of the seventeen hospitals.)

The Selection of Patient Categories

An important charge to our group was to study the types of treatments and outcomes for hospitalized patients and to characterize differences other than those that could be explained by variation in the health status and stage of disease of the patients. For this reason we adopted a "tracer" method for characterizing patient care, studying a few types of diagnostic and surgical procedures in depth and using the set of categories as a whole to represent the quality of care and services provided to patients at the hospital.

Attention was focused on surgical patients in part because of our historical background of studying surgical anesthesia (i.e., the National Halothane Study) and because patients grouped by surgical procedure tended to be relatively homogeneous compared with those grouped by diagnosis, and because assessing outcomes of patients after relatively short periods, such as seven days after treatment, was generally more appropriate for surgical treatment than for medical stays in the hospital.

In addition to the need, as far as possible, to keep IS patient categories parallel to those of the ES, several considerations were taken into account in selecting the fifteen categories. First, since we wanted to study surgical care carried out in most hospitals, we focused on relatively common procedures. Second, in order to study variation in outcomes, we needed to have a sufficient number of complications (postsurgical morbidity or mortality) occurring in each hospital and each category, since the power or sensitivity of the statistical tests depends principally upon the number of patients with complications rather than upon the total number of patients per se. Thus we could select procedures

Table 5.7. Characteristics of the seventeen hospitals in the IS

	Acute-care beds	Occupied acute-care beds[a]	Total employed staff	Expenses per patient-day[b]	Teaching[c]
	638	529.54	2352	147.80	1
	585	473.85	2002	122.96	1
	433	342.07	1031	105.34	1
	426	340.80	910	97.32	0
	377	297.83	731	132.62	1
	310	257.30	910	115.47	1
	299	209.30	633	87.18	0
	290	214.60	879	134.78	0
	271	184.28	586	77.93	0
	252	199.08	939	108.79	0
	248	213.28	775	132.79	0
	240	201.60	503	81.63	0
	193	140.89	445	76.56	0
	179	127.09	558	142.80	1
	172	151.36	478	100.91	0
	149	93.87	470	154.40	0
	99	57.42	192	99.72	0
Mean	303.59	237.30	848.47	112.88	.35
Standard deviation	147.92	126.56	550.10	25.03	.49
National average in 1973[d]	163.62	124.27	395.79	115.47	.28

Note: Data for 17 hospitals in 1973 were supplied by the administrator at each hospital.

[a]Computed by multiplying the number of acute-care beds by the occupancy rate for 1973.

[b]Computed by dividing the total annual expenses by the product of the number of occupied acute-care beds times 365.

[c]*1* indicates an active residency program.

[d]National averages come from AHA 1974a (p. 18, table 1) for nonfederal not-for-profit, short-term general and other special hospitals. The national average for teaching comes from AMA 1973.

with high complication rates or high volume. Third, since we wanted to have a fairly representative sample of surgical procedures and patients, the set needed to involve a number of organ systems and treat a variety of ages and physical conditions and both sexes. Fourth, since an important patient variable was the stage of the disease, we wished to choose diseases that were amenable to staging.

For the most part, we chose surgical procedures performed for a single type of disease and for which the indications were fairly standardized. However, we included some surgical procedures for which the indications were more controversial or varied, such as hysterectomy and craniotomy. Except for a few situations in which patients with local cancer or carcinoma *in situ* were included and in cases of craniotomy, where all malignant diagnoses were studied, patients with a diagnosis of cancer were excluded. This decision was made because the goals of surgical therapy may change for advanced cancer, and we wished to have the stage of the disease directly reflect the seriousness of the outcomes and the difficulty of the surgical procedure performed. In contrast, for advanced cancer patients, the primary therapeutic goal is often palliation, rather than cure or correction, and surgical intervention is often more limited in scope; and the model for our use of staging that includes an assumption of more extensive surgery is therefore inappropriate. The selection of the study categories was made by physicians at the SCHCR in consultation with general and specialist surgeons at Stanford and several other sites throughout the country. (The final study patient categories are listed in table 5.8.)

The Collection of Patient Data

Specially trained technicians on site at each hospital, usually with a background in nursing or medical records, collected designated data about the patients from several sources and at specified times before and after surgery. (The actual forms used are reproduced in SCHCR 1974, 438–502.) The measures are described in more detail below, but briefly, they were used to characterize the patient's health status prior to surgery, to provide basic demographic and financial background data, to stage the extent of the patient's disease and the difficulty of the surgical procedures, and to assess his or her health status at seven days following surgery and forty days following surgery. These data were sent to the SCHCR, where they were checked for completeness and returned for correction when necessary. Copies of the surgical logs were also monitored by the Center to check for qualifying patients and reasons for not being entered into the study. (The number of final-study patients in each hospital by study category is noted in table 5.8.)

IS Measures of the Quality of Care

Measures of outcome in the IS differed from those in the ES in four important respects. First, they were collected *at two designated times* following surgery so that we would be able to characterize short-term and follow-up outcomes. The period of seven days was chosen because it would take us past the immediate transient results of surgery (e.g., postsurgical fever) and was long enough to allow appraisal of the effects of most types of surgery; the majority of patients in the study would still be in the hospital at seven days; and a uniform period of seven days for all categories would ease data collection and

Table 5.8. The number of patients in the IS final study, by operation category for each hospital

Hospital[b]	01	02	03	04	05	06	07	08	09	10	11	12	13	14	15	Total
1	5	56	5	25	1	34	56	0	0	0	0	2	0	17	0	201
2	7	106	13	72	6	67	48	8	10	33	7	34	9	47	2	469
3	9	103	19	31	1	69	1	0	9	29	0	6	5	22	2	306
4	19	113	16	27	9	32	24	11	8	36	8	37	26	99	7	472
5	25	134	24	70	7	120	78	27	2	52	11	137	10	85	3	785
6	45	168	36	26	9	137	26	20	9	50	1	85	38	104	8	762
7	10	70	6	47	0	15	97	1	8	18	1	1	6	69	2	351
8	25	83	23	84	1	131	36	10	4	50	3	38	6	59	2	555
9	30	157	23	64	7	299	317	38	6	51	28	98	5	115	18	1,256
10	29	77	21	81	31	76	54	26	54	54	12	4	26	92	5	642
11	11	13	6	14	2	22	25	6	2	21	12	23	0	31	4	192
12	1	16	0	0	0	9	3	0	3	4	1	0	0	2	0	39
13	30	148	27	74	4	175	265	12	18	49	8	67	9	69	10	965
14	11	73	11	50	6	152	44	5	15	30	6	65	20	18	18	524
15	18	85	12	34	2	65	35	8	7	30	46	49	52	22	21	486
16	15	79	21	34	4	33	10	1	5	32	0	3	4	41	1	283
17	14	88	7	54	5	59	7	0	5	31	0	1	3	30	1	305
Total	304	1,569	270	787	95	1,495	1,126	173	165	570	144	650	219	922	104	8,593

[a]
01 Gastric surgery for ulcer
02 Selected surgery of the biliary tract
03 Surgery of the large bowel
04 Appendectomy
05 Splenectomy

06 Abdominal hysterectomy
07 Vaginal hysterectomy
08 Craniotomy
09 Amputation of lower limb (ankle to hip)
10 Repair of fractured hip

11 Arthroplasty of the hip
12 Lumbar laminectomy, with or without fusion
13 Pulmonary resection
14 Prostatectomy
15 Selected surgery of the abdominal aorta and/or iliac arteries

[b]To preserve the anonymity of the hospitals, the hospital numbers below have been randomly assigned and do not correspond to the order in which any structural data are provided.

minimize the need to collect on weekend days. Forty days was chosen as a reasonable amount of time for patients to recover from the effects of surgery and as a time frame for attributing death to the surgical treatment.

Second, patients were *followed beyond the single hospital episode*. Eligibility rules included a determination of rehospitalization and/or additional surgical procedures within forty days of the study operation. In addition, most patients (99 percent) were discharged by forty days, so that assessment of outcome at forty days required follow-up outside the hospital. This longer time frame presented both practical difficulties in locating the patients and theoretical ones, since it introduced the possibility of care outside the hospital affecting the patient's outcome and, for dying patients, of different patterns of practice in discharging patients without full recovery to die at home or in another care setting.

Third, *mortality within forty days* was considered to be the most important outcome to determine. We reasoned that the importance of measuring death within forty days for all our study patients made up for the practical and theoretical difficulties involved in following patients over this period, and special efforts were made (e.g., review of official death notices and contact with the patient's family or surgeon) to determine the dead-or-alive status of all study patients at forty days. Virtually all (99.3 percent) were so characterized. These decisions regarding assessment of death resulted in important differences in characterizing the mortality of our study patients; among 224 study-patient deaths within forty days, 25 percent occurred after discharge from the initial hospitalization, and 62 percent occurred after seven days.

Fourth, information to characterize *morbidity* was systematically collected from several sources. At seven days, the medical record and the nurse responsible for the patient's postsurgical care were consulted to provide the following types of information: the types of monitoring devices and "tubes" being used; body temperature from the day of surgery to seven days postoperative; the extent of ambulation and location of the patient (e.g., in an intensive-care unit); and the presence or absence of seventy-three specific morbidities, arranged by seven organ systems. The nurse was then asked to rate the overall extent of physiological difficulty the patient was experiencing in each organ system using a scale from 0 (no difficulty) to 4 (life-threatening). Finally, the nurse rated the overall physiological difficulty of the patient, using the same scale.

Because of the central importance of outcome as a measure of care in our study, special efforts were made to secure information designated as minimally acceptable for inclusion in the study. As a consequence of this research design procedure, ratings, used in the primary seven-day outcome measures for analysis, were available for all final-study patients; the availability of other seven-day outcomes ranged from about 85 percent (specific morbidities) to 98 percent (body temperature).

We asked the nurse responsible for the patient's postoperative care at seven days, rather than the surgeon, to rate the patient because we felt that the nurse would be a consistent, objective, and more readily available source to rate the patient's status at seven days. Nurses were more likely to have had frequent and current patient contact, could be more readily located on the patient's ward, and would be able to use a broader standard for comparison, at least within a hospital, since they would be rating patients from many different surgeons.

At forty days, morbidity was assessed by patient questionnaire, obtaining information on the functional status, the extent of ambulation, the presence of specific signs or symptoms, and comparisons of their forty-day status with their health prior to surgery. Morbidity at forty days was available for about 85 percent of the final-study patients. We asked the patients (or their family) to provide information at forty days because we felt that the patient would be better able to assess his or her health on a specific day after surgery and could be a reliable source of reporting selected specific indications of morbidity such as the extent of ambulation and the presence of incontinence, persistent cough, and so on.

Death as an Outcome

Since we regarded death within forty days to be the most important outcome and the best time frame for assessing mortality associated with the study surgical procedures, all measures of outcome include whether death occurred within forty days—even those measures including morbidity assessed at seven days.

Morbidity as an Outcome

As already noted for both seven- and forty-day morbidity, we obtained several types of information (e.g., objective indications or specific signs and symptoms and subjective ratings of the physiological difficulty) from several sources (e.g., the patient's medical record and nurse) and used this information to perform validity and reliability tests for our measures and to examine for biases across institutions and by surgical procedures. In general, we found the seven-day overall rating, collapsed from five to three categories of morbidity, to be the best measure for most analyses. Table 5.9 presents the definitions and weightings of the primary measures we used. Three measures involve dichotomized versions of outcomes at seven days, suitable as dependent variables in logistic regression (reported in chap. 6). Three involved weightings all of which preserve the order of severity implied by the ratings but differ in the extent to which they emphasize death and morbidity as important outcomes; these were used in linear regression models (reported in chaps. 6 through 9).

Table 5.9. Primary seven-day outcome measures in the IS

Outcome Measures	Weights Associated with the Overall Physiological Rating			
	Death within 40 days	Severe or Life-threatening Morbidity	Moderate Morbidity	Mild or No Morbidity
Dichotomous for logistic models				
Outcome A	1	0	0	0
Outcome B	1	1	0	0
Outcome C	1	1	1	0
Scaled for linear models				
Mortality emphasized	9	2	1	0
Intermediate	9	5	2	0
Morbidity emphasized	9	7	5	0
Overall percentage of final-study patients	2.65%	2.0%	15.65%	79.8%

Standardizing Variables

The basic philosophy for selecting the IS standardizing variables paralleled that of the ES, and included demographic variables, general indicators of the preoperative physical status, and staging information specific to each disease. However, in the IS we were not restricted to data available in the medical chart abstracts. An important consideration in designing data to be collected was the ease and reliability of the assessments and their validity to characterize the preoperative physical status. When possible, we adopted measures whose validity and reliability had been established and that were in common use by health professionals, such as cardiovascular ratings from the American Heart Association (AHA) and physical-status ratings from the American Society of Anesthesiologists (ASA) (Dripps, Lamont, and Eckenhoff 1961; *Anesthesiology* 1963). A social-stress score, ordered into three levels, uses the number of recent life-change events reported by the patient. This measure is based on the work of Holmes and Rahe (1967), and its application to these data is discussed in detail in Rundall 1978. We also wanted to obtain the information at a uniform time and from standardized sources. The selection of measures was generally made by physicians at the SCHCR in consultation with other physicians.

Staging of malignant disease was fairly well developed and in widespread use at the time we designed the study, but staging of nonmalignant disease (such as for our study categories) was seldom reported. Even inflammatory diseases such as cholecystitis did not have uniformly accepted stages for reporting purposes but were simply categorized as acute or chronic or gangrenous. Since then, several groups (Gonnella and Goran 1975; Gonnella, Hornbrook, and Louis 1984; Horn et al. 1985) have also argued for the importance of staging nonmalignant disease and have developed staging schemes (Gonnella 1982; Horn, Sharkey, and Bertram 1983).

For our purposes, we developed fifteen separate staging algorithms, one for each study category, based on the prediction of postsurgical morbidity and mortality due to either the severity of the disease itself or the surgical procedures performed. A panel of surgeons whose area of practice and expertise was relevant to the category being staged met with staff physicians several times to develop and finalize the specific information to be collected and the sources (medical record, operative notes, pathology report, or surgeon) for collecting it. Based on this information collected for study patients a staging algorithm was subsequently created and validated using thirty to fifty patients in each category from a pilot hospital (see SCHCR 1974, 447–95, for data-collection forms and algorithms for staging each category). For these patients, staff physicians rated the severity of the disease and procedures performed independently from the algorithm. The interrating correlations between the scoring algorithms and the independent ratings were .7 or higher for each category. Forrest et al. (1978, 282–86) reported details of the significance of the original staging score for predicting seven-day morbidity for study patients. Additional work on the stage of disease has been reported for cholecystectomy patients (Flood et al. 1985a and 1985b, for example, analyze the accuracy of the preoperative stage to predict the stage observed postoperatively).

We collected most of the standardizing information as soon as the hospitalized patient was scheduled for a qualifying operation and agreed to participate. Demographic information was obtained from a patient questionnaire filled out prior to surgery or from the medical record. Information concerning the patient's preoperative physical status was obtained from the patient's anesthetist. Information for staging the disease and concerning the difficulty of the surgical procedures was obtained from the medical record and the patient's surgeon prior to surgery for some types of information (e.g., preoperative diagnosis and procedures performed and the extent and length of a history of the disease) and following surgery for others (e.g., pathological confirmation of the stage of the disease and information on all related and unrelated surgical procedures performed at the operation).

Using the Logistic Model to Predict Outcomes

Analyses to test the null hypothesis that there are no differences among hospitals in the outcomes of patients after standardizing for patient mix used a logistic model of regression in predicting outcomes. The logistic model was chosen because of the skewed distribution of the dependent variable (i.e., most patients did not experience adverse outcomes, particularly death and serious morbidity); because it modeled the relationships among patient characteristics in a clinically desirable model (i.e., patient characteristics were modeled as having a multiplicative effect on outcomes, not simply additive ones, permitting, for example, old age to be modeled as increasing the effects of poor physical status); and because it constrained the predicted outcomes to be between 1 and 0. Its primary disadvantage was that it required a binary dependent variable, forcing the decision to equate morbidity with mortality in measures that included both types of outcomes.

For the logistic-model analyses, several types of binary-outcome measures were created. In addition to the three main measures noted in table 5.7, two others were created: (1) death within forty days or any catheters, monitors, or breathing assistance at seven days; and (2) death or poor health status at forty days. A total of seventy-five regressions were run, one for each of the five binary outcomes for each of fifteen study categories of patients. For these analyses, the predictor variables were age, sex (unless not relevant, such as for hysterectomy), the AHA cardiovascular rating, the ASA physical-status rating, an emergency indicator, the staging score, the extent of hospital care covered by insurance, and the stress-level index. Quadratic versions of age, physical status, and stage were included to allow fitting of curvilinear relationships. The full complement of variables was used except where the number of adverse events was too small to yield statistically reliable prediction equations.

Tests for Differences among Hospitals in Adjusted Outcomes

In order to examine the impact of differences among hospitals, medical staffs, and physicians on these adjusted surgical outcomes, it behooved us to determine first whether there were any differences among hospitals to explain. It can be argued that the major differences in outcomes among hospitals are to be attributed not to differences in the quality of care provided but to the types of patients treated. We sought to determine whether there were significant differences in outcomes among hospitals after differences due to patient mix were taken into account. If there were, we needed to regard these differences as reflecting the quality of care provided. These are the differences we shall attempt to explain.

The tests for differences in the performance of hospitals based on the dichotomous patient outcome measures, which used the logistic model for standardization, paralleled those already described for the ES and used the same statistics developed for testing the null hypothesis in the larger study. (These results are presented in chap. 6). Basically, we found that there were significant differences, even after standardizing.

Tests for Provider Characteristics That Explain Differences

After first establishing that hospitals do differ in their performance as measured by standardized outcomes following surgery, we wished to be able to address several types of questions regarding these differences. For example: Do hospitals that perform well in avoiding serious outcomes also perform well in avoiding moderate morbidity? Do hospitals that differ in outcomes at seven days still demonstrate differences at forty days? Do hospitals tend to perform uniformly well for all study categories? Do surgeon characteristics explain the standardized differences in outcomes? Which, if any, hospital-level characteristics explain differences—for example, those associated with power and control in the medical staff organization, the hospital administration, or the nursing staff organization? The need to answer these questions led to the development of an alternative standardization that retained the ability to rank the severity of the outcomes (thus we shifted to using linear regression to standardize the outcomes). Testing these hypotheses also led to the characterization of outcomes that could compare the effects of different levels of providers, such as measures of individual surgeons versus those at the hospital level (thus we shifted from using ISMRs to a patient-level model).

Two methodological issues had a major impact on the operationalization of our measures and the design of our analyses. Briefly, they related to the appropriate level for analysis and the use of measures at more than one level of analysis.

The Level of Analysis

Four different levels of analysis were employed in the IS research reported here: (*a*) the hospital level; (*b*) the ward level; (*c*) the physician level; and (*d*) the patient level. As already noted, the analyses for the ES were conducted at only two levels: the hospital level and the patient level. Most of the analyses reported here were conducted at the patient level. In our view this was the most appropriate level of analysis, given the nature of the variables employed and the types of arguments to be tested. Patients in hospitals are not "treated" by the entire organizational structure and its associated staff but receive care from specific physicians and the nursing staff in particular units. In attempting to explain differences among outcomes of surgery, in all our analyses we took into account differences due to the characteristics of individual patients. Similarly, in the IS, the data we collected allowed us to assess which physician carried out the surgery and in which ward the patient received his postsurgical care. In moving to the patient level, not only was the sample size increased for certain analyses but more specific and accurate data could be utilized. Moving to the patient level of analysis also enabled us to avoid some of the possible statistical biases associated with the use of aggregated data (see Robinson 1950; Alker 1969; and Hannan 1971), but patient-level analyses could tend to overestimate the significance of relationships for variables not at the patient level. Overestimation can occur because ordinary regression analysis at the patient level ignores the covariance among patients being treated by the same provider. That is, there will be a systematic component in the patients' error terms if there are provider influences on outcomes that are not included in the regression model. It is difficult to assess the magnitude of these biasing effects.

Structural or Compositional Effects

Sociologists such as Blau (1968) and Davis, Spaeth, and Huson (1961) noted that a given variable can sometimes exert an effect at more than one level of analysis simultaneously. They suggested that it is often possible and useful to examine the influence of attributes both at an individual and at an aggregated level. In our data we distinguished the impact of attributes of individual surgeons (e.g., whether each was board certified or the extent of residency training) from the importance of the qualifications of the surgical staff as a whole for affecting the quality of surgical outcomes. We expected a highly qualified (or highly committed or highly specialized) medical staff to have a positive impact on the quality of care that was above and beyond the impact expected on the basis of the level of qualifications of the particular surgeon. This expectation was founded on the importance of collegial evaluation and normative support for professionals and the consequent impact on their professional efforts.

Tannenbaum and Bachman (1964) and Blalock (1967) discussed the appropriate operationalization of a test of structural effects. Tannenbaum and Bachman identified conditions necessary for avoiding spurious structural effects or spurious individual effects. These conditions include the characterization of each variable as continuous whenever appropriate. It is also important to examine the structural effect after controlling for individual effects. Therefore, we examined structural effects on outcome in our model by characterizing both the individual and the aggregate variables measured as continuous variables (if possible) and by partialing out the effect of the individual attributes before determining the impact of the aggregate measure.

Using the Linear Regression to Predict Outcomes

The linear approach involved different measurement assumptions from those of the logistic method. It assumed that each patient could be characterized by an outcome following surgery—little or no morbidity, mild morbidity, severe morbidity at the seventh day, or death before the fortieth day—and that these outcomes were ordered such that scores might be assigned to them to represent the increasing degree of their undesirability. The measure we used was an ordinal ranking of four categories and was certainly not a variable scaled with a true zero and with equal distance between intervals. Yet we intended to use it as a dependent variable in a linear regression. Purists will correctly point out that such a dependent variable does not meet the necessary assumptions for linear regression analysis. But other analysts have argued that the direction of analysis and the strength of the conclusions of analyses performed on ordinal data—using both linear regression and nonparametric techniques—are substantially the same (see Abelson and Tukey 1959; Labovitz 1970; and Verba and Nie 1972). We believe that the benefits derived from using linear regression to predict the outcome expected on the basis of patient variables and the familiarity with the associated statistics in evaluating its strength justify its use.

To try to assess the importance of the weighting scheme on our standardization, we examined three versions of weighting the four categories of outcome (see table 5.9). In practice we found few differences and have focused on the Intermediate Scale for reporting most results. The same patient data used in constructing the adjusted outcome measures for the logistic approach were employed in the linear approach. However, because of the differences in measures and approach, we describe the linear method briefly.

We used six basic health-related characteristics to assess the patient's condition prior to surgery: age, sex, physical status, stage, cardiovascular status, and emergency status. (The mean scores for patients in each category for each of these health-related attributes are presented in Forrest et al. 1978, 281.) We also wished to consider those interactions among the variables that could prove to be important predictors of outcome, independent of the direct effects of the variables. For example, the effect of stage on predicting outcome could vary as a result of the overall physical status. We performed some preliminary analyses on the 304 patients who had undergone gastric surgery for an ulcer. Based on these results and on medical considerations, we included three interaction terms: stage and physical status, emergency status and physical status, and age and physical status. Each individual component of the interaction term was converted into a standard Z score before multiplying in order to better assess the importance of the interaction term separately from the effects of its individual components.

A separate linear regression was performed for each operation category and for each of the three outcome scales. The linear regression used a least-squares solution. In each case the regressions were performed using Statistical Package for the Social Sciences (SPSS), employing the methods and estimates as presented in Nie et al. 1975. Since each patient category was analyzed independently, the importance of each type of variable for predicting surgical outcomes could vary from one category to another. (These results are included in Forrest et al. 1978, 282–86.) The results for overall predictability and for the relative importance of each individual predictor of outcome were generally consistent across all three outcome scales within each of the fifteen operative categories. Moreover, for the fifteen categories using each of the three outcome scales, the forty-five resultant regressions were each significant overall at $p \leq$ .001. The influence of each predictor variable varied depending on the surgical category. Generally speaking, however, physical status, age, and stage of disease, together with the interaction term combining age and physical status, were the more powerful variables.

To obtain the adjusted outcome scores, we first standardized each health-related characteristic and each outcome score based on the mean and standard deviation of each characteristic observed in our data, for a given operative category and a given outcome scaling. For each variable, the standardized value was obtained by subtracting the group mean for the variable from the original value and then dividing this difference by the group standard deviation for the same variable. In this case, the "group" was the set of all patients in a given operative category. Next, we obtained the level of outcome we expected for the patient on the basis of his or her age, sex, stage of disease, type of operation, and so on. This expected outcome score was computed by using the above-described linear regressions to obtain estimates for the effect of each patient-related characteristic in predicting outcome. We then multiplied the patient's actual standardized score for each attribute by the standardized regression coefficient for that attribute and summed these products to obtain a single value. For example, for each appendectomy patient, his or her actual standardized age was multiplied by the standardized regression coefficient for age; his or her actual standardized stage was multiplied by the standardized regression coefficient for stage; and so on for all the independent variables in our original regression equation. Then these products were summed to obtain the patient's standardized expected outcome, for a given outcome scaling. In this manner we obtained three expected outcome scores for each patient in the study, one for each outcome scale. Last, for each of the outcome scalings, we subtracted the expected outcome—representing the standardized outcome expected on the basis of the patient's attributes—from the patient's actual standardized outcome score. This difference score was what we called the adjusted surgical outcome for each patient. Each patient had three such adjusted surgical outcome scores—one for each outcome scale: the Mortality, Morbidity, and Intermediate scales.

These scores of surgical outcomes were "adjusted" in several important senses. First, our scores took into account, within each category, the patient's condition on a set of key health-related characteristics. Thus the organizational unit or individual treating patients who were in poorer health (e.g., patients who had a worse cardiovascular status, had a more advanced stage of disease, were older, or had a worse physical status) were not penalized; at least, to the extent that our adjustment was successful in measuring all the appropriate aspects of presurgical health, they were not penalized. Since a universal standard of health is lacking, these adjustments were made on the basis of the usual experience of patients in our entire sample for each category. This procedure assumed that the sample of patients was large enough to provide a secure basis for estimating the average outcome. This type of adjustment paralleled that carried out by the logistic approach, as detailed earlier. Second, and unlike the procedure used in the logistic approach, this procedure took into account the types of outcomes usually experienced by patients who have had the same kind of surgical intervention. This helped to adjust for differences among individuals or units that might vary in their relative concentration of types of surgical patients. Surgeons, too, differed in the variety of patients they treated. Since the scores standardized for surgical category, the organizational unit or individual under examination was not faulted for treating patients undergoing operations that more frequently result in undesirable outcomes.

As with the logistic equation, coefficients from the linear equations were employed to arrive at predicted outcomes for each patient. The choices for presenting these scores at a hospital level were the same as for the logistic scores already discussed. We chose to work with the average difference score and to emphasize the Intermediate Scale.

An Overview of Structural Hypothesis-Testing Procedures in the IS

Procedures for Testing Hypotheses

Most of the analyses reported in following chapters were conducted at the patient level. As already noted, given the nature of the data collected and our conception of the causal processes linking structural characteristics with patient outcomes, we believed that the patient level of analysis was best suited to our purposes. In particular, the approach taken enabled us to avoid errors in specification due to analyses performed at the wrong level. To avoid such errors, it was not enough to measure surgical outcomes for each patient. If we argued that surgeon attributes impacted on the quality of care, then we had to be able to associate each surgeon's attributes with the outcomes of patients he or she had treated. And where we argued that aggregate attributes of the medical staff, other structural measures of the medical staff, or other features of the hospital impacted on the quality of outcomes observed in patients, then we also needed to associate these attributes with the patients treated by these staffs or in these situations. Unless we could make all these attributions, then our analyses could be said to suffer from errors of specification.

Weighted Means of Structural Measures

It is necessary to call attention to one important consequence of our decision to focus primary attention on the patient level of analysis. For each structural measure, every patient in the hospital had the same value attached to his or her record. Similarly, for each physician measure, every patient for a given physician exhibited an identical value. The result of this approach was to create weighted means and standard deviations for all structural and physician variables; they were weighted because not all hospitals or surgeons had the same number of patients. Some tables reporting descriptive statistics and zero-order correlations based on these weighted measures naturally differ somewhat from others in which the structural measures were examined at the hospital level. The weighted measures were not the most efficient predictors of the true means, standard deviations, and correlations among variables at the hospital level, but in all cases, the direction, patterns, and conclusions drawn were consistent with those based on an unweighted approach. We report these weighted values for consistency because they were the basis of the later analyses at the patient level. Note that a similar approach was used in the ES.

The Regression Model

In each of the following steps, we used the adjusted measures of surgical outcomes based on the linear regression model with the Intermediate Scale as the dependent variable (referred to as step 1). At each subsequent step, we introduced, in hierarchical fashion, a new class of variables to explain differences in adjusted surgical outcomes. In this way our design could be argued to avoid aggregation errors. We believe this to be a conservative approach to the examination of the impact of the hospital and medical staff and its organizational characteristics on the quality of outcome following surgery in the sense that it allowed classes of control variables involving patient characteristics, surgeon attributes, and hospital characteristics to "explain" all the variance in surgical outcomes that each set could. We briefly outline the hierarchical steps employed.

There is a body of literature that suggests that in addition to a patient's health and certain demographic characteristics, his or her socioeconomic level and recent life stresses can have important effects on the outcome of surgery. Therefore, in the second step, we associated each patient's socioeconomic level and a measure of recent life stresses with adjusted surgical outcome. In the third step, we examined the effect of the individual surgeon's attributes on the adjusted surgical outcome. Because of the hierarchical introduction of each class of variables, the examination of the surgeon's characteristics on adjusted outcomes was conditioned on the patient's socioeconomic status and stress. In the fourth step, we introduced the three control variables for the hospital: size, resources, and teaching status. Finally, we introduced into the regression analysis the measures used to test the major hypotheses presented in chapter 1.

Undoubtedly, this approach did not eliminate all possible specification errors. The approach ignored the impact of individual nurses and organizational subunits such as the postsurgical wards. (We reported in Forrest et al. 1978 [232–79], however, an analysis suggesting that postsurgical wards did not have a significant effect on outcome independent of hospital effect.) In our view, the approach selected is both conservative and reasonable as a method of testing predictions of organizational factors affecting the quality of surgical care at the patient level of analysis.

Tests for Significance

In considering tests for the statistical significance of the results, it is important to recall the sample size for the various levels of analysis. There were approximately 8,000 patients, 500 surgeons, and 17 hospitals. In spite of the care taken to select hospitals that would be somewhat representative of the large population of CPHA hospitals, the small number of total hospitals studied necessitates viewing this study as exploratory. In examining our hypotheses, we placed great emphasis on the consistency of patterns of explaining variables and on the relative ability of classes of variables to predict adjusted surgical outcomes rather than on isolated relationships.

In presenting tests of significance, we based the degrees of freedom on 8,000 cases when analyzing patient variables, on 500 when analyzing individual physicians, on 17 when analyzing hospitals, and on 15 when analyzing medical staff characteristics. When more than one level was being examined, we used the smaller number of cases in testing the significance of the correlation coefficients.

(Mis)Interpreting the Amount of Explained Variance

Throughout our study, because many of our analyses were performed at the patient level, the amount of explained variance (R^2) was small, even when statistically highly significant. The small amount of explained variance was an artifact of our model and should not be construed to mean that our results have no real import in explaining hospital or physician performance.

The argument that the R^2 is constrained to be small when the dependent variable is dichotomous and highly skewed (such as for patient deaths) is adapted from Gordon, Kannel, and Halperin 1979. In this example, we compare death rates for hospitals classified as treating a high or low volume of patients, such as we report for the ES in chapter 11. Let

$$y_{ij} = \begin{cases} 0 \text{ if alive,} \\ 1 \text{ if dead,} \end{cases}$$

where $i = 1, 2$ types of hospitals (HV) and $j = 1, \ldots, n$ patients in each type of hospital, assuming, for simplicity, that $n_1 = n_2$. Let

$$x_{ij} = \begin{cases} x_{1j} \equiv -1 \text{ for } HV \text{ type 1 (e.g., low-volume hospital),} \\ x_{2j} \equiv 1 \text{ for } HV \text{ type 2 (e.g., high-volume hospital).} \end{cases}$$

Simplify by assuming that all cases have the same probability except due to x_{ij}. Then

$$E(y_{ij} \mid x_{ij}) = \mu + \tau x_{ij} = \begin{cases} \mu - \tau \text{ if } i = 1, \\ \mu + \tau \text{ if } i = 2, \\ \mu \text{ overall,} \end{cases}$$

where τ is the effect of interest (e.g., surgical deaths due to volume). The overall variance of y from the binomial distribution is Var $(y_{ij}) = \mu (1 - \mu)$. Within an HV class, the within-group variance is Var $(y_{ij}|x_{ij}) = (\mu + \tau x_{ij})(1 - \mu - \tau x_{ij})$. If Var $(y_{1j}|x_{1j})$ and Var $(y_{2j}|x_{2j})$ are pooled as in an analysis of variance (ANOVA), the pooled average is $\overline{\text{Var } (y|x)} = \mu (1 - \mu) - \tau^2$.

Substituting these quantities,

$$R^2 \leftrightarrow \frac{\text{Var } (y) - \overline{\text{Var } (y|x)}}{\text{Var } (y)} = \frac{\tau^2}{\mu(1 - \mu)}.$$

In our example, we take 4.5 percent as the overall death rate (approximately that of our ES surgical patients) and assume that low volume accounts for a doubling of death rates; that is, $\mu = .045$ and $\tau = .015$, so that the death rate is either .03 or .06, a twofold increase in the one HV class:

$$R^2 = \frac{(.015)^2}{(.045)\,(.955)} = .0052 \cong (.07)^2.$$

To get a higher R^2, μ must be nearer to .50, with a large τ.

METHODS USED TO MEASURE SERVICE INTENSITY IN THE SEVENTEEN HOSPITALS

The volume of research reports on the cost and the quality of medical care has increased spectacularly over the past two decades. Interest has been spurred by the need to understand the tremendous increase in national health costs, by the need to anticipate the impact of health insurance legislation recently enacted, and by a growing preoccupation with health and the quality of health care. Considerable interest has centered on the hospital which is both a major focus of health care delivery in this country and a locus of escalating costs.

Although our earlier interest focused on the quality of surgical outcomes, the data we collected demanded study of the related questions of the intensity and the cost of care for hospitalized patients. If hospitals differ in the quality of outcomes they produce, do they also differ greatly in the intensity of care they provide to their patients, and are these two factors—the quality of outcome and the intensity of service—related? As discussed in chapters 3 and 4, few studies of the relation between the intensity of care and outcomes have been reported, and the results have not been clear or persuasive. Important limitations of previous work include a lack of effective techniques for taking into account differences among patients affecting both the types of services consumed and the outcomes observed, and lack of attention to the development of output measures that distinguish the quality of care received from the quantity of services delivered or the qualifications of health care personnel. Our research approach was designed to deal with both of these difficult issues. Patient data for the SIS came from detailed discharge information contained in PAS abstract files on over 600,000 patients treated in the seventeen IS short-stay, acute-care hospitals during the four-year-period 1970–73.

Measures of Service Intensity and Outcome

Service intensity was defined as the number or amount of selected services received by a patient during a hospitalization. The focus was on actual services received; services such as blood chemistry tests, use of the intensive-care unit, and number of types of drugs received were examined. By focusing on units of actual services provided in each hospital, the approach facilitated comparisons over time and across hospitals by minimizing differences due to inflation or to regional differences in the dollar costs of care. Hospitals offer a broad range of services to patients, and no attempt was made to assess all of the services provided to patients. Rather seven types of service were assessed, representing important categories of diagnostic and therapeutic care, and we counted the number of consultations with other physicians and the patient's length of stay. In order to assess the overall service mix that a given patient received, two summary measures were analyzed: (1) an index of specific services based on the seven indicators of individual diagnostic and therapeutic services, after weighting each according to the relative cost of the class of service represented, and (2) an index of routine services, based on length of stay, for assessment of those nursing and basic services received regardless of any specific treatments utilized.

Parallel to in the ES, the quality of health care was indicated by patients' health status at discharge (dead or alive). By utilizing measures of quality defined by the outcomes of care rather than by the intensity of services received, we could examine the relation of utilization of services and outcomes (reported in chap. 7).

Standardizing Service Intensity and Outcome

Measures of service intensity and outcome were adjusted to take into account differences in the patients treated, using the technique of indirect standardization as described for our ES and IS methodology. While the general approach can be described simply, the specific procedures and measures developed were rather complex. Since the data source was the PAS abstract, many of the standardizing variables were identical to those used in the ES. The major difference between the two studies had to do with the staging and operation-specific variables in the ES, which were replaced in the SIS by the approximately 350 List A diagnostic categories developed by CPHA to report length of stay and outcomes (CPHA 1975, 1977). In the original SIS report (Forrest et al. 1977), thirty-one separate models for standardization were developed, involving the service-intensity and outcome measures described above and four varying sets of standardizing variables to adjust for (1) admission condition, (2) receiving surgery, (3) discharge status, and (4) an indication of inhospital complications. Since in practice these varying sets made little difference, we report only ten models and the summary measures in this volume. (Additional detail on these methods is contained in chapter 6.)

Assumptions about Service Intensity in Our Methods

Before examining hospital-level measures of services, let us comment briefly on two additional considerations incorporated into our approach: the focus on the entire hospital episode in assessing intensity of services and the assumption of the independence of sets of services.

During a hospitalization, a patient can receive varying amounts of several different types of services. Some authors point out that the *rate* of services consumed during a single hospitalization is not constant but varies by day of stay, usually being higher at the beginning of the stay. In defining the intensity of services, we chose not to focus on the rate at which a patient consumed services; instead, we examined two different measures summarizing the total amount of services received during the entire stay. We called the total amount of a given specific service consumed the *intensity* of that service delivered to the patient. The total length of stay we called the *duration* of routine services. The duration of services reflects the total amount of routine nursing and hotel services consumed. (Note that intensive nursing care was treated as a specific service, and variations in nurse/patient ratios were examined as a hospital structural measure.)

For purposes of defining the "need" of the patient for each service, the second assumption incorporated into our approach was the independence of services consumed. In defining each specific medical service, we took care to group interdependent services to the extent possible. Thus, categories of drugs were grouped together as one type of service; radiographic examinations for diagnostic purposes were grouped; and so on. In this manner, we assumed that each of the seven types of services could be delivered independently of the other types. For example, we assumed that the number of drugs did not depend on blood use, and so on. Therefore, the "need" for each service could be derived independently. The one major exception to this assumption was the belief that surgery (a class of service) was interdependent with the other services, so that, for example, the need for intensive care, blood, and drugs did depend on whether the patient underwent surgery. We handled this interdependence by using surgery as one of the predictor sets in assessing the need for other services.

Hospital Measures of Service Intensity

Although adjustment procedures were applied at the level of the individual patient, patients were aggregated to carry out analyses based on service intensity and outcomes. Parallel to the methods using linear regression discussed for the IS, standardized hospital-level measures were based on the difference between the actual services received and those predicted on the basis of patient characteristics (observed-predicted). Ordinary one-way ANOVA was used to examine the extent of variation. We estimated the between-hospital component of variance assuming a random-effects model (Forrest et al. 1977, 165–73).

Service Intensity as an Indicator of Hospital Efficiency

Efficiency is a concept with many definitions, and some of the definitions themselves involve the identification of several components or dimensions (see Pauly 1970; and McClure 1976). Most definitions revolve around the comparison of the amount of inputs expended (in terms of labor, supplies, or other forms of capital) during the production of a given unit or amount of output. If amounts of inputs are to be compared, it is obviously of critical importance to be certain that the outputs are truly comparable in terms of amount and/or quality. When the output compared is the health status of patients, it is important to control for both the level of outcome achieved and the patient's condition on admission. These controls were effected by our standardization approach, which independently took into account patient characteristics affecting service intensity, as well as the quality of the outcome achieved. Thus, comparisons among hospitals in terms of their tendency to provide patients with higher or lower levels of services than expected may be regarded as a measure of the relative efficiency of a hospital to achieve a given level of outcome with the expenditure of more or fewer services. This measure of hospital efficiency is closely related to McClure's (1976) concept of "service efficiency." The summary measures of service intensity were particularly appropriate in this regard, since they took into account not only the amount of a given service utilized (as did the individual service measures) but the relative costliness of these services. Further, by focusing on a variety of services, the summary measures allowed for the interchangeability of service ingredients and thus permitted the substitution of less expensive for more expensive types of services.

Since our study was designed, many others have written on hospital efficiency. For example, Donabedian, Wheeler, and Wyszewianski (1982) distinguished between *hospital production efficiency,* which compares hospitals with regard to expenditures for providing a service (taking into account such factors as overqualified staff or delays in reporting laboratory findings), and *clinical efficiency,* which involves the appropriateness of the service for the patient and thus relates to the quality of clinical decision making. Our SIS indicators attempted to measure clinical efficiency rather than production efficiency. Note that the weighting scheme, which combined measures of services by their relative expense, was applied to all patients in all hospitals and did not reflect the actual charges or expenditures by the hospital. A hospital that provides more services than typical has not necessarily spent more money on them; they could have been produced at lower costs owing to production efficiencies.

Finally, it is important to note that the measures of efficiency in this study examined the relative ability of hospitals to use their resources to provide care to patients. They did not address the question of whether the patients could be treated as effectively but more efficiently in a different care setting than a hospital. For example, Luft (1981a) argued that the major mechanism by which prepaid health organizations achieve their savings is providing more service on an outpatient basis. We could not address this important question in our data base. On the other hand, one of the important rationales for prospective payment of hospitals or other regulatory attempts to control hospital costs is that the variation in costs for hospitalized patients is due largely to production and service inefficiencies, which could be eliminated through proper economic incentives to hospitals, without harm to patient care quality. This important question we can begin to address.

6 · Tests for Differences among Hospitals in the Quality of Surgical Outcomes and Service Intensity

Ann Barry Flood, W. Richard Scott, Wayne Ewy,
William H. Forrest, Jr., and Byron W. Brown, Jr.

The issues and problems surrounding the assessment of the quality of health care in hospitals have been the subject of much research, dating back to 1913 with Codman's work at the Massachusetts General Hospital in Boston (Codman 1916). Subsequent published work on the quality of hospital health care spans a broad spectrum of theoretical and practical issues, ranging from the assessment of the efficacy of alternative modes of treatment to comparisons of the effectiveness of the individuals or organizations delivering the care. Within this spectrum of research and depending on the purpose, many indices of quality have been used. Taking into account Donabedian's admonition that "outcomes, by and large, remain the ultimate validators of the effectiveness and quality of medical care" (Donabedian 1966, 169), we chose to measure quality by observing outcomes in our study of differences in surgical care among short-term hospitals in the United States.

Relevant studies conducted prior to the initiation of our study that attempted to make hospital comparisons of the quality of health care were generally compromised by one or more of the following weaknesses:

1. Assessments of quality based on evaluations of the process of delivering care in which the standards for good process of care were not verified by proof of better outcome for the patients (Rosenfeld 1957; Trussell, Morehead, and Ehrlich 1962; Fine and Morehead 1971).
2. Comparisons of patients within a single diagnostic or operative category that did not allow sufficiently for differences in outcome due to variations in the general health status or the severity of disease of the patients

Preliminary results from the IS and ES studies were published in SCHCR 1976 and reported in Scott et al. 1976. Some final results for the ES were included in Flood, Scott, and Ewy 1984a.

(Lipworth, Lee, and Morris 1963; Bunker et al. 1969; Eckles and Root 1970; Posner and Lin 1975).

3. Comparisons of hospitals based on one disease entity only (Ashley, Howlett, and Morris 1971).

4. Comparisons of patients involving multiple groups of diagnostic or operative categories that did not allow sufficiently for differences in outcomes due to the variety of diseases treated (Helbig, O'Hare, and Smith 1972).

5. Assessments of outcome limited to information obtained during the patient's stay in the hospital, ignoring morbidity and mortality following discharge (Lipworth, Lee, and Morris 1963; Bunker et al. 1969; Posner and Lin 1975).

6. Comparisons of outcomes based only on death (even though death rates are not sufficiently sensitive indicators to discriminate among levels of care quality of many surgical diseases) or based on indirect measures of morbidity such as length of stay in the hospital (even though hospital differences in the average length of stay may be due to variations in regional patterns of practice or to the availability of extended-care facilities or nursing homes) (Roemer 1959; Roemer, Moustafa, and Hopkins 1968).

7. Data sources of questionable reliability and validity for making sound evaluations regarding the quality of care (Bunker et al. 1969).

In developing our methodology we tried to meet these objections to past studies and develop a means by which meaningful comparisons of the quality of hospital care could be made.

Our original study, the Institutional Differences Study (IDS), was planned specifically to follow up an incidental finding of the National Halothane Study (Bunker et al. 1969): its thirty-four participating hospitals had markedly different overall surgical mortality rates, even after corrections were applied for differences in types of operations and some patient characteristics. The importance and implications of this result and the limitations of the study for establishing that hospitals are truly different in quality were discussed by Moses and Mosteller (1968), who called for further investigation of differences among hospitals in the outcome of surgical care. Accordingly, the IDS was designed with four major objectives: (1) to develop a method for measuring the quality of surgical care in individual hospitals, using postoperative morbidity and mortality as outcome criteria and using a comprehensive set of patient variables to take into account differences in patient mix in the individual hospitals; (2) to determine whether hospitals do differ in the quality of surgical care they deliver and to estimate the magnitude of this variation among hospitals; (3) to develop and apply methods of characterizing individual hospitals with regard to their organizational characteristics, including physicians and nurses; and (4) to obtain some leads as to what the principal organizational factors affecting variation in surgical outcome might be.

The research design, methods, and rationale developed to implement these first two objectives are presented in detail in chapter 5. The first section of this chapter presents an overview of these methods and provides some intermediate-level results from our work to illustrate the discussion. The reader already familiar with chapter 5 may wish to skip to the second section (The Results of Hospital Tests for Differences in Outcomes), which details the major findings of our study regarding the extent to which U.S. voluntary hospitals do differ significantly in the quality of care they provide, focusing on outcomes of surgical care and making detailed and careful adjustment for differences in the mix and health levels of patients treated. These results are based on the ES, a retrospective study of patient abstract records in a large number of hospitals, and the IS, a specially collected prospective patient data set collected in a much smaller sample of these hospitals. In presenting these basic results, we also illustrate some practical differences that arise from the choices made as to how to measure outcomes of surgery and how to adjust for differences in patients. In the third section, we compare and contrast these ES and IS studies and methods. The primary task of this section is to evaluate whether an assessment of quality based on data that are routinely collected and relatively available could be a useful tool for health services researchers and for health policy planners who need to assess the impact of programmatic changes or structural evolution in our nation's hospitals. Last, in the fourth section, we briefly review tests for hospital differences in the length of stay and services received by patients, using patient abstract records in the small sample of hospitals.

The results presented in this chapter are important to our research because they establish the need to examine structural differences in hospitals that can explain why some hospitals perform better than others. These results also have important implications for today's health care scene because they provide some evidence of real and continuing differences in the quality of care and clinical services received during a period in which major federal and state programs (e.g., Medicare and Medicaid) were attempting to alter the "two-class" structure of medicine, whereby the amount and quality of medical services and the facilities available depended upon the patient's ability to pay. The hospital structures associated with better care during this period can help us to understand and predict some of the consequences of organizational changes in response to more recent programs such as Medicare's Prospective Payment System (PPS) and trends toward increasingly complex corporatization of health care (Starr 1982). The methods we used could be adopted or adapted to examine whether and to what extent there still is large variation in the quality of care in hospitals, not just in terms of structural amenities like modern buildings and the latest capital equipment but in outcomes experienced by patients as well. Today there is great concern for increasing the efficiency of health care delivery and for reducing its costs. These changes and their assessment require assessing the simultaneous effects on quality as well.

RESEARCH DESIGN

Overview: Two Overlapping Studies

The overall objective of the methodology discussed here was the assessment of the quality of surgical care in hospitals as indicated by the outcome of surgery. We were interested in examining hospital performance in a variety of types of surgery. To ensure—or at least increase—the validity of the final measures of outcome, the methods used had to remove the effect of the patient's initial condition on the observed outcome so that any remaining systematic variation in outcome could be reasonably attributed to the quality of treatment. Therefore, the methods had to assess the effect on outcome of various factors, such as the specific disease and operation, the extent or stage of the disease, and the general health or physical status of the patient. The strategy employed was to empirically estimate the outcome that could be expected for each patient. Then a comparison of actual outcomes and expected outcomes for patients in a given hospital provided a basis for contrasting the performance of the hospital with that of the others.

In order to allow generalization of our results and obviate certain weaknesses of earlier investigations, we conducted two overlapping studies. The Extensive Study (ES), involved summary data from 1,224 short-term U.S. hospitals that participated during all of 1972 in the Professional Activity Study (PAS) system of the Commission on Professional and Hospital Activities (CPHA). The data furnished by CPHA did not reveal the identity of any hospital. PAS abstracts contain various data on each patient, such as results of laboratory tests, demographic characteristics, operations received, final diagnoses, and condition at the time of discharge. This data base reflects a substantial portion of all U.S. inhospital care in 1972, since at that time PAS discharge abstracts were prepared for all patients in about one-fifth of the short-term hospitals in the United States, serving about one-third of the patients in this country.

From the 1,224 hospitals in the ES, a subset of seventeen hospitals was studied in a second investigation, the Intensive Study (IS). Specially trained personnel collected data for the IS from several sources, including the patient, the surgeon, the anesthetist, and the nurse on the postsurgical ward; approximately 8,500 patients were studied over a nine-month period from May 1973 to February 1974.

The overlapping design of these two studies had several advantages. The greatest advantage for the ES came from the large number of hospitals and patients involved, which allowed for greater statistical precision and a broader base for generalization to all U.S. short-term hospitals. However, since the data for the ES were based on discharge abstracts, they were subject to variations in the quality of collection among the member hospitals. The PAS abstract data cannot include information on deaths that occur after discharge to other institutions or to home care. Further, PAS data are not collected specially for the purpose of assessing presurgical physical status, extent of disease, or surgical outcome and are thereby limited and subject to imprecision and bias in such an application. For these reasons, the smaller IS was essential as a source of more detailed information specially collected for measuring the quality of surgical outcomes.

The overlap of the two studies constituted the Little ES conducted in the seventeen IS hospitals. With the permission of those hospitals, we obtained PAS data for all patients discharged from May 1970 through December 1973— from three years prior to the beginning of the IS extending through two-thirds of the period of on-site data collection. Time constraints prevented obtaining PAS data for the entire IS period. The logistic functions developed on the 1,224 hospitals in the ES were applied to patients in the ES categories from this PAS data set for the seventeen IS hospitals, which made it possible to compare the relative adequacy of the two approaches in an independently gathered data set and independently standardized predictions for a corresponding set of patients in the seventeen hospitals. These analyses provided important evidence of the consistency and reliability of the two study methods and for the usefulness of a retrospective data set based on medical record abstracts. Finally, the full set of PAS records in the seventeen hospitals was used in the Service Intensity Study (SIS) to assess variation in selected clinical services and length of stay.

Hospital Selection

ES hospitals. The ES included 1,224 short-term hospitals in the United States that had participated in the PAS for the entire year of 1972. These hospitals discharged about 11 million patients that year, or approximately one-third of the patients discharged from all U.S. short-term hospitals. Compared with all nonfederal, short-term U.S. hospitals, the 1,224 ES hospitals were similar in size and the percentage that were teaching hospitals but tended to have lower expenditures than the national average. Nearly all states were represented, although most hospitals were located in five of the nine major geographic regions (see chap. 5 for details).

IS hospitals. The IS hospitals were selected randomly from a stratified sample of all short-term voluntary hospitals participating in the PAS system of CPHA. Variables used in stratifying the sample included size (measured by the average census), teaching status (measured by the presence of a residency or internship program or affiliation with a medical school), expenses (cost per patient-day), and a crude estimate of surgical mortality (age- and operation-adjusted mortality for selected types of surgery from previous PAS data).

Three additional requirements were included in order to ensure that reliable estimates and long-term comparisons of surgical outcome could be made: the hospitals had to have had at least 3,000 discharges annually, they had to have been enrolled in the PAS for the preceding three-year period (beginning May 1970), and they had to have performed certain minimum numbers of the selected surgical procedures. From the final stratified random sample of thirty-two hospitals, sixteen agreed to participate. A seventeenth hospital, associated with one of the sixteen, asked to take part in the study at its own expense. The final set of seventeen hospitals may contain the more self-critical hospitals, as exemplified by their willingness to participate in this research. The final set were significantly larger than the national average for short-term voluntary hospitals but tended to be similar in terms of expenditures and the percentage that were teaching hospitals. Ten states and seven major regions of the United States were represented.

Patient Categories and Data Sources

ES categories. The categories of surgical patients were chosen to cover a range of organ systems and surgical specialties; to include both sexes and a range of ages and physical conditions prior to surgery; to permit estimation of the extent of surgical disease; to include some operations for which indications are relatively well established and others for which indications are not so clearly defined; and to maximize the number of complications and deaths that would be observed either because of a large volume of operations or because of the high risk of the disease and procedure. Two medical categories, corresponding to two surgical study categories, were included in order to be able to compare medical and surgical hospitalizations for the same basic diagnostic category. In addition, a subset of nine ES surgical categories, the selected surgical categories, was identified on the basis of their relative diagnostic purity. "Purity" indicated that patients in these study categories were likely to share the same diagnosis and, if operated upon, to have had the study surgical procedure. This subset has been used especially in ES analyses investigating hospital characteristics associated with performance, as reported in chapters 11 and 12. Additionally, these selected surgical categories represent all of the ES categories having corresponding categories in the IS.

Table 6.1 shows the fifteen surgical and two medical patient categories studied through detailed analysis of the discharge abstracts of the 1,224 hospitals in the ES. Altogether, 331,749 surgical patients and 227,107 medical patients were included in the detailed analysis of patients in the ES; these represented about 5 percent of patients discharged during the study year from these hospitals.[1] Table 6.1 also displays and summarizes the selected surgical categories for the ES and their corresponding IS categories. The original design

---

1. For some analyses reported briefly in chapter 12 only, the remaining 95 percent of the patients' abstract records were summarized by hospital, providing indicators of their unadjusted death rates and relatively crudely adjusted mortality ratios, taking into account age and primary diagnosis (or major operation code when limited to surgical patients).

Table 6.1. The study categories, number of patients, and incidence of adverse outcomes in the ES and the IS

	ES (1,224 hospitals)	
Category[a]	Number of Patients	Inhospital Death (%)
Selected surgical categories		
Intraabdominal artery operations	9,532	15.5
Arthroplasty of the hip	13,424	1.5
Biliary tract operatons	130,749	1.1
Stomach operatons—ulcer	26,688	4.3
Large bowel operatons—specified diagnoses	16,110	3.2
Hip fracture diagnosis with other trauma	6,925	8.0
Hip fracture diagnosis without other trauma	52,368	9.1
Amputation of lower limb with no current trauma	10,267	14.4
Amputation of lower limb with current trauma	881	8.5
All selected surgical categories	266,944	4.4
Additional surgical categories[b]		
Stomach operations with cancer diagnosis	1,500	10.7
Stomach operations with other diagnosis	7,148	8.1
Large bowel operations with cancer diagnosis	17,872	6.5
Large bowel operations with other diagnosis	6,575	12.4
Fracture of the pelvis	18,033	3.8
Fracture of the shaft of the femur	13,677	4.1
All surgical categories	331,749	4.7
Medical categories	227,107	2.5
Biliary tract diagnosis—nonsurgical	88,839	2.8
Ulcer diagnosis—nonsurgical	138,268	2.4

[a]Categories are ordered, within each subset, by their decreasing complexity as assessed by an independent panel of surgeons (Forrest et al. 1978, 287).
[b]Noncorresponding in the two studies.

called for all surgical categories in the ES and the IS to be nearly identical and corresponding, but time and financial constraints prevented the full implementation of the ES categories. The correspondence is only approximate because of differences in definitions and in methods for collecting data to determine eligibility in the two studies.

IS categories. The fifteen patient categories chosen for on-site study in the

	IS (17 hospitals)			
Category[a]	Number of patients	Death within 40 days (%)	Severe Morbidity at 7 days (%)	Moderate Morbidity at 7 days (%)
Corresponding IS categories				
Intraabdominal artery operations	104	16.3	4.8	34.2
Arthroplasty of the hip	144	1.4	6.3	54.8
Biliary tract operations	1,569	1.0	1.3	10.4
Stomach operations—ulcer	304	3.3	3.0	19.3
Surgery of large bowel	270	4.4	3.4	30.7
Hip fracture diagnosis	570	9.6	4.7	44.6
Amputation of lower limb	165	17.6	8.5	48.9
Additional surgical categories[b]				
Craniotomy	173	15.0	10.4	30.7
Pulmonary resection	219	5.0	4.1	32.0
Lumbar laminectomy	650	0.3	1.5	14.5
Vaginal hysterectomy	1,126	0	0	6.9
Prostatectomy	922	3.5	2.2	13.3
Splenectomy	95	6.3	4.2	26.3
Abdominal hysterectomy	1,495	0.3	0.9	7.0
Appendectomy	787	0.1	0.3	7.2
All surgical categories	8,593	2.6	2.0	15.6

seventeen hospitals of the IS and the number of patients actually studied in each category are noted in table 6.1 also. The 8,593 study patients represent approximately 8 percent of admissions to the seventeen hospitals during the nine-month study period and roughly 16 percent of those who had surgery.

ES data. All PAS patient records for discharges from the 1,224 hospitals during 1972 were examined in order to select patients whose final diagnoses and operation codes qualified them for one of the ES surgical categories. For these study patients, data indicating presurgical physical status were obtained from the PAS abstract. The items included age, sex, several routine admission findings such as urinalysis and white blood count, and diagnosis or operation codes additional to the qualifying diagnosis and operation. Using predetermined weights, we used additional diagnoses and operations to quantify the extent of the surgical disease and the preoperative health status for each patient. The PAS records for study patients were the only source of information on outcome in the ES.

IS data. Data pertaining to patients were collected by specially trained technicians in each hospital, using seven different forms developed for this study. These data were collected for description of the patient at three points in time: just prior to surgery, seven days after the operation (or at discharge, if earlier), and forty days after the operation.

Information describing the patient prior to surgery permitted prediction of the outcome that would be expected on the basis of the preoperative status and the extent of the disease. These data came from several sources. Patients were interviewed by the study technician to obtain their consent and to collect personal health-related information such as age, sex, marital status, income, education, ethnic origin, insurance status, and recent stressful events. The majority of these interviews were conducted the day before surgery. Special procedures were used to obtain information for patients undergoing non-scheduled surgery and for patients excluded by the technician but later judged appropriate for the study by continuing central review of photocopies of the surgical log from each hospital. The anesthetist recorded the patient's preoperative physical status, cardiovascular status, and the urgency of the procedure. Based on their findings during surgery, surgeons answered questions on the extent of surgical procedures performed and the stage of disease for each patient. To optimize recall, these questions were asked immediately following surgery. Additional routinely available but category-specific information concerning the preoperative extent of the disease was later obtained from the patient's chart. Data forms to stage the disease were developed in consultation with specialists in each type of surgery and varied for each study category.

Assessing the Quality of Surgical Outcomes

The statistical method used in both the IS and the ES yielded a measure of the quality of surgical outcome based on the rate of adverse outcomes (death and, for the IS, postsurgical morbidity) for each hospital, adjusted to remove the effects of variations in the characteristics of patients receiving surgery. The method depended on estimation of the outcome expected for each patient, based on the experience of similar patients in all study hospitals. Then, actual and expected outcomes for patients in a hospital could be compared.

Measures of Patient Outcome

The ES. Outcome in the ES was limited to a single measure: inhospital death. This outcome measure differed from that of the IS in two important ways: no reliable morbidity data were available, and all inhospital deaths were considered. That is, the ES picked up all inhospital deaths, including those occurring later than forty days after operation, which were not counted by the IS; the IS recorded all deaths that occurred within forty days, including deaths after discharge. Table 6.1 displays the percentage of deaths for the seventeen ES patient categories and groupings of study patients. The overall death rate for the ES surgical categories was 4.7 percent, nearly 2 percent higher than that for the IS, primarily because of the proportion of high-death rate patient categories included in the ES.

The IS. Data describing the patient's postoperative condition were used to assess the outcome of surgery. As in most previous research, death occurring after surgery was a basic measure. However, we did not limit our study to those deaths that occurred in the hospital. The use of only inhospital deaths would have created an important potential measurement bias if some hospitals transferred their patients to other institutions, where they might die, while other hospitals provided extended care for their patients. We made a vigorous effort to ascertain survival status of patients in the study forty days after operation. It was felt that the forty-day period was long enough to cover most deaths attributable to the study surgery and short enough to assure a high response rate to questionnaires. Information regarding survival or death on or before the fortieth day after operation was obtained for 99.7 percent of all study patients.

Although death is an easily defined and widely accepted measure of postsurgical outcome, it is a relatively rare event: in the IS sample, 2.8 percent of the patients died within forty days of surgery. Therefore, postsurgical morbidity was included for outcome measurement, both to increase the statistical power of the study and to provide a more sensitive measure of the quality of surgical care. The level of morbidity for all surviving patients was assessed at two discrete points in time: seven days after operation (or at discharge, if earlier) and forty days after operation. To detect a large portion of the major morbidity attributable to the surgical procedure, and for ease in data collection, the seventh day was chosen for short-term assessment to ensure that most study patients would still be hospitalized. The seven-day health-status report was based on information provided by the ward nurse. Data analyzed for this report included an overall rating of the patient's physiological difficulties. Additional data on complications by organ system, support devices needed or used, and health status at forty days were obtained but are not reported here.

Several levels of surgical outcome were developed for the IS. We report three: (1) death within forty days of surgery, (2) severe morbidity on the seventh postoperative day, and (3) moderate morbidity on the seventh postoperative day. Table 6.1 presents the observed frequency for each level of outcome in each study category. There was considerable variation in the percentage of patients experiencing each outcome by surgical category; for example, although the mean death rate for study patients was 2.8 percent, the range was from 20 percent for amputation of a lower limb to no deaths for vaginal hysterectomy.

In our study patients, those categories that tended to have a high death rate were in general more likely to exhibit a high morbidity rate for both severe and moderate morbidity. (Spearman rank order correlations between these three types of outcomes within each category were .8 or higher, and all were significant at $p \leq .001$.) Two categories tended to be exceptions to this general tendency: hip arthroplasty patients experienced a relatively low death rate but had high morbidity at seven days; craniotomy patients tended to have high death rates and severe morbidity rates (about five times higher than average) but a relatively lower moderate morbidity rate (twice the average). These exceptions could be due in part to random variation as a result of our small sample sizes, but they raise the issue of when postoperative morbidity should be measured and, in particular, whether a short-term morbidity such as seven days is appropriate for all surgical procedures. They also demonstrate the need, when selecting a uniform time period for assessment, to adjust outcomes to take into account what would be typical at that time for patients receiving a specific surgery.

Prediction of Patient Outcome

The ES. The first step in predicting surgical outcome (death during hospitalization) in the ES was to analyze all the study patients in each category, disregarding hospital. Patient characteristics used to calculate the probability of an inhospital death included sex; age; admission findings regarding blood pressure, temperature, hemoglobin, hematocrit, urine sugar, and albumin; an index comparing height to weight; and several specially developed "severity scores" for diagnoses and extent of surgery in addition to the qualifying diagnosis and operation. Performing separate regressions for each operation category ensured a better methodological fit in making predictions about outcomes. Analyses by operation group also better mirror medical beliefs that the individual predictors can have differential importance for predicting outcome. For example, the aging process can have a different impact on recovery depending on whether the patient had a fractured hip or an appendectomy. Some specific findings relevant to such variations in the importance of factors by surgical category are reported below, in the section on the Little ES.

The parameters estimated by the logistic equations derived in this manner were then used to arrive at a predicted outcome of each type for each patient. This predicted outcome was the outcome the patient would be expected to experience with average or "standard" care, given his or her particular type of operative procedure and preoperative physical condition. Our standard for assessing the outcomes, then, was empirically derived and based on the collective experience of patients receiving care for the study disease and operation in the 1,224 ES hospitals. To arrive at a measure of the quality of care rendered to the patient in the hospital, we examined the disparity between the outcome the patient actually experienced and the "standard" outcome expected for that patient in an average hospital.

The IS. The basic model for predicting surgical outcome in the IS was parallel to that employed in the ES. The following patient characteristics were used for predicting surgical outcome: age, sex, extent of insurance coverage, level of stress, physical status, cardiovascular status, whether or not the operation was an emergency, and the extent of the surgical disease. In the IS both a logistic function and a linear regression were fitted. For the logistic function, dichotomous measures of outcomes were used that combined mortality and the two types of morbidity: Outcome A, death within forty days; Outcome B, death within forty days or severe morbidity at seven days; and Outcome C, death within forty days or severe or moderate morbidity at seven days. In the linear regression, moderate and severe morbidity at seven days and mortality within forty days were combined into a scaled measure. Three versions of scaling were analyzed, but the few observed differences had essentially no effect on the conclusions drawn. For simplicity's sake, only the Intermediate Outcome is presented: death (9), severe morbidity (5), moderate morbidity (2), and no or mild morbidity (0). The patient predictors used in the linear regression were similar to those in the logistic function but included some interaction terms and quadratic versions of variables that were identified as important predictors in preliminary analyses. The influence of each predictor variable varied depending on the surgical category. Generally speaking, however, physical status, age, and the stage of the disease, together with the interaction term combining age and physical status, were the more powerful variables. Overall, each of the resultant regressions for each IS category was significant at $p \leq .001$.[2] As a final step in the linear regression, each patient's actual outcome and predicted

2. Details of these analyses are in Forrest et al. 1978, 281–86. In more refined analyses of the IS data for biliary tract disease (Flood et al. 1985a, 1985b), data for staging were separated into data for the preoperative stage of the disease and data for the postoperative stage, with additional measures to indicate the difficulty of the biliary tract procedures performed. These measures of the stage of the disease, although less powerful than measures of physical status, had a significant and independent effect in predicting LOS and the outcome at seven days. Interestingly, we found that almost 50 percent of our patients did not have the extent of postoperative biliary tract disease (i.e., confirmed by a pathology report) predicted prior to surgery. Further, when the patient's stage was misdiagnosed (either worse or better), this measure was a significant predictor of a longer LOS and a worse outcome, controlling for the other major patient variables. These refined analyses suggest that at least for some nonmalignant diseases, stage is an important variable for predicting outcome, but that a simple measure that combines patient history, laboratory and x-ray studies, postsurgical pathological reports, and procedures performed tends to mask the importance of stage.

outcome were presented as standardized scores (by subtracting the mean and dividing by the standard deviation) to further eliminate differences in outcomes that could be due to treating a disproportionate mix of patients in high mortality or high morbidity categories.

Hospital Performance Measures

Thus far we have discussed our methods for assessing the quality of outcome at the patient level. For each outcome measure we defined, we had two pieces of information about each patient: the patient's actual outcome and the predicted outcome, which took into account health-related reasons for variations in outcomes. We still had to decide how to aggregate these two pieces of information in order to portray the quality of outcomes at the hospital level. We chose two basic ways, both based on summing, for each hospital, the observed and the expected outcomes for the set of patients of interest. For the tests of differences among hospitals in adjusted outcomes, the first and most important hospital measure was a ratio of the sums of the actual outcomes to the predicted outcomes. Such ratios are similar to indirectly standardized mortality ratios, commonly used to correct for population risk differences in mortality comparisons. If all the differences among hospitals were due to differences in the characteristics of their patients, these ratios would have a value of 1.0, except for the effect of simple random variation and imperfections in the method of adjustment.

In the ES, one standardized mortality ratio, based on death at discharge, was computed for each of the seventeen patient categories and for the various sets of categories in each of the 1,224 hospitals. In the IS, three basic outcome ratios based on the logistic regressions were calculated for each hospital—one for each of the three outcome measures, summed over all fifteen categories. (Ratios were calculated for individual categories as well, but the small number of adverse outcomes per category made these tests relatively insensitive.) A ratio based on a small sample size is, of course, statistically less reliable than one based on a larger sample. Since the seventeen IS hospitals differed widely as to their sample size, the IS ratios were further adjusted by an empirical Bayesian procedure (see chap. 5), which theoretically provides better estimates in the sense of smaller mean square error of predictions. With the Bayesian adjustment the less reliable estimates, based on the smaller samples, are moved relatively more toward the average, that is, toward 1.0.

The second hospital-level measure we used to test for hospital differences was based on a difference score, subtracting the sums of the predicted outcomes from the actual outcome. This measure was used for the IS only and was limited to the Intermediate Scaled Outcome and the linear regression analyses. Since most of our subsequent IS analyses of hospital characteristics influencing hospital performance were based on the linear regression analysis of the Intermediate Scaled Outcome, we briefly present the test for hospital differences for this hospital-level measure as well.

As argued in chapter 5, these hospital-level measures have been "adjusted" in several important ways. First, within each category, our scores took into account the patient's condition on a set of key-health related characteristics. In this way, organizational units or individuals that had worse outcomes because they treated patients in poorer health were not penalized; at least, they were not penalized to the extent that our adjustment was successful in measuring and standardizing for all the appropriate aspects of presurgical health. Lacking a universal standard of health, we made these adjustments on the basis of the usual experience of patients in our entire sample for each category. We assumed that the sample of patients was large enough to provide a secure basis for estimating the average outcome. This type of adjustment was parallel for both the IS and the ES and for the logistic and linear approaches. Second, and unlike the procedure used in the logistic approach, the linear procedure in the IS took into account the types of outcomes usually experienced for patients having had the same kind of surgical intervention. Since the outcomes were presented as standardized scores within categories, the organizational unit or individual under examination was not faulted for treating patients undergoing operations that more frequently resulted in undesirable outcomes. In comparing the linear and the logistic approaches, below, we discuss the implications of this additional adjustment of the linear scores.

The effects of choices of hospital-level measures. Even though the focus of our research on the quality of surgical care in hospitals was relatively narrow, we developed a number of specific measures, and many more could be generated. Like the choice of which activities to evaluate (see chap. 4), the selection of which measures to emphasize affected our conclusions: results varied depending on which measure was selected, and the relative score of a hospital or a surgeon can be determined by this choice. For example, one important methodological question was the extent to which death and morbidity, adjusted for initial patient health, reflect the same underlying quality of care, so that a measure of hospital performance based on death alone is also an indicator of the quality of care that tends to result in increased morbidity for patients at the hospital as well.

To further illustrate the effects of selecting measures, it is instructive to examine the relationships among the outcome measures in the IS generated by the two somewhat different methods employed to assess outcomes and adjust for patient differences. Table 6.2 presents the interrelationships among four different hospital-level measures as assessed by Spearman rank order correlations. It is important to recall that only 2.6 percent of the patients experienced an adverse outcome of type A; 4.6 percent, an adverse outcome of type B; and 20.2 percent, an adverse outcome of type C. Not too much confidence should

Table 6.2. Correlation of selected standardized outcome ratios based on 8,593 IS patients for the seventeen hospitals

	Outcome A[a]	Outcome B[b]	Outcome C[c]	Intermediate Scaled[d]
Outcome A		.45	−.10	.30
Outcome B			.34	.67
Outcome C				.82

Note: Entries are Spearman rank order correlations among the hospital-level measures.
[a]Dead vs. alive.
[b]Dead or severe morbidity vs. else.
[c]Dead or severe or moderate morbidity vs. else.
[d]Dead (9); severe (5) or moderate morbidity (2); else (0).

be placed in the results for Outcome A because of the small number of adverse events involved. Nevertheless, in view of the nesting of adverse outcomes involved in A, B, and C, we were surprised to observe a negative association between measures A and C and only a small positive association between measures B and C. The construction of these measures was such that Outcome A was dominated by the outcomes on a few surgical procedures, such as the amputation of a lower limb, craniotomy, and selected surgery of the abdominal aorta, while Outcome C was dominated by other types of operations, such as prostatectomy and biliary tract surgery, where the outcome of mild morbidity is fairly common, and large numbers of cases are available. Thus, one explanation of the inverse correlation between rankings of hospitals using measures of care quality based on Outcome A in contrast to measures based on Outcome C is that hospitals performing well on types of surgery associated with relatively high mortality or severe morbidity rates may not perform as well on types of surgery in which moderate morbidity is the most severe adverse outcome. It is also possible that hospitals that succeed in obtaining a low death rate for a given operation may fail to prevent a high rate of morbidity among their patients.

The measures developed for the linear-regression approach reduced the effects of variations among surgical categories in the levels of observed outcome in two ways. First, these measures did not focus on any one particular outcome or combination of outcomes, but allowed each possible level of outcome (mortality, severe morbidity, moderate morbidity, no or little morbidity) to have some (varying) weight in each measure. Second, unlike the approach followed for the logistic equations, the outcome measures and predictor variables were standard scored within each operation. This approach allowed the emphasis to be on any "poorer than expected" outcomes, even though for some operations poor outcomes might be at most mild morbidity, while for others they might refer to mortality as well.

Which standardized measures of outcome and methods of aggregating them are better? The answer depends on the questions being asked. If one cares more about locating and preventing the relatively more serious problems suffered by patients undergoing surgery, such as excessive amounts of mortality or severe morbidity, then the procedures for combining operations should give greater weight to these outcomes regardless of whether they characterize the outcome of patients undergoing most operations. Outcomes like A and B and the methods used to combine the logistic results have this effect. If one wishes to evaluate the quality of surgical care in general, however, then as much may be learned from standardized outcomes experienced by patients undergoing less serious operations as from standardized outcomes experienced in connection with the more serious and life-threatening procedures. Outcome C, the Intermediate Scaled Outcome, and the aggregation used in the linear model reflect these objectives.

The actual scores and rankings of the seventeen hospitals for Outcome B and the Intermediate Scaled Outcome are displayed in table 6.3. While table 6.3 reveals broad similarities in the four outcome measures developed, there are also important differences. For example, the Pearson correlation between the two difference measures from table 6.3—Outcome B treated as a difference score (col. 6) and the Intermediate Scale (col. 7)—was only .56 (the Spearman correlation was .67). This suggests that the choices represented by these two different hospital-level measures—one based on a logistic model of prediction and a binary outcome and other based on a linear model of prediction and a normalized interval outcome measure—can have an important impact on any results we report or conclusions drawn with respect to the quality of surgical care in the study hospitals.

THE RESULTS OF HOSPITAL TESTS FOR DIFFERENCES IN OUTCOMES

The ES Results

Standardized mortality ratios were calculated for all 1,224 hospitals for each patient category. Some hospitals had only a few patients in a particular category, and the resulting ratios exhibited wide variation. For instance, deaths associated with biliary tract surgery averaged slightly more than 1 per hospital, and 218 of the 1,224 hospitals (17.8 percent) had standardized ratios greater than 2, meaning that they had at least twice as many deaths for this procedure as would be expected given their mix of patients. On the other hand, 489 hospitals

Table 6.3. The IS outcome rates for death at forty days or severe morbidity at seven days (Outcome B) and for the Intermediate Scale based on 8,593 IS patients

Hospital	Number of Patients	Unstandardized Outcome B — Percentage of Patients with Adverse Events	Measures of Standardized Outcome B — Standardized Ratio[a]	Measures of Standardized Outcome B — Bayes-adjusted Standardized Ratio[a]	Measures of Standardized Outcome B — Average Difference[b]	Standardized Intermediate Scaled Outcome — Average Difference[b]
1	201	0.5	0.37 (1)	0.71 (2)	−.008 (5)	.042 (12)
9	1,256	2.7	0.72 (3)	0.73 (3)	−.010 (3)	−.029 (8)
14	524	2.7	0.80 (5)	0.83 (5)	−.007 (6)	−.132 (3)
2	469	3.4	0.83 (7)	0.85 (7)	−.007 (7)	−.073 (5)
16	283	3.5	0.88 (8)	0.91 (9)	−.005 (9)	−.098 (4)
4	472	3.6	0.74 (4)	0.77 (4)	−.013 (2)	−.167 (1)
8	555	4.1	0.82 (6)	0.84 (6)	−.009 (4)	−.041 (7)
11	192	4.1	0.49 (2)	0.54 (1)	−.004 (1)	−.166 (2)
7	315	4.5	0.95 (10)	0.96 (10)	−.003 (10)	−.014 (9)
13	965	4.9	1.45 (16)	1.43 (16)	.015 (16)	.075 (15)
12	39	5.2	3.73 (17)	1.56 (17)	.038 (17)	.078 (16)
17	305	5.2	1.22 (14)	1.20 (14)	.009 (13)	.031 (10)
6	762	5.4	1.16 (12)	1.15 (12)	.007 (11)	.069 (14)
15	486	5.6	0.90 (9)	0.91 (8)	−.006 (8)	.236 (17)
5	785	5.9	1.32 (15)	1.31 (15)	.014 (15)	.041 (11)
3	306	6.2	1.12 (11)	1.12 (11)	.007 (12)	−.068 (6)
10	642	9.0	1.17 (13)	1.16 (13)	.013 (14)	.054 (13)
Total	8,593					
Mean	505.4	4.8	1.07	0.99		
Standard deviation	306.7	3.4	0.62	0.25		

Note: Numbers in parentheses indicate the rank of hospital from best (1) to worst (17) for each measure. Hospitals are ordered by the unstandardized Outcome B.

[a] The ratio is computed as the total number of adverse outcomes divided by the total number of expected adverse outcomes.

[b] Average difference is computed as the average number of adverse outcomes minus the average number of expected adverse outcomes.

(40 percent) had no deaths at all. The total deaths, standard deviation, and significance levels of hospital differences in mortality ratios for each surgical category are summarized in table 6.4. Statistical tests are, of course, better able to identify differences in hospital mortality ratios for these single categories when there are more deaths. Five of the six categories with more than 1,000 deaths demonstrated highly significant differences among hospitals ($p < .001$), and the sixth was significant at the .05 level. When the patient categories were combined into sets such as selected surgical categories and all study categories, hospitals were found to be strongly significantly different in their mortality ratios. For each of the groupings, even after careful adjustment for patient mix, hospitals were found to differ by more than twofold[3] in the likelihood of a given patient's experiencing inhospital death if treated in the hospital with the poorest performance instead of the best.

The IS Results: The Logistic Model

Table 6.3 also shows standardized outcome ratios (col. 4) and their Bayesian adjusted counterparts (col. 5) for death within forty days after surgery or severe morbidity at the seventh day; the ratios are calculated on all patient categories combined for each hospital in the IS. These ratios range from 0.37 to 3.7 among the hospitals. This tenfold spread reduces to an almost threefold difference (0.54 to 1.56) between the best and worst ratios after the Bayesian adjustment. The variation among hospitals is much more than would be expected by chance: a normal deviate test, based on the chi-square formulation, indicates that they differ significantly, with $p < .001$.

Similarly, the test based on Outcome C (not reported here), death within forty days or moderate to severe morbidity at seven days, was strongly predictive of differences ($p \le .001$). The hospitals also varied on the outcome measure based on death alone, but this variation was not statistically significant. This result may be partly due to the small number of study deaths (238) and does not necessarily indicate lack of true variation in mortality ratios, since a test of the more populous categories of the ES did indicate that significant differences exist.

The IS Results: The Linear Model

Table 6.3 also displays, for each hospital, the average difference based on the Intermediate Scaled Outcome (col. 7). To examine the extent of differences among hospitals based on outcomes adjusted with the linear model, we per-

---

3. Estimates of magnitude reported are based on one standard deviation. Thus, with a standard deviation of .37, hospitals at one standard deviation from the mean (1.0) will have ratios of 1.37 and 0.63, respectively, or a 2.17-fold difference.

Table 6.4. The results of the ES: Observed incidence of inhospital death in 1,224 hospitals, by study category based on 558,856 ES patients

Category	Observed Deaths	Standard Deviation of Mortality Ratios[a]	Significance Level[b] of Differences among Hospitals (p)
Surgical categories			
Intraabdominal artery operations	1,441	0.81	<0.001
Arthroplasty of the hip	196	—	0.341
Selected biliary tract surgery	1,444	0.48	<0.001
Stomach operations—ulcer	1,135	0.97	0.017
Large bowel operations—specified diagnoses	520	—	0.046
Hip fracture diagnosis with other trauma	542	0.31	0.371
Hip fracture diagnosis with no other trauma	4,773	0.37	<0.001
Amputation of lower limb with no current trauma	1,457	0.58	<0.001
Amputation of lower limb with current trauma	49	—	0.508
Stomach operations with cancer diagnosis	128	1.33	0.291
Stomach operations with other diagnosis	560	.60	0.119
Large bowel operations with cancer diagnosis	1,151	0.59	<0.001
Large bowel operations with other diagnosis	802	—	0.179
Fracture of the pelvis	681	0.54	0.179
Fracture of the shaft of the femur	557	0.33	0.184
Selected surgical categories (9)	11,653	0.38	<0.001
All surgical categories (15)	15,618	0.37	<0.001
Medical categories			
Biliary tract diagnoses	2,479	0.53	<0.001
Ulcer diagnoses	3,299	0.20	<0.001
All medical categories (2)	5,776	0.37	<0.001

[a]Derived from the square root of the hospital component of variance ($\hat{\sigma}^2$) in observed/expected mortality ratios (see chap. 5).

[b]Based on the Z statistic (see chap. 5).

formed a two-way analysis of variance (ANOVA). We introduced a hospital-identification measure as a dummy variable to test for differences in the outcomes measures at the hospital level. We also introduced a measure of the relative difficulty of the surgical procedure undergone. This measure was based on the ratings of surgical procedures provided by the panel of surgeons, with the operations trichotomized into those regarded as relatively easy, those regarded as moderately difficult, and those regarded as difficult procedures. Relatively easy operations included appendectomy and amputation of a lower limb, involving 952 patients in all; operations judged to be of moderate difficulty included gastric surgery for ulcer, selected surgery of the biliary tract, surgery of the large bowel, splenectomy, abdominal hysterectomy, vaginal hysterectomy, repair of a fractured hip, lumbar laminectomy, pulmonary resection, and prostatectomy, involving 7,220 patients in all; and operations judged to be relatively difficult included craniotomy, arthroplasty of the hip, and selected surgery of the abdominal aorta and/or the iliac arteries, involving 421 patients.

The measure of the relative difficulty of the operations was included for two reasons. The adjustment procedures applied to outcomes should, if effective, preclude our finding any remaining direct effect of the level of difficulty of operation in explaining outcome. For this variable, then, we do not expect to find significant differences. But we are, in addition, interested in examining the consistency of the quality of care in each hospital across these three levels of difficulty in performing operations. Thus we looked for the possibility of interactions between the hospital and the difficulty of operations performed to discover whether the quality of care delivered by a hospital depends upon the difficulty of the procedure being studied.

As expected, in the two-way ANOVA tests, the main effect of hospitals for explaining variation in adjusted surgical outcome was significant at the .001 level, while the main effect of the difficulty of the operation was not significant; however, the interaction effect of the hospital and the level of difficulty of the operation did reach a significance level of .025. This suggests that hospitals may not perform equally well for all kinds of operations but tend to perform poorly or well depending upon the difficulty of the procedure.

We performed a related analysis entering hospital identification, the extent of operation difficulty, and the interaction between these as a series of dummy variables in a linear regression, with the adjusted outcome scores as the dependent variable. Again, hospital effect was consistently apparent. With each hospital dummy variable entered, the step was significant at the .001 level, with an R^2 of .010. Inclusion of the extent of difficulty of the operation and all the interaction terms between hospital identification and the level of difficulty of the operation only boosted this R^2 to .016. The change in R^2 resulting from the addition of the interaction terms and the main effects of the difficulty of the operation was not significant at the .05 level.

These analyses support the conclusion that there are significant differences among hospitals in adjusted outcome measures, a finding that is consistent across all of the scales based on the linear model and the outcomes used in the logistic model and across the two overlapping studies. There was some evidence in the IS to suggest that a fruitful examination could be made of the differences in the quality of care, within each hospital, that occur across groups of operations varying in level of difficulty. Yet these differences are not large, and a cursory examination of these interaction effects showed no hospitals performing very well in one group and very poorly in another.[4] Thus we feel justified in examining our hypotheses involving structure using these adjusted outcomes in the IS combined across all operative categories as an important first approach to testing them.

COMPARING THE IS AND ES DATA IN THE SEVENTEEN HOSPITALS (THE LITTLE ES)

The overall intent of the Little ES was to learn the extent to which these rather different data sources and standards of good performance led to similar results when applied to an identical set of hospitals and to an identical set of patients. It was not strictly a study of the "validity" of the PAS data, comparing them with the prospectively collected IS data.[5] Rather, it was an examination of the consistency of the two data sources, with important implications for the feasibility and adequacy of applying the ES methods and data sources to assess the quality of care, since they were more readily and economically obtained and applied to hospitals.

Obtaining the Matched Sample of Cases

For the Little ES, we wished to isolate that set of patients for whom both IS and ES variables would be available for comparison. In order to be in both studies, the patient (1) had to have qualified for inclusion in one of the surgical categories that corresponded in the ES and IS (see table 6.1, selected surgical categories) and (2) had to have been hospitalized and operated upon during the 7½-month period of overlap between the two data bases.

As a first step in identifying matched patients, since we had available the PAS records for a 3½-year period including the entire time during which IS and ES data were collected, we attempted to match all 8,593 final-study IS patients. We succeeded in matching records for 97.7 percent of these patients; records for

---

4. These issues are addressed in chapter 11 for the ES, with similar conclusions.

5. We did conduct a validation study of a random sample of PAS records in the seventeen hospitals, reabstracting the data from the medical records. The results of this study are reported in Forrest et al. 1977, 260–98.

the remaining 2.3 percent apparently contained transcription errors in the medical record number (the initial matching variable) in either the PAS abstract or the IS data base. From these matched patients, 2,064 cases met the criteria for inclusion in both data bases.

Comparing the IS and ES Patient-Selection Rules

Of the 2,064 matched cases, 98.1 percent were placed in the appropriate corresponding study categories in both studies. The forty cases not matched appropriately were examined individually; thirty-eight patients were found to have had multiple procedures, and the differences in classification arose because of different category-assignment rules in the two studies or because of the order in which the different operations occurred (which was considered in the IS but not in the ES). The remaining two patients were biliary-tract-diagnosis patients who were called surgical in the IS but medical in the ES, probably due to operation codes inadvertently omitted on the PAS record.

Comparing the IS and ES Results at the Patient Level

Death as an Outcome
Death as an outcome of surgery was measured differently in the two studies: for the ES, any inhospital death was counted; for the IS, any death within forty days of surgery, including those occurring after discharge, was counted. Thus some discrepancy between the two measures was expected for definitional reasons. For this reason, we first compared the discharge status in both studies. The two sources agreed exactly in reporting seventy deaths at discharge but differed in destination for live patients (i.e., to home or some other facility) in 2.5 percent of discharged patients. This difference had no effect in determining the dead-alive status at discharge; however, the definitional differences in death resulted in some potentially important differences for assessing hospital performance. Two patients died inhospital after forty days, and an additional twenty-three patients died within forty days but after discharge. Among those deaths that occurred after discharge, 83 percent of the patients had been discharged to an extended-care facility or other hospital. Thus, the death rate of study patients discharged routinely was 0.2 percent, whereas among those transferred to some other facility the death rate was 9.5 percent, or forty-two times higher.

These postdischarge deaths could potentially seriously bias the use of inhospital death as a surrogate for forty-day death, for example, if hospitals differed in their postdischarge death rates due to differences in patterns of transferring patients to other facilities. Using one-way ANOVA, we were unable to find any evidence of significant differences in postdischarge death rates among our seventeen hospitals, but with such a small sample of deaths, the test had little statistical power to detect any but the largest deviations. One insight that might be drawn from these comparisons in assessing death is that since most of the additional deaths occurred among patients discharged to another facility, a future study might profit from a follow-up for only those patients, rather than for all patients. Alternatively, discharge with incomplete recovery could be used as an additional indicator of outcome, as in our studies of service intensity and outcome.

Predicting Death for Patients

Table 6.5 shows the probability of dying based on the logistic predictions from the ES and from the IS for each of the 2,064 matched patients. In addition, we present the IS probabilities for logistic regression on Outcome B (death within forty days or severe morbidity at seven days) and Outcome C (death within forty days or moderate to severe morbidity at seven days). The correlations were reasonably high (.62 for Pearson and .76 for Spearman) considering the differences in the definitions of death in the two studies and the types and methods for collecting information on patient status to use as predictors. Taking the IS probabilities of death within forty days as the standard (acknowledging that it is likely to be more perturbed by random estimation error due to a more limited sample size), we conclude that the ES probability of inhospital death provides a reasonable but certainly not perfect approximation for predicting a given patient's postsurgical death.

Comparing the IS and ES Measures at the Hospital Level

Comparisons at the patient level primarily give us information about the exact correspondence of the methods. When measures are aggregated to the hospital level, other factors come into play that may increase or decrease the extent to which the two data bases and methods agree about the ranking of a hospital with regard to deaths, expected deaths, and their standardized mortality ratios. Table 6.6 presents these hospital-level correlations for the matched patients, using only sixteen hospitals, since one hospital had only ten patients in the Little ES. Concentrating on the ES measure and Outcome A, we observe that the average outcome probabilities (or the expected number of deaths) were correlated .80, compared with .62 at the patient level; the crude outcomes correlated .88; and the standardized ratios, .75. Similar to the results reported for the entire IS sample in table 6.2, the standardized ratios based on Outcomes A, B, and C do not demonstrate strong intercorrelation despite the overlap in defining outcomes among the three measures at the patient level.

We find it encouraging that the correlations among the hospital measures of death in the ES and IS were so high, especially in view of the differences in defining death and the different standard populations used to estimate the "average hospital's experience." Due to the relative unreliability of the IS

Table 6.5. Comparison of the results from the ES and IS methods to assess each patient's probability of having a poor outcome, using patients from the Little ES

Outcome Measures	Extensive Study	Intensive Study		
	Inhospital Death	Outcome A	Outcome B	Outcome C
ES Death		.621	.631	.549
		(.763)	(.794)	(.795)
Outcome A			.901	.583
			(.872)	(.764)
Outcome B				.689
				(.861)

Note: Main entries are Pearson product-moment correlations of a patient's probability of having each type of poor outcome; Spearman rank order correlations are in parentheses. All are significant at $p \le .001$.

estimates of death, which involved so few patients, the disagreement between the methods may be related more to random noise than to systematic or "true" differences.

The Importance of Prospective, Specially Collected Data for Assessing Quality

In the next set of results from the Little ES, we sought to determine the additional predictive information for standardizing outcomes gained by having the prospectively gathered, specially defined data (i.e., the IS data) over what is more routinely available in medical abstracts (i.e., the ES data). We used two different approaches, both based on regression analyses.[6] First we looked at the change in predictive power as measured by the R^2 when the IS variables were added to a regression model already containing the ES variables. This approach examined prediction at the patient level. Second, we used hospital indicator variables ("dummy" variables), whose regression coefficients served as outcome scores for each hospital. We then wished to discover how these hospital coefficients would change if sets of variables were added. That is, the extra variables may indeed have had substantial predictive power for patient-level outcome, but if hospitals did not differ sufficiently in their mean for these extra variables, adjusting for these extra variables would not affect the relative outcome scores for the hospitals.

These analyses used some or most of the predictor variables from the IS and the ES; they also included one predictor, diuretic drugs, available in the ES

6. Details of these analyses and results are contained in Forrest et al. 1978, 398–413.

Table 6.6. Correlations among measures at the hospital level, derived by ES and IS logistic regression methods ($N = 16$)

Outcome Measures	Intensive Study		
	Outcome A	Outcome B	Outcome C
1. Average probability of adverse outcome			
ES: Inhospital death	.80	.78	.74
IS: Outcome A		.98	.90
IS: Outcome B			.94
2. Average crude outcome			
ES: Inhospital death	.88	.62	.35
IS: Outcome A		.77	.48
IS: Outcome B			.58
3. Standardized ratios			
ES: Inhospital death	.75	.48	−.06
IS: Outcome A		.64	−.17
IS: Outcome B			.02

Note: Hospital 12 was omitted because it had only 10 patients in the sample. Hospital measures were aggregated, using the remaining 2,054 patients in the Little ES. Pearson correlations among these variables are presented.

but not used, since it could reflect postoperative complications as well as preoperative physical status. The methods differed slightly too, employing a linear regression and pooling all the 2,064 patients together. These changes were compromises necessary because differences in the definitions and methods, as well as the data base, made interpretation of these results difficult, and the sample size was too small for separate regressions by category.

We used four outcome measures: the ES inhospital death and, from the IS, Outcome A, Outcome B, and the Intermediate Scaled Outcome. In the first set of regressions we entered "all" of the ES predictor variables and then used stepwise regression to enter seven specially created IS predictor variables (e.g., stage, preoperative physical status, cardiovascular status).

For all regressions, the first step (using the ES predictors) was always highly significant. The R^2 ranged from .16 (for inhospital death) to .27 (the Intermediate Scaled Outcome). When the IS variables were added, the change in R^2 was quite small (around .01) but significant at the .001 level. When we examine the step breakdown for the IS variables, preoperative physical status[7]

7. Throughout the discussion of predictor variables in the Little ES, the IS indicator of physical status refers to two variables, both assessed by the patient's anesthetist and both based on the ASA definition of preoperative physical-status ratings (*Anesthesiology* 1963).

was uniformly the first to be selected. The IS staging variable was significant at the .05 level only for the regression on inhospital death (ES outcome).

When we examined the impact on the ranking of hospitals of adding the IS measures, we found it to be small but significant. Most of the change in hospital ranks, of course, occurred in assessing hospitals first by their crude outcomes and then by outcomes adjusted by the ES variables alone. The Spearman correlation among hospital-level measures based on inhospital death, for example, was .48 between crude death rate and ES adjusted ratios and .94 between ES adjusted and ES-IS adjusted ratios.

Which Is "Better"—the IS or the ES?

The final set of analyses from the Little ES asked a slightly different question: Which predictor model was better—the IS or the ES? The predictor variables and outcomes used for these analyses were identical to those used in the above analyses. The major difference was that the ES variables were not forced into the regression but competed with the IS variables in a stepwise regression. For all four outcome measures, the first variable chosen was the IS preoperative physical-status rating. The ES indicator diuretic drugs was the second variable entered in three regressions, while age was selected as the second variable in the fourth regression.

For all four outcomes, the IS measures of preoperative physical status and the ES measures of diuretics, white blood count, and diastolic blood pressure were always represented among the ten "best" predictors chosen by the stepwise regression. Three other ES variables were among the ten best in three out of four outcome regressions: age, the rating of the most difficult operation, and an indicator of one ES study category, nontraumatic amputation of a lower limb. Although one or two variables indicating the disease category or stage or the operation type or difficulty (from either the IS or ES) were always selected among the ten best, we had expected these variables to be more powerful than that (although see n. 3).

We also found one other surprising result: for each regression, the predictive power (R^2) of the ten best variables as a set, from either the IS or the ES, was less than or equal to a regression in which the only predictor entered was the probability of inhospital death from the ES. Given that data on inhospital death are easier to collect than data on deaths following discharge and more reliable than data on morbidity, it is important to find that the ES probability based on the experience of 1,224 hospitals predicts care quality as well as or better than the probability based on specially collected IS data for the same patients.

One is a five-point scale, and the other is an "urgency" indicator that the patient is relatively worse off than most patients in the given physical-status category.

RESULTS OF TESTS FOR HOSPITAL DIFFERENCES IN SERVICE INTENSITY

Overview of Methods

Chapter 5 briefly summarizes the methods used in the Service Intensity Study (SIS), which examined the variation in clinical services received and outcomes achieved by all patients discharged from the seventeen IS hospitals during the study period 1970–73. The measures of services and outcomes were based on the approximately 600,000 PAS medical record abstracts of these patients. Using the PAS records, we identified several classes of clinical services that each patient could receive: consultations with other physicians, diagnostic and therapeutic services, and lengths of stay. Wherever possible, the measures included the amount of each service that the patient received (see table 6.7 for definitions of the services). In order to measure the mix of services, we created two indices of service intensity: the *specific services index,* which was based on the diagnostic and therapeutic services received, weighted by their relative costliness, and the *routine services index,* which was a weighted measure of the length of stay. Outcomes were measured by inhospital death, as in the ES.

Parallel to the standardizing methods in the IS and ES, we used the entire set of patients as a standard against which we could estimate the services the patient would receive in the typical, or "standard," hospital. We created four classes of standardizing variables: the patient's admission variables (including diagnosis), the operative procedures performed, the discharge status, and inhospital complications incurred. The types of standardizing variables selected were very similar to those used in the ES, the major exception being that the SIS used the List A diagnostic categories developed by CPHA for reporting length of stay and outcomes (CPHA 1975, 1977) as the basis for categorizing patients by diagnosis; the SIS also did not develop staging variables for the disease and operations specific to each group as we had done in the ES. We tried a number of different sets of standardizing variables for each dependent variable, some chosen for theoretical reasons (e.g., while we always adjusted *consultations received* to take into account the patient's diagnosis, admission status, and operations, we sometimes included inhospital complications to reflect the quality of care received during the hospitalization) and some for methodological reasons (e.g., when we used *the number of operative procedures* as a dependent variable, we did not want to adjust for operations). In practice we found that essentially all of the explainable patient variation was due to the diagnosis and admission set of standardizing variables and, where appropriate, the operations received.

Tests for Hospital Differences Based on All Patients

Table 6.7 displays the measures we used to assess service intensity and outcomes in the SIS and the standardization sets included in the models we present. For dichotomous dependent variables, the means can be interpreted as the percentage of patients receiving the service (e.g., 7.4 percent of patients received intensive care and 65.3 percent of patients had normal blood test results). For most other services, the majority of patients received no such service, while others received varying amounts of the service (e.g., an individual patient could have no diagnostic procedures recorded or up to 7). For drugs and length of stay, virtually all patients received at least one unit of such services, so these means can be interpreted as the average number of classes of drugs each patient received (1.06 out of 14 classes) and the average number of days stayed (8.4). The overall means for the specific services index and the routine services index reflect the relative weightings of these two measures, based on the proportion of expenditures for these types of services on a typical patient bill. Specific services, for example, represent just under half of a typical bill.

Table 6.7 also presents the test for hospital differences for each service and for outcomes, using all study patients combined. The estimates of the magnitude of the between-hospital standard deviation are based on a one-way ANOVA of the standardized measures of each dependent variable (expressed as the difference: observed minus expected services for each patient), with hospital as the criterion variable. For every comparison in table 6.7, the F statistic in the ANOVA was significant at $p \leq .001$. The final columns present the ratio of the estimate of standardized services for hospitals at one standard deviation above the mean compared with one standard deviation below the mean and the corresponding ratio for two standard deviations from the mean.

Assuming a normal distribution (which, though not completely appropriate, provides a useful guide for interpreting our results), 32 percent of hospitals would be outside the one-standard-deviation limits—16 percent lower and 16 percent higher—and 5 percent would be outside the two-standard-deviation limits. Thus, using *consultations received* as an example, there is an 80 percent higher number of consultations, after standardizing, for patients at the upper 16th percentile of hospitals than for those at the lower 16th percentile. Taking the more extreme limits of the distribution, we estimate that patients at the upper 2.5th percentile of hospitals receive about four times as many consultations as patients at the lower 2.5th percentile.

A recent study by Luke and Thomson (1980) also reported large variation in consultation use for patients who were insured by fee for service (higher use) compared with prepaid patients. Recall, however, that all our hospitals were voluntary hospitals, and all were reimbursed by fee-for-service insurance, including the versions of Medicaid and Medicare then in practice, or by charity

Table 6.7. Definition of standardized measures of service intensity and outcome and results for tests of hospital differences in the SIS

Class of Dependent Variable	Model[a]	Dependent Variable[b]	Standardization Sets Employed				Overall Mean	Between-Hospital Standard Deviation[c]	Ratio of Limits for 1 Standard Deviation	Ratio of Limits for 2 Standard Deviations[d]
			Admission Condition	Operations	Discharge Status	Complications				
Consultations	11	Number of kinds of M.D. specialists from which consultations were received (0 to 7)	X	X	X	X	.316	.095	1.85	3.98
Diagnostic care	1	Total number of diagnostic procedures performed (0 to 7)	X	X			.217	.067	1.28	1.65
	8	Blood tests with normal results given (yes or no)	X	X	X	X	.653	.119	1.45	2.15
Therapeutic care	13	Number of nondiagnostic surgical procedures performed (0 to 7)	X				0.545	.056	1.23	1.52
	15	Intensive care received (yes or no)	X	X	X	X	.074	.018	1.67	3.01

18	Number of different classes of drugs received (0 to 14)	X	X	X	X	X	1.066	.101	1.21	1.47
20	Blood given (yes or no)	X	X	X	X	X	.054	.030	3.44	—
21	Physical therapy (yes or no)	X	X	X	X	X	.051	.031	4.04	—
22	Number of days of stay (0.5 to 100)	X	X	X	X	X	8.399	1.275	1.36	1.87
Length of stay										
Indices of service intensity										
(RS)	Routine services summary index; weighted version of model 22						51.1	1.275	1.36	
(SS)	Specific services summary index (0 to about 50) (weighted sum of diagnostic and therapeutic measures)						47.3			
Outcome										
27	Inhospital death (yes or no)	X		X			.032	.005	1.33	1.80

Note: Statistics reported here are based on all 603,580 patients discharged from the 17 hospitals during the 3½-year study period.

[a] The original model numbers are given, out of 31 analyzed and reported in Forrest et al. 1977. All original service-intensity variables are represented; those models omitted differed slightly in definition or in standardization sets used; in practice, these variations had little effect on our results.

[b] Numbers in parentheses represent the potential range of the variable.

[c] Standard deviations reported are based on an ANOVA with hospital as the criterion variable. All tests were significant at $p \leq .001$.

[d] Where ratios are not computed, it is because the standard deviation was so high relative to the mean that the lower limits produced negative estimates.

[e] These represent "very great" differences among hospitals. The exception is for the specific index, where the analysis for hospital differences was not performed due to computational complexity.

and self-pay. Even though the comparison is limited to hospitals all reimbursed by fee for service, we found strong evidence of variations in consulting rates.

Several services show sizable variations after adjusting. While variation in LOS has already been well documented (Lave and Lave 1971; Fetter et al. 1980), we found evidence of an even greater variation for most of the specific services indicators, in particular for blood tests with completely normal results, the number of M.D. consultations received, the use of intensive-care units, blood units given, and provision of physical therapy. The remaining services— diagnostic surgical procedures, nondiagnostic surgical procedures, and the number of different classes of drugs—indicate at least a 25 percent increase in use for hospitals at the upper 16th percentile, and a 50 percent increase for hospitals at the upper 2.5th percentile, compared with hospitals at the corresponding percentiles of lower use. Moreover, these particular services involve a substantial proportion of the expenditures and costs, so that even a 25–50 percent increase in use translates into an annual expense of many millions of dollars in "above-standard" services nationwide.

Outcomes also differed significantly, showing about a 1.3-fold difference in the limits. While we have already demonstrated significant differences in adjusted outcomes in the IS and ES, here we include *all* patients during the study period, about half of them nonsurgical (in contrast to our concentration on surgery in the ES and IS). We address the important question of whether above-standard services are associated with or "buy" better outcomes in the next chapter.

COMPARING THE PERFORMANCE OF HOSPITALS FOR SURGICAL AND NONSURGICAL PATIENTS AND OVER TIME

We turn last to a brief report on our analyses to examine, using our standardized measures, the consistency of each hospital's performance in treating surgical versus nonsurgical patients and over the 3½-year period. We note first that there were, of course, important and major differences in the use of services and the outcomes achieved, even after standardization, between surgical and nonsurgical patients (e.g., surgical patients used more blood and nonsurgical stayed longer) and over time (e.g., specific services increased and length of stay decreased). The question we wished to address was different: Do hospitals that provide above-standard services for surgical patients also tend to provide above-standard services for nonsurgical patients? Do hospitals that provide above-standard services one year tend to continue to be above-standard in other years (i.e., after taking into account general time trends occurring in all hospitals)? The simple answer is yes: these seventeen hospitals tended to provide service intensity and outcomes that were similar for surgical and nonsurgical patients and over the 3½-year period of our study. (Details of these analyses are in Forrest et al. 1977, 146–64, 194–200.)

SUMMARY

We conclude that hospital abstract data can be used to measure the quality of surgical care in hospitals. The degree of variation in quality is large enough to constitute an important public-health problem, warranting further work toward a methodology that will allow each hospital to place itself on a continuum of performance quality.

It is clear that a great variety of patient characteristics have a direct effect on the outcome of medical or surgical care. It is essential that such systematic effects be removed from measures of the quality of hospital care if these are to be used to evaluate performance of hospitals or other health care providers. Our results suggest that despite the pervasive and preponderant influence of patient characteristics on outcome, carefully standardized measures can be used as valid indicators of provider performance.

While no claim is made for comprehensiveness in our sets of standardization variables, and while we do not claim to have developed an ideal methodology, we did attempt to go beyond what had been done in previous studies comparing institutions by outcome. In the IS, the ES, and the SIS, we carefully assessed the specific procedures performed, the nature and extent or severity of the patient's disease, and other concomitant conditions affecting the patient's health status, and we supplemented these direct measures of preoperative or admission status by indirect measures such as age and sex.

The specific variables used for risk assessment differed markedly among the three studies, primarily because of the nature of the basic patient information available. In the IS, very specific information regarding the nature and extent of disease was collected on forms especially constructed for each type of operation. Overall health level was obtained from the anesthetist's rating of physical status. In the ES, the primary sources of information for preoperative health status were admission laboratory tests and a coded listing of the patient's diagnoses. Numerous status indicators were defined using this information. The ES counterpart of IS disease categorization involved using diagnosis codes both to indicate the principal disease and to score or stage selected complicating conditions (for example, pancreatic involvement in gall bladder disease). Any additional conditions present, such as diabetes or hypertension, were first scored and then combined into indicators corresponding to the IS physical-status measure. The laboratory results allowed additional sensitivity in risk assessment. Despite the differences in source data, the overall predictive power of the ES models was similar to that of models based on the IS data. The predictive power of the ES logistic model was satisfactory, yielding a method of calculating the probability of death for the individual patient that was close to actual experience.

More detailed comparison of the two methods—or precisely, of the two types of patient data—is certainly warranted before further application of these methods is undertaken. However, the agreement between our on-site results and results based on PAS data suggests that the abstract data, with a small number of additional items to allow risk assessment of initial health status, may provide a valid and reliable basis for the measurement of quality, using the method of adjusted rates described here.

For actual measurement of outcome, the on-site data were clearly superior to those obtainable from routine abstract sources. Salient features were the postdischarge follow-up for death before forty days and the collection of seven-day morbidity estimates. After additional development and testing to verify their validity and sensitivity, outcome measures such as these would be valuable additions to routine abstracts, if these data sources are contemplated for use in assessing the quality of outcome.

In the SIS, we again found substantial differences (about twofold) in outcomes, standardized for patient health, for both surgical and nonsurgical patients. Using standardized LOS as an indication of routine services, we found significant differences that could not be explained by patient diagnosis and health-related characteristics. What is more important, we found evidence of even greater differences (up to fourfold) in some of the specific clinical services, perhaps due to less scrutiny of these services compared with LOS. For several of the most expensive services and for the summary measure of specific service intensity, we found evidence of significant differences that, though not of great magnitude, translate at a national level into millions of dollars more spent in the high-use hospitals for the same kinds of patients treated elsewhere for less. Whether there is a measurable benefit in terms of the quality of outcome for these additional dollars is an important question addressed in chapter 7.

7 · The Relation between the Intensity and the Duration of Medical Services and Outcomes for Hospitalized Patients

Ann Barry Flood, Wayne Ewy, W. Richard Scott, William H. Forrest, Jr., and Bryon W. Brown, Jr.

Much recent literature on the operation of the health care systems has concentrated on the issues of cost containment and the assurance of quality care. There is widespread agreement on the importance of these problems both as political issues and as research topics. But too frequently these problems have been addressed independently: proponents of higher-quality care fail to assess the impact of changes in the intensity of services on costs, and those searching for ways to reduce costs do not measure the impact on care quality of reductions in the amounts and types of services.

The cost and quality of care are inextricably linked to one another: both are a function, at least in part, of the intensity and duration of medical services. When policy makers attempt to change one of these factors without considering the other, serious malfunctioning in the health care system may result. Similarly, when researchers give exclusive attention to cost variables or to quality variables, serious distortions or omissions in the analysis of health care systems can occur. In the Service Intensity Study (SIS) we attempted to avoid this error, examining variations in the services and the quality of care in a sample of seventeen acute-care hospitals in the United States. This chapter reports a portion of that study, focusing on the relation between the intensity and duration of medical services provided to hospitalized patients and the resulting differences in the quality of their outcomes.

PROBLEMS IN ASSESSING SERVICES AND OUTCOMES

Before proceeding to describe the data base and methodology employed, we briefly discuss the general problems to be solved in assessing services,

For an earlier version of this chapter see Flood et al. 1979.

outcome, and their interrelationship (see chap. 4 for details). At the most general level, a hospital provides widely disparate types of services. While its primary service relates to inpatient care, most hospitals also provide varying amounts of education, research, community service, and outpatient care. Each of these services presents problems in measurement, for example, which indicators to choose and whether to focus on the quantity or the quality of services delivered.

In this research, we restricted ourselves to examining services provided to inpatients. Even though this decision eliminated the need to contrast or combine, for example, measures of education and inpatient care, complex problems in assessing services to patients still remained. In particular, the types of services provided and the amounts of each service differ vastly among hospitals. These differences arise chiefly from the varying requirements for services of the patients in each hospital, depending on their disease and general physical condition, but they can also arise from variations in the modes of treatment. The first source of variation is not of primary interest, since it only addresses the question, Do sicker patients receive more services? The second source has more interesting implications. Differences in services that are not due simply to patient condition can affect the total cost of the treatment and the quality of the services provided. Here we can address such questions as, Do more costly services lead to better-quality care? Several researchers have established that patient populations do differ significantly among hospitals (Feldstein 1967; Lave and Lave 1971; chap. 6 in this volume). Not to take these variations into account is to fail to acknowledge differences in the medical care demands placed on hospitals, for example, treating a fractured arm versus a fractured skull or appendicitis versus advanced cardiovascular disease. Thus the first requirement of research to compare the amount and the effectiveness of services provided to hospitalized patients is to take into account differences in the needs of the patients to be treated.

The next problem is to decide how to measure the amount and the quality of the services provided. Many approaches for assessing the output of health care services have been pursued. For the purposes of this discussion we identify five variations: (1) the use, as an indicator of services, of the amount and type of facilities available, assuming that the availability of more and better facilities implies that more and better services are in fact provided (Cohen 1970; Morse, Gordon, and Moch 1974); (2) the measurement of the quality of the services provided by evaluating whether or not the services provided match some predetermined standard set by physicians for treating the disease (Trussell, Morehead, and Ehrlich 1962; Payne et al. 1976); (3) the assessment of the amount of services provided by examining the length of stay for patients (Eckles and Root 1970); (4) the examination of costs of services, concentrating on costs either per patient-day or per patient episode (Carr and Feldstein 1967); and (5) the use of measures of outcomes to assess the quality of care (Roemer, Moustafa, and Hopkins 1968; Brook et al. 1977; chap. 5 in this volume).

The strengths and limitations of each of these solutions for characterizing the outputs of health care organizations have been enumerated many times before (Donabedian 1966; Scott 1977; chaps. 3 and 4 in this volume). The use of some of these measures requires researchers to make untenable assumptions. For example, to use the quality or quantity of the institutional facilities as a measure of the quality of care requires the assumption that quality care is obtained wherever facilities for good care exist, regardless of patient needs. To use adherence to current practice standards as the measure of care quality requires the assumption that these standards are themselves correct and invariably associated with better outcomes. Several attempts to establish the connection between performing the "correct" services and better outcomes have, however, failed to support this assumption (Brook 1973; Payne et al. 1976; chap. 12 in this volume). While measures of care based on length of stay (LOS) permit the consideration of differences in services based on patient condition they focus on the duration of services rather than either the quality or the quantity. Medical care services tend to be concentrated most heavily in the initial days of an episode rather than spread uniformly throughout. Thus, each additional day of stay is not an adequate index of additional intensity of services provided. Regional variations in LOS for the same types of patients further compromise the ability to compare LOS from hospital to hospital (Fuchs 1974). Measures of patient costs per day or per episode are a function not only of the differences in the quality and the quantity of services delivered but also of regional variation in prices as well as variation in the technical efficiency of a given hospital to provide low-cost services (see chap. 3, above). Finally, measures of outcome both permit the adjustment for differences in patient mix and avoid the assumption that the correct services imply that better outcomes will result. However, because such measures emphasize differences in the final outcomes obtained, they indicate only indirectly the quantity or the quality of the services provided.

The greatest single limitation of past research for examining the relation between the quantity of services provided and the quality of care obtained derives from the failure to provide independent measures of both concepts. Without independent measures, the question of the relation between the intensity and duration of services and the outcomes is handled only by inference rather than by empirical examination.

DATA AND METHODOLOGY

The SIS data used in this study were from the records of the over 600,000 patients treated during the period 1970–73 in seventeen acute-care hospitals in the United States. We have already described the selection of hospitals and methods for the SIS (see chap. 5) and the basic results for establishing that hospitals do differ significantly in services and outcomes, even after adjustment for patient mix (see chap. 6). Recall that ten states and all major geographic regions within the continental United States were represented in this sample. It should also be noted that the short-term hospitals from which this sample was drawn did not include any federal or proprietary hospitals.

The Measures

Data from the patient's PAS abstract record provided the basis for the measures of service intensity, including the types and amount of diagnostic and therapeutic services received during the hospitalization and the duration of services indicated by length of stay, as well as for the measure of patient outcome—death inhospital. In addition, information relating to the patient's disease and physical condition was used to adjust measures of service intensity and outcome for differences in patient mix.

Outcomes of Care

In order to examine the quality of services provided to patients in hospitals, the outcome of care (inhospital death) was measured.[1] The outcome measure was adjusted to take into account patient disease and physical condition, as described in chapters 5 and 6.

Measures of Service Intensity and Duration

Service intensity refers to the quantity of services received by a patient during a hospitalization episode. While many kinds of patient-care services provided by hospitals could be enumerated, we were limited to those services recorded on the PAS abstract. From these data we identified nine independent measures of service. Seven of these measures indicated important diagnostic and therapeutic services. The eighth was based on the number of consultations received during the hospitalization from physicians in different departments. The ninth, duration of services, was based on the number of days of hospitalization. Whenever possible, the amount of each individual service consumed, for example, the number of classes of drugs received or the number of operative procedures undergone, was assessed. In some cases, information was limited to the use or nonuse of service.

1. In the full set of analyses, three other outcome measures were developed. Two of these measures were based on inhospital death within a specified time period, seven days and forty days, respectively. Neither of these measures substantially altered any relationships reported here and so were excluded from this chapter. The third, inhospital complication, was found to be subject to substantial underreporting, which varied by hospital, so it too was dropped as an outcome measure.

In addition to these individual measures, two composite measures of services were developed. The intent of the first composite measure, the intensity of specific services, was to reflect the total amount of specific medical services provided to a given patient. To estimate this total, we considered three important aspects of the intensity of these services: (1) the total mix of different types of specific medical services received, (2) the amount of each type of specific service received, and (3) the relative costliness of each of the different types of services used. The components of this composite measure were the seven previously mentioned diagnostic and therapeutic services received during the hospitalization episode, including the use of intensive-care units. These components as a set represent, within the constraints of the data base, the total mix of diagnostic and therapeutic services a given patient received and, whenever data permitted, the actual amount of each service received. The third aspect of intensity, relative costliness, was reflected in a weight assigned to each individual component before combining them into the composite measure. These weights were based on the average proportion of total charges for a hospitalization episode associated with each type of specific service being measured. The weights were obtained from data on hospital charges supplied by a nonstudy hospital. They do not reflect the actual variations in charges in each study hospital but were uniformly applied for all hospitals. They do reflect the average relative costliness of providing a given type and amount of service. The individual measures used for this composite measure and their respective weights[2] are summarized in table 7.1.

The intent of the second composite measure,[3] the duration of services (length of stay) was to reflect the total amount of basic nursing care and hotel services provided to each patient. This total was estimated entirely on the basis of the number of days of hospitalization and did not take into account any variations among hospitals in the quality or quantity of these basic services.[4]

It is important to note that for each of these composite measures of services, the basic unit of analysis was the hospitalization episode for a patient. Other analysts have utilized a hospital day as the unit of analysis (Neuhauser

2. Since we used the actual amount of each diagnostic and therapeutic service whenever possible, the final weighting of the relative costliness of each service consisted of the proportion of charges for each service, as reported in table 7.1, divided by the amount of each type of service provided to study patients during a hospitalization. For example, since the average number of operations for study patients was 0.545, the final weight for the relative costliness of surgery was 14.27/0.545, or 26.183, applied to each operative procedure for a given patient.

3. The measure of duration of services was not strictly a *composite* measure, since it was based on only one individual measure.

4. In chapter 10 we attempt to measure variation in the quality and quantity of basic nursing services provided, such as the nurse–patient ratio, the proportion of the nursing staff who were registered nurses, and the average expenditures per patient-day.

Table 7.1. Components of the service intensity and duration indices and their weights

Items from the PAS Abstract	Class of Services Being Estimated	Proportion of Patient Charges (%)[a]	Weighting Factor of the PAS Item for Each Patient[b]
Components of the index of service intensity			
Diagnostic services			
Number of radiographic procedures performed	Radiological services	7.08	32.627 per procedure
Number of blood tests	Laboratory	8.48	12.676 per test
Therapeutic services			
Number of operative procedures	Surgery	14.27	26.183 per procedure
Administration of any blood or blood parts	Laboratory	2.83	52.407 if any blood given
Physical therapy	Therapy	2.66	52.157 if physical therapy given
Number of classes of drugs	Medical supplies	8.52	7.992 per class of drugs
Use of intensive-care unit	Special-care units	4.21	56.892 if special unit used
	Subtotal	48.05	
Component of the index of service duration			
Number of days in hospital	Hotel services Routine nursing care	51.95	6.185 per day
	Total	100.0	

[a]Based on the proportion of the average patient's bill attributable to a given service class, using 1973 figures from a nonstudy hospital.

[b]To obtain the weighting factor, the proportion of charges for the class was divided by the mean number of corresponding services on the PAS abstract actually used by patients in the study (see n. 3).

and Andersen 1972; Blumberg and Gentry 1978), which allows the investigation of variations in the level of services across the hospitalization episode. The approach in this chapter emphasizes the overall amount of services rendered. For the remainder of this chapter, analyses of services are restricted to the composite measure.[5]

5. A third composite measure, overall services, was developed to reflect both aspects of total services for a patient—specific medical services and duration of basic services—and was based on these two composite measures. The resultant standardized measure of overall services bore a very strong relationship to the measure of duration of services ($r = .90$). Since this measure added little to the understanding of the relation between intensity of services and outcome, we have dropped it from our presentation.

Standardization: The Rationale and the Procedure

The rationale and the procedure for standardization were essentially the same for both the intensity and the duration of services and outcomes. For simplicity's sake, we use services as the primary example. In the analyses reported in this chapter, the primary concern was to assess the impact on the outcome of care for patients of providing more or fewer services. How best to assess intensity of services is a difficult question, both theoretically and practically. As discussed earlier, one of the most important determinants of the amount and types of services is the nature of the disease and the general condition of the patient upon admission. Whether the patient is a surgical or medical patient is a second important determinant of the likelihood of his or her receiving specific amounts and types of services—use of blood being an obvious example. Third, complications arising during the hospitalization (intermediate outcomes) also increase the likelihood of requiring more services. Fourth, a patient who leaves the hospital before he or she is completely recovered not only receives fewer days of basic services but also is likely to forgo some specific medical services that might otherwise have been provided to achieve a satisfactory status at discharge. Death inhospital is, of course, the extreme example of incomplete recovery and brings an immediate cessation of need for further diagnostic and therapeutic services.

As described in chapter 6, the first step in measuring the level of intensity of services, then, is to define a set of measures that indicates the patient's status with regard to these four patient-related determinants of the intensity of services. We therefore defined four basic types of standardization sets: (1) admission status, including the major diagnosis explaining admission to the hospital (any of 332 diagnostic groups), several indicators of the patient's physiological status (such as additional diagnoses, admission test findings, and severity of the disease), and several demographic characteristics (such as age, sex, and height-weight index); (2) surgical or medical treatment, including the number of (nondiagnostic) operations and the severity of operations undergone; (3) complications, including inhospital infection or other complications; and (4) discharge status, including death at discharge, transfer to another facility, or discharge with incomplete recovery. In all, over forty different measures were defined in these four standardization sets.

We always used admission status to standardize the intensity of services and outcomes. In the full analyses we used various combinations of the other three types of standardization variables to estimate the intensity of a given type of service expected for a patient (Forrest et al. 1977). In the analyses reported here, however, the primary concern was the relation between the intensity of services and outcomes. Thus we did not want to include outcome or even intermediate outcomes such as complications as predictors of the intensity of services.[6]

In the standardization procedure, data from the detailed records of all 603,000 patients were pooled across hospitals within each of the 332 major diagnostic groups. Through linear regression, an estimate was obtained of the impact of each of the standardization variables (e.g., all those reflecting admission status) on the amount of medical services of a given type received by a patient. Then, multiplying these estimates (the unstandardized coefficients) by the patient's actual values on each standardization variable (e.g., age, admission-test findings, number of operations) and summing their products, we obtained the amount of services predicted for that patient. This predicted level of service was based on the typical experience of similar patients in the "standard hospital," which in this case was all the hospitals combined. We thereby knew both the amount of services predicted for a patient and the amount of services he or she actually received. We used the predicted amount as the baseline for a given patient against which we could observe whether he or she actually received more or fewer services than expected on the basis of his or her health status.[7]

In a similar fashion we obtained both the likelihood of dying in the hospital and whether or not the patient died. Again we used the comparison between these two to assess whether the patient had an outcome better or worse than expected. The greatest disparity occurred, of course, when a patient with a low likelihood of dying actually died or when a patient with a high likelihood of dying lived.

Because our primary interest was not whether sicker patients received more services or whether sicker patients were more likely to die, we did not conduct the critical comparison of outcome and service intensity at the patient level. What we were interested in was the impact on outcome of different modes of treating the same type of patient, that is, whether or not hospitals that tended to provide a higher or lower intensity of services compared with what would be typical also tended to produce better or worse outcomes compared with what would be expected. The final step, then, was to aggregate the standardized measures of intensity of specific services, duration of services, and outcomes for all patients in each study hospital.

6. The one major exception was duration of services, wherein we included discharge status as a predictor. As reported elsewhere, the inclusion of the additional sets of standardization variables made little empirical impact on the estimates, but we prefer to use the theoretically most appropriate set available.

7. It should be noted that the phrase "expected on the basis of health status" used throughout this chapter refers to this empirical prediction based on statistical analysis, and not on clinical judgments.

RESULTS

Before examining the relation between services provided and outcomes, we note the interrelationship among the standardized composite measures of services for hospitals using Pearson correlations (table 7.2). There was a slight tendency for more specific services than expected to be associated with a shorter duration of services (−.27). To indicate the impact of the standardization procedure, table 7.2 also presents, in parentheses, the Pearson correlations for the unstandardized measures. We note that a higher crude number of specific services bore a slight positive association with a longer duration of services (.18).

Table 7.2 also reports the correlation of standardized service intensity and duration measures to standardized outcomes. Here we note that a greater number of specific services was associated with a lower death rate (−.43). In contrast, a longer duration of services was associated with an increased death rate (.64). All correlations between standardized services and outcome were significant at the 10 percent level or less for a sample size of seventeen.

These results can be restated: hospitals that provided an excess amount of specific services to their patients had better than expected outcomes for those patients. But patients in hospitals that tended to keep patients in hospitals longer than expected experienced worse outcomes than expected. The implications of these results for policy decisions and for future research are important enough to justify additional examination of these data to ensure that the observed relations between services and outcomes were not artifactual.

Before presenting these additional analyses, we examine the relation between the composite measures of services and outcomes before standardizing for patient mix. These correlations, presented in parentheses in table 7.2, revealed no relation between crude rates of specific services and death rate (−.03 in contrast to .43 for the standardized measures). The relation between duration of services and death rate was in the same direction as seen in the standardized measure but smaller in magnitude (.59 compared with .64). Again we see that the results were strongly influenced by whether the analysis was performed on standardized or crude data. Taking into account the condition of the patients treated did affect the nature of the relations observed between service intensity, duration, and outcomes.

In table 7.3 the standardized death rates for the seventeen hospitals are displayed, classified according to whether the specific service intensity was greater or lower than expected and whether the duration of services was longer or shorter than expected. Looking first at the marginal effects, the eight hospitals providing more specific services than expected had a mean standardized death rate of −.28, in contrast to a mean of .28 for the nine hospitals with fewer specific services than expected. (The overall mean standardized death rate for

Table 7.2. The relation between service intensity, duration, and outcomes

Composite Measures of Service Intensity	Service Intensity		Outcomes
	Specific Services	Duration of Services	Inhospital Death
Specific services		−.27 (.18)	−.43* (−.03)
Duration of services			.64*** (.59)**

Note: Entries are zero-order Pearson product-moment correlations among hospital-level averages based on 603,580 patients treated in the 17 hospitals. Main entries are measures standardized to remove differences in patient mix. Entries in parentheses are crude rates of services and outcomes.
  $*p \leq .10$ $**p \leq .05$ $***p \leq .01$

the seventeen hospitals was .01, with a standard deviation of .52.) The hospitals that provided a shorter duration of services than expected had a mean standardized death rate of −.35, in contrast to a mean of .43 for the eight hospitals with a longer duration than expected. These marginal effects followed the findings reported in table 7.2.

Turning to the main cell entries of table 7.3, the two effects of services appeared to combine strongly: the four hospitals with the best (lowest) standardized death rates were among the five hospitals in the cell with more specific services and shorter duration of services. And the five hospitals with the worst (highest) standardized death rates appeared without exception in the cell with fewer specific services and longer duration of services. Consistent with the effect reported in table 7.2 and in the margins of table 7.3, the effect of standardized duration of services was stronger than that of specific services. That is, the hospitals ranked fifth, sixth, seventh, and eleventh best in terms of their standardized outcomes were in the cell with shorter duration and fewer specific services, while the hospitals ranked ninth, tenth, and twelfth best were in the cell with longer duration and more specific services. These two dichotomized measures provided nearly perfect discrimination of hospitals into the four cells of increasing standardized death rates.

In table 7.4 we present formal statistical tests of significance for these results using an ANOVA approach. We choose an ANOVA approach in order to be able to estimate the two basic sources of variability in our measures: random variation of patients within hospitals and error in the fit of the model relating variation in the measures of service intensity to variation in standardized outcomes. Estimates of both types of variability were derived from the differences among the hospitals' means. The first two sets of ANOVAs in table 7.4 examined the effects on the standardized outcome (i.e., death rates) associated with classifying the hospitals into high or low standardized service intensity. They

Table 7.3. Standardized outcomes at the hospital level, classified by standardized service intensity and duration

Specific Services	Duration of Services					
	Shorter Than Expected		Longer Than Expected		Ignored	
More than expected	5 hospitals	−0.27	3 hospitals	−0.02	8 hospitals	
		−0.44		−0.06		
		−0.47		0.14		
		−0.55				
		−0.58				
	Mean	−0.46	Mean	0.02	Mean	−0.28
	S.D.	0.12	S.D.	0.11	S.D.	0.27
Fewer than expected	4 hospitals	−0.27	5 hospitals	0.31	9 hospitals	
		−0.35		0.34		
		−0.35		0.51		
		0.09		1.14		
				1.07		
	Mean	−0.22	Mean	0.67	Mean	0.28
	S.D.	0.21	S.D.	0.40	S.D.	0.56
Ignored	9 hospitals		8 hospitals		17 hospitals	
	Mean	−0.35	Mean	0.43	Overall mean	0.01
	S.D.	0.20	S.D.	0.46	Overall S.D.	0.52

Note: Entries represent the standardized inhospital death rate for each hospital. A negative score indicates fewer deaths than expected. The hospitals have been dichotomized on the basis of their standardized service intensity for specific services and for duration of services.

correspond directly to the marginal effects observed in table 7.3 and to the correlational analyses in table 7.2, except that service intensity was treated here as a dichotomized variable. For both standardized duration of services and specific services, there was strong evidence that service intensity was related to outcome. As before, the evidence was stronger for standardized duration of services, with a p value of less than .001 and an R^2 of .593. For standardized specific services, the p value was .023, and the R^2 was .301.

The final set of ANOVA results in table 7.4 presents a two-way analysis of the death rate measures corresponding to the two-way classification in table 7.3. The impact of the main effects of each measure of standardized service intensity was clearly demonstrated. We expected these main effects to appear even stronger because any interactive effect of the other measure of service intensity had been removed; the p value was .005 or less for each main effect.

Table 7.4. ANOVAs of standardized death rates for hospitals, classified by high or low standardized service intensity and duration measures

	Degrees of Freedom	Mean Square	F Ratio	p Value
	One-way ANOVA classified by high or low standardized duration of service			
Duration of services	1	2.607	21.9	$<.001$
Residual	15	0.120		
R^2 of .593				
	One-way ANOVA classified by high or low standardized specific service intensity			
Specific services	1	1.321	6.5	.023
Residual	15	0.205		
R^2 of .301				
	Two-way ANOVA classified by high or low standardized duration and specific service intensity			
Main effects	2	1.684	25.7	$<.001$
Specific services	1	0.761	11.6	.005
Duration of services	1	2.047	31.2	$<.001$
Interaction	1	0.171	2.6	.131
Main effect and interaction	3	1.179	18.0	$<.001$
Residual	13	0.066		
Total	16	0.274		
Multiple R^2 of .767				

Testing for an interaction effect did not reveal a significant nonadditive effect of service intensity on outcome (the p value was .123). The amount of variance in the standardized death rates accounted for by this two-way ANOVA of the effect of service intensity was .767.

Another factor may account for these results. It is well documented that length of stay in hospitals is influenced in part by regional differences in medical practices. There is also evidence to suggest that the types of patients, as well as the types of services and outcomes, vary by region. Since our study hospitals were sampled from a national set of acute-care hospitals, we can investigate the possibility of regional variations' accounting for the relationship between the hospital-level measures of services and outcomes. All four major census regions of the continental United States—Northeast, North Central, South, and West—were represented by our sample of seventeen hospitals. (Since only one hospital was located in the North Central region, in table 7.5 we present the information for this hospital combined with the hospitals in the

Table 7.5. Regional variation in measures of services and outcomes

Region	Number of Study Hospitals	Duration of Services		Specific Services		Outcome: Inhospital Death	
		Crude	Standardized	Crude	Standardized	Crude	Standardized
North[a]	9	9.27(1.20)	0.84(0.60)	46.31(3.31)	−1.00(2.35)	4.03(1.21)	0.34(0.50)
South	3	7.06(0.80)	−0.54(0.11)	42.01(9.80)	−3.73(5.61)	2.88(0.44)	−0.39(0.14)
West	5	7.15(1.28)	−1.58(0.91)	52.19(7.93)	1.63(2.46)	2.57(1.13)	−0.33(0.26)
Total	17	8.26(1.56)	−0.11(1.27)	47.28(6.82)	−0.70(3.42)	3.40(1.25)	0.01(0.52)
From ANOVA							
F ratio		7.168	22.018	2.797	2.953	3.175	6.247
p value		.0072	.0001	.0951	.0851	.0729	.0115
Multiple R^2		.506	.759	.285	.297	.680	.500

Note: The main entries for this table are the means and, in parentheses, the standard deviation for hospital-level crude and standardized measures of duration (in days), specific services (in weights as detailed in table 7.1), and outcome (in the percentage of inhospital deaths).
[a]*North* combines both the Northeast (with 8 hospitals) and the North Central (1 hospital) region.

Northeast region, resulting in three regions for examination: North, South, and West.)

If we examine the crude average length of stay for hospitals in each region, the hospitals appear to vary by region, with the northern hospitals keeping patients the longest (9.27 days) and the southern hospitals, the shortest (7.06 days). However, when patient disease and physical condition were taken into account in the standardized measures, the northern hospitals still kept their patients the longest (nearly a day longer than expected), but the hospitals in the West kept their patients the shortest (a day and a half less than expected). A one-way ANOVA testing for regional effects was significant at less than .001 for crude duration of services and at less than .0001 for standardized duration of services.

Specific services revealed a somewhat different and less distinct pattern: the western hospitals provided on the average the highest crude specific services per patient, and the southern hospitals, the lowest. Taking patient disease and physical condition into account did not alter this relationship: the western hospitals provided more specific services than expected, and the southern hospitals provided fewer than expected. A one-way ANOVA was significant at less than .01 for both hospital-level measures of specific services. For outcomes, measured by inhospital mortality, hospitals in the North had on the average the highest crude death rate, with 4.03 percent of patients dying, and the West had the lowest, with a death rate of 2.57 percent. This relationship was preserved for the standardized measures of outcomes as well, but the ANOVA for regional effects was more pronounced for the standardized death rate (significant at less than .01) than for the crude rate (significant at less than .1).

Having found evidence of regional effects for standardized measures of the intensity of specific services, the duration of services, and outcomes, we then investigated their relationship within each region. Directly paralleling the procedure used in table 7.3, we divided the entire set of hospitals into (*a*) those with longer than expected duration of services versus those with shorter than expected and (*b*) those with less specific services than expected versus those with more than expected. Then we inspected the standardized death rate for hospitals within each region as cross classified by specific services and duration of services. For the nine hospitals in the North, only one hospital had shorter lengths of stay than expected. This hospital also had fewer specific services than expected and was the top-ranked hospital in terms of its outcomes (i.e., it had the best care, measured by the lowest standardized death rate) of all the hospitals in this region. Of the remaining eight hospitals with a longer duration of services than expected, the three providing more specific services were the three next best hospitals (with a mean standardized death rate of 0.02), and the five with fewer services were the five poorest hospitals (with a mean of 0.67). Thus, among the eight hospitals with longer duration, the intensity of specific services perfectly partitioned the hospitals into the three best (with more specific services) and the five poorest hospitals (with fewer services).

Among the five hospitals in the West, none provided a greater than average duration of services to its patients. Four of the five hospitals provided more specific services than expected; the one that did not was ranked fifth among these hospitals in terms of its standardized death rate. Again, the intensity of services perfectly partitioned the hospitals, with the four best (having a mean standardized death rate of -0.44) providing more services and the poorest (0.09) providing fewer specific services.

This pattern was repeated for the three hospitals in the South. None of these hospitals provided a longer duration of services than expected. The one hospital providing more specific services than expected had the best outcomes (-0.55), and the two hospitals providing fewer services than expected had a mean standardized death rate of -0.31.

In general, it would appear that most of the impact of duration of services (i.e., length of stay) on outcome was due to regional variation. However, within each region, the intensity of specific services provided perfect discrimination among the standardized death rates of the hospitals, with more specific services being associated with better outcomes.

SUMMARY

We found strong consistent evidence that after careful standardization to estimate the amount of services and the level of outcome typically expected for each patient, the outcomes obtained by patients in hospitals were associated with the intensity and duration of services provided. In particular we found that hospitals providing more specific services than expected to their patients exhibited better outcomes than expected, conversely, hospitals that provided shorter duration of services than expected had better outcomes than expected.

Since our study hospitals were drawn from a national sample of hospitals, we investigated the possibility of regional variations in (1) duration of services, (2) specific services, and (3) outcomes. Using three major regions of the United States, we found strong evidence to support the claim of regional variation in medical practices, particularly for length of stay in hospitals. And for both measures of services and for outcomes, regional effects were more pronounced after we adjusted for patient mix. Thus, regional effects could not be explained away by differences in the health of patients in each region but indicated real differences in modes of treatment. Given the strength of the findings regarding regional variation in length of stay and outcomes for patients in hospitals within each region, the relation between duration of services and outcomes observed in the entire set of hospitals was probably due to regional variations in medical practices rather than to hospital differences. These results also led us to conclude that the interpretation of length of stay either as a measure of basic services provided or, as some authors have suggested, as a surrogate for outcome is seriously compromised by variations among hospitals due simply to regional differences in modes of treatment. On the other hand, the apparent strength of the findings regarding specific services and outcomes, coupled with consistent results within regions, encourages us to seek to examine outcome benefits associated with each of the component measures of specific services. For certain specific diagnostic categories, we would expect to find that certain classes of services are more highly associated with outcome.

These results are consistent with the intuitive belief that for any given patient, providing a higher level of services is associated with a better health status. By the same token, they are inconsistent with contemporary claims that medical care services bear little or no relation to health outcomes. It is important to note that such conclusions from our results must assume an association at the patient level—a patient was less likely to die if he or she received a higher level of services—although our analyses were conducted at the hospital level. Thus, our data really showed that the *set* of patients in hospitals that provided greater intensity of services than typically provided tended to have better outcomes than would have been expected for that *set* of patients. Since these relationships were observed at the hospital level, it is possible that the relationship at the level of the individual patient differs; for example, it is conceivable that increasing the intensity of services for most patients in a hospital would not significantly alter their chances for a better outcome (see chap. 4 for a discussion of aggregation effects).

Since these analyses were limited to inhospital death as the only reliable measure of outcome, the strength and consistency of the relationship we observed may pertain only to life-threatening situations. A more restricted interpretation of our results may be in order: for patients at risk of death, a higher level of services, such as more use of the intensive-care unit, appears to have been a crucial determinant of whether or not they survived. We had no way of establishing whether the relationship also held for less serious outcomes. Unfortunately, we had no reliable measures of morbidity in the PAS data base, nor did the type of analysis carried out permit a "split half" approach to examining whether or not the association was stronger for patients who were sicker initially.

Having gone to much expense and effort to standardize services and outcomes for patient characteristics, we emphasize the impact of these procedures on the results observed. Crude service and death rates exhibited relationships that were quite distinct from those observed following standardization. Careful standardization to take into account the effect of differences among the patient groups served is essential if the relation between care processes (services) and outcomes is to be validly examined. Also, independent indicators of services and outcomes are necessary if we are to meaningfully evaluate the relation between care processes and outcomes.

Turning to health policy concerns, the methodological implications of our work may be more important than the substantive findings. Our research demonstrated that data obtained from patient abstracts, if treated in enough detail and with very careful statistical adjustment for variations in case mix, can be successfully employed to examine differences in services provided by hospitals and the quality of care delivered.[8] The implications of this approach for the feasibility of establishing large-scale monitoring systems to evaluate the costs and quality of health care in hospitals can be of the greatest importance for national health policy.

8. The SCHCR conducted an independent study of the reliability of PAS abstract data. Selected patient records from the study hospitals were reabstracted and the results compared to the original PAS abstract for the same patient. While there was substantial evidence of errors in recording data, these errors were randomly distributed across hospitals and so did not bear directly on the conclusions of this chapter. They would indicate, however, the need for stronger data quality control if these data were to be adopted for national health care monitoring.

PART III

Effects of Surgeons and Surgical Staff Organization on Hospital Performance

8 · Effectiveness in Professional Organizations: The Impact of Surgeons and Surgical Staff Organizations on the Quality of Care

Ann Barry Flood, W. Richard Scott, Wayne Ewy, and William H. Forrest, Jr.

Throughout the decade of the 1960s, students of organizational structure focused their energies on discovering the determinants of varying structural arrangements. Differences in size, goals, technologies, and environments were examined to determine their impact on organizational structures such as coordination mechanisms and differentiation (Woodward 1965; Pugh et al. 1968; Blau and Schoenherr 1971). During the 1970s, organizational theorists began to turn their attention to discovering the consequences of varying structural arrangements. What characteristics of organizations and their environments are predictive of more efficient functioning or better performance? A growing literature on organizational effectiveness addresses these questions (Friedlander and Pickle 1968; Goodman and Pennings 1977; Steers 1977; and Shortell and Kaluzny 1983).

In our study we sought to examine the determinants of effectiveness in general hospitals. The major theoretical decisions we confronted involved defining and choosing appropriate indicators of effectiveness and conceptualizing hospital structure. Both types of decisions become quite complicated when the subjects of study are professional organizations as complex as hospitals.

THEORETICAL ISSUES

Chapter 4 contains a detailed discussion of the conceptual and methodological issues involved in assessing hospital performance. Here we briefly review some of these problems from an organizational-theory perspective.

For an earlier version of this chapter see Flood et al. 1982.

Conceptualizing Effectiveness

Effectiveness may be defined as the extent to which an organization is successful in reaching its goals. This deceptively simple definition becomes very complex when it is recognized that (1) definitions of goals vary depending on the theoretical perspective used (e.g., output goals would be emphasized in a rational-system perspective, while system or maintenance goals would be stressed in a natural-system perspective) (Yuchman and Seashore 1967; Gross 1968); (2) organizations are recognized as pursuing multiple and sometimes incompatible objectives simultaneously, so that an assessment of overall effectiveness is always somewhat arbitrary and incomplete (Simon 1964); and (3) multiple constituencies can and do vary in evaluating the importance of different goals and in choosing the criteria necessary to determine "success" at reaching the goals, so that organizational assessment is often a controversial political action supported by some interested parties and resisted by others (Goodman and Pennings 1977).

Assessing effectiveness is difficult and controversial in any professional organizational setting.[1] Law firms, hospitals, universities, and research organizations are often "multiproduct" firms, serving diverse groups and interests. Hospitals, for example, provide a wide array of services to a diverse set of patients and often engage in teaching and research. For the analyst, deciding which aspects of performance to emphasize is difficult, since the resultant measure of effectiveness can vary according to the aspects examined. For this study, we focused on the quality of inhospital surgical care as one aspect of hospital effectiveness. We recognized that this was a restricted focus, but our purpose was to direct attention to one of the important services offered by hospitals, as viewed by both organizational participants and clients.

Evaluating the effectiveness of professional organizations is problematic for another reason. Professional work is allegedly more complex and uncertain than other types of work; correct performance does not invariably produce successful outcome. As a consequence, measures of professional work emphasize the work process—for example, in the hospital, the thoroughness of a diagnostic workup of a patient or student-contact hours—rather than work outcomes—such as improvements in a patient's condition or changes in students' knowledge or abilities—as appropriate indicators of effectiveness (Hughes 1958; Freidson 1970; Dornbusch and Scott 1975). Process measures evaluate effort or conformity to established practice norms but do not directly assess the effectiveness of the activities performed (Suchman 1967). In the few studies that have attempted to examine whether or not good performance im-

---

1. These general issues surrounding the assessment of effectiveness are discussed in more detail in Scott 1977; Scott et al. 1978; and chap. 4 in this volume.

proved the chances for successful outcome, such evidence was lacking or unconvincing (Brook et al. 1971; Brook and Appel 1973).

Several articles and books have addressed the limitations and strengths of measures of both outcome and process (Donabedian 1978, 1980, 1982; McAuliffe 1978; chap. 4 in this volume). These authors have argued that the choice of the most appropriate measure depends on the aims of the research. In the absence of support that good performance and improved outcomes are closely linked, we believe that research seeking to understand the impact of organizational and individual variables on health care should be based on outcomes. Process measures invariably focus on a subset of the health care professionals involved. The question becomes, Were nursing or physician or administrative procedures correctly followed? Outcome measures have the benefit of summarizing actions by all units and health care professionals involved in the treatment.

The level of outcome achieved does not depend solely on the quality or the quantity of professional service offered; it is responsive to a variety of other factors as well. The work is more difficult in some cases than in others; for example, some surgery is more difficult than others, and some subjects taught are more abstract and complex. The patient's or student's initial status, given the same degree of improvement, also influences the final level of outcome achieved. To be valid indicators of effectiveness, outcome measures need to take into account both of these factors. Thus, in the case of surgical care for hospitalized patients, outcome measures, such as morbidity or mortality, need to be adjusted so that hospitals and surgeons who treat more seriously ill patients or perform more complex surgical procedures are viewed equitably when outcome results compare their patients with patients less ill. We think such adjustments are possible for surgical care; in chapter 5 we detail our procedures for adjusting surgical outcome evaluations to take into account patient differences. As a further advantage, our measures of adjusted outcomes do not require the determination of a universal standard for evaluating the quality of outcome. Instead, we make comparisons of quality relative to the distribution of outcomes experienced by comparable groups of patients in all of the hospitals surveyed.

Conceptualizing Organizational Structure

Organizations are complex systems, and relatively little theoretical work has emphasized the problem of identifying those structural features most salient for performance. Professional organizations represent especially complex systems because many units may contribute toward the performance output. One might attribute the performance of a typical organization to the entire organization—in our case, the hospital. In a professional organization, the professional staff is often granted autonomy to organize and exercise considerable control over the conduct of professional work; in the case of surgical care, the responsible organizational unit may be the entire professional staff of surgeons. Alternatively, the individual practitioner may be allowed to exercise a great deal of discretion in the work conducted on his or her own patients. In this case the relevant performance unit accounting for the quality of surgical care may be the individual surgeon. Thus, the quality of work performed within these settings can variously be attributed to the characteristics of (1) the larger organizational context; (2) the corporate structure by which the professionals organize themselves; or (3) the individual practitioners, either individually or in aggregate, depending on the level of analysis utilized. Since all of these alternatives can possibly account for the quality of surgical care, and their relative importance can vary across organizations, we have developed measures for all three types of organizational units: the hospital, the surgical staff, and individual surgeons. Our research, however, places particular emphasis on the characteristics of the latter two. Only a few measures of hospital context are considered in this chapter, and they are treated primarily as control variables, allowing us to evaluate broad differences in hospital characteristics before examining the effects specific to surgical staff organization or individual surgeons. (Chap. 9 presents analyses involving more hospital characteristics.)

Previous studies of organizations have suggested the relevance of several classes of structural variables in accounting for differences in effectiveness (Lawrence and Lorsch 1967; Neuhauser 1971; Roemer and Friedman 1971; Khandwalla 1974). The primary structural variables examined in our study were power, differentiation, coordination, staff qualifications, and commitment. These variables are applicable to each type of organizational unit just identified; and measures for most of them are available for each unit in the IS data base. Since predictions relating these structural variables to effectiveness vary somewhat according to organizational unit, our hypotheses are described below in association with the specific organizational measures.

We begin by introducing new measures from the IS used in this chapter. Next the principal measures for hospital, surgical staff, and surgeons are described and operationalized. Finally, the relation between measures of the professional organizational units and of effectiveness are examined and discussed.

DATA SOURCES AND THE SIZE OF THE SAMPLES

The IS data base was collected as part of the larger investigation of factors affecting the quality of surgical care in hospitals. Hospital selection, patient outcomes, and methods for standardizing outcome to adjust for patient health are detailed in chapter 5. Here we use the Intermediate Scaled Outcomes, with the standardized version expressed as the difference between the outcome achieved and the outcome expected based on patient health.[2] Seventeen hospitals were surveyed for the original study, but only fifteen were included in this analysis because data on surgeon characteristics for the remaining two were incomplete.

Chapter 1 details the methods and measures for the organizational data in the IS. We briefly review those measures used in the analysis reported in this chapter. Information on organizational characteristics relating to both hospital context and the corporate organization of the medical/surgical staff was obtained through interviews with key personnel acting as expert informants on the structure and operation of their units. Most of the data utilized in this analysis were based on interviews with hospital administrators and chiefs of surgical services.[3]

Data on the characteristics of individual surgeons came from three sources. First, working with a number code to ensure the surgeons' anonymity, information on the education and board certification of all surgeons treating study patients was obtained from either the records of the AMA or those of the study hospital. Second, since surgeons often practice in more than one hospital, our technician asked each surgeon to estimate the proportion of his or her practice carried out in the study hospital. Third, PAS patient records were utilized to develop measures for each surgeon for the total number of operations and the proportion of specialized operations performed during the study period. These data relate to all patients treated by these surgeons in the study hospitals during 1973, not just to the study patients. The average number of operations performed annually by study surgeons in the fifteen hospitals and at least some of the types of information just described were available for 98 percent (544) of them.[4]

2. Postsurgical status was measured in terms of the short-term outcome, which was defined as the extent of morbidity occurring seven days after surgery or any death occurring within forty days after surgery. The nurse on the patient's postsurgical ward was asked a variety of questions regarding the patient's health status, but we analyzed here only the overall assessment of the patient's condition using the weighted Intermediate Scaled Outcome, defined in table 5.9.

Information on the patient's educational level, income level, marital status, ethnicity, and the number of recent life crisis events was included in preliminary analyses, but when the health characteristics of the patient were taken into account, only a lower income level was significantly predictive of more postoperative morbidity. Income level was included in subsequent analyses but did not influence any of the findings. Consequently, all socioeconomic and personal variables have been dropped from the analyses reported in this chapter.

3. As previously noted, two of the hospitals were operationally linked. While representing different contexts, they shared the same surgical staff organization. Thus, data on fifteen hospitals and fourteen surgical organizations were employed in this analysis.

4. Since two of the hospitals shared the same surgical staff, for some analyses examining the impact of surgeon characteristics on patient outcomes, surgeons treating study patients in both hospitals were included and in this sense were counted twice. For this reason the N for surgeons in some analyses is 605 rather than 544.

In the analyses we report here, it was important to distinguish between the impact of the individual practitioner and that of the hospital context of the surgical staff organization on outcomes. To do these comparisons properly, it was necessary to relate the relevant characteristics of each surgeon to the outcomes for specific patients treated by that surgeon within the hospital. Thus, the analyses were performed at the patient level, matching the patient's outcome with descriptions of his or her surgeon and with the hospital in which the operation occurred, which allowed us to examine directly the importance of the individual surgeon for predicting outcome, avoiding possible biases in interpreting aggregated data only.[5] We also related aggregated versions of surgeon's characteristics to patient outcomes, which allowed us to test whether there was an effect on outcome due to a collegial context as measured by the qualifications of the average surgeon at the hospital.[6]

MEASURING THE CHARACTERISTICS OF THE HOSPITAL, THE SURGICAL STAFF ORGANIZATION, AND THE SURGEON

As discussed previously, the primary structural variables examined were power, differentiation, coordination, staff qualifications, and commitment. A large number of measures within each of these variables were developed, and data were collected across several functional units within each hospital, including the larger hospital context, the surgical staff organization, and the individual surgeons. For present purposes, we have selected only one or, at most, two measures from each variable, measures that (a) were theoretically meaningful; (b) were among those determined to be most valid and reliable; and (c) related as expected to alternative indicators of the same variable. We briefly describe these selected measures here. (See Flood 1976; Forrest et al. 1978; and chap. 1 in this volume for further detail.)

The Hospital Context

Three measures were employed to assess hospital context. As already noted, measures of the hospital context served primarily as control variables in

5. For a more detailed description of the biases that can arise from analyzing data at the wrong level of analysis see Hannan 1971; Hannan, Freeman, and Meyer 1976; and chap. 4 in this volume.
6. Consistent with the patient-level approach employed, the characteristics describing each surgeon and each hospital were duplicated for all patients being treated by that physician or in that hospital. Thus, the means and correlations used in this analysis were weighted by the number of relevant observations, in this case the number of treated patients. Throughout this

this study. Size was measured as a product of the number of beds and the average occupancy rate for each hospital. This indicator was highly correlated with other measures of size, such as the number of employees; it was also strongly and positively correlated with measures of differentiation, such as the number of different departmental units or occupations present in the hospital. Other things being equal, we expected larger hospital size, because of its association with increased specialization, to be associated with higher-quality surgical care.

Expenditures for patient care were measured by dividing the total annual hospital expenditures by the number of patient-days. For hospitals in our sample, this measure was positively associated with both differentiation and coordination indicators. Because of these associations and because money allows the purchase of more and better facilities and equipment and attracts more and better-qualified staff, we expected more expenditures to be associated with higher-quality care.

The teaching status of a hospital was indicated by the presence of an active residency program. Like size and expenditures, teaching status was positively correlated with differentiation within the hospital. Previous research suggested that teaching hospitals deliver higher-quality medical care, although most of these studies were based on process rather than outcome indicators of quality (see reviews in Goss 1970; and chap. 3 in this volume). For the fifteen hospitals, teaching status was positively correlated (.53) with expenses per patient-day. The other control variables were not significantly intercorrelated.[7]

Surgical Staff Organization

The measures used to assess the power of the surgical staff over its own members were based on the strictness of admission requirements for new members of the surgical staff. Based on information supplied by the chief of surgery in each hospital, four indicators were given equal weight and combined into a single index: the average length of the probationary period; the probation waiver (1 if waived, 0 if not); the probation difference by specialty (1 if different, 0 if not); and the number of review bodies that must pass on the appointment. It was our expectation that better surgical care would result from the exercise of more control by the professional staff over its own members (see chap. 9 for more on this).

Differentiation within the surgical staff was measured by the number of surgical specialties listed and actively used by each hospital, based on the report

---

chapter, the means and correlations presented are the weighted versions used in these analyses. For this reason, they differ slightly from reports based on unweighted data.

7. For these hospital measures and for all measures of surgical staff organization for which the *N* was fifteen, only intercorrelations significant at the .1 level or lower are reported.

of the chief of surgery. Our expectation was that the more specialized the surgical care, the better the quality of the care.[8]

Several different types of coordination measures were collected and analyzed in our original design. Based on the selection criteria noted earlier, we found one of the most important mechanisms for coordination within the physician staff to be the presence of contractual or salaried physicians. We argue that these physicians provide coordinating activities through two mechanisms. They are most likely to serve in specialties such as anesthesia, pathology, and radiology, where they consult frequently with other physicians, or as clinical administrators or chiefs of services, where they serve on committees and perform other administrative services.

We used as our indicator for coordination the proportion of the medical staff who were contract physicians (reported by the hospital administrator). This type of indicator was first used by Roemer and Friedman (1971), who regarded it as the best simple index of the extent of organization of the medical staff. This indicator correlated positively with the measure of admissions requirements for new members (.41). We expected that the higher the level of coordination (reflected in contract physicians), the better the quality of care.

As an indicator of the general level of qualifications of the surgical staff, we used the proportion of surgeons who were board-certified. Board certification—given after successful completion of an examination testing one's competency in a medical specialty—is widely used as a measure of a physician's competence. We expected that the greater the proportion of board-certified surgeons on the staff, the better the quality of care.

Finally, to measure organizational commitment, we asked surgeons to report, via questionnaire, the percentage of their overall practice conducted at the study hospital. The average percentage of practice at the study hospital was used as the measure of the general commitment of the surgical staff. Higher average commitment by the surgical staff to the hospital was expected to be associated with better care.

The Individual Surgeons

Measures were developed to assess individual surgeons for three of the five variables: differentiation (i.e., specialization at the individual level), qualifications, and commitment. Several of these measures were simply the individual counterparts of the aggregate measures used to characterize the surgical staff. To measure the specialization of the work of individual surgeons, we used

---

8. More complex contingent predictions were investigated, for example, that differentiation was associated with high-quality care only if coordination needs were met; however, these analyses are not reported here.

information from medical abstract records reflecting all the surgery performed by an individual surgeon in the study hospital during 1973. Each nonminor operation was coded into one of twelve specialty groups. The measure of surgical specialization was the number of types of surgery performed subtracted from twelve—the total possible. As might be expected, this index correlated negatively with the number of years in practice (−.17). It also correlated negatively with the percentage of the surgeon's practice conducted at the study hospital (−.14), suggesting that some surgeons might be specialized, not necessarily in their entire practice, but in their surgery conducted at the study hospital.[9] Other things being equal, we expected higher levels of surgeon specialization to be associated with better outcomes.

Three measures of qualifications were used: (1) whether or not the surgeon was board-certified, (2) the number of residencies completed, and (3) as an indicator of experience, the number of years in practice after completion of any residency training. The three measures were not significantly related except that the number of years in practice was negatively associated with the number of residencies, which may be the result of the recent trend toward completing more, shorter, and more specialized residencies. We expected that greater length of training and experience (at least up to some point) would be associated with better-quality care.[10]

To measure commitment, we used the percentage of each surgeon's practice conducted at the study hospital, an individual counterpart of the surgical staff measure previously discussed. In addition to correlating negatively with surgical specialization (as already noted), this measure also correlated negatively with the number of residencies (−.25). As before, we expected greater commitment to be associated with better-quality care.[11]

9. For measures of individual surgeons with an *N* of over 500, only intercorrelations significant at the .001 level or lower are reported.

10. Several authors have reported a curvilinear relation between physician experience and quality (see chap. 3); that is, both very recent graduates and those trained many years previously tend to produce poorer-quality care. Recent examination of the IS data, limited to surgeons performing biliary tract disease, did not find support for a curvilinear relationship (Sharp 1986).

11. The percentage of the surgeon's practice conducted at the study hospital was related but not identical to the volume of cases treated by that surgeon. For surgeons with the same total volume of procedures performed annually in any hospital, the percentage of their practice conducted at the study hospital can serve to indicate which surgeons were more "committed" to the study hospital. We observed, in our results, a higher percentage of practice at the study hospital was strongly predictive of a higher total volume of cases across all hospitals (an estimated measure based on the surgeon's report). See Sharp (1986) for an examination of the effects of volume of similar cases on the quality of care (carried out at the level of the individual surgeons and at a hospital level in the IS, using patients undergoing biliary tract surgery).

RESULTS

To evaluate the impact of various facets of organizational structure on the quality of surgical care, we used two approaches. First, we used ANOVA to compare the importance of hospital organization (including surgical staff organization) with that of individual surgeons for explaining differences in the quality of care. Second, we carried out regression analyses in order to assess and compare the impact on adjusted surgical outcomes of measures of hospital context, surgical staff organization, and individual surgeons.

The Hospital Effect versus the Surgeon Effect

ANOVAs in adjusted surgical outcomes were based on those patients in the fifteen hospitals for whom we could identify the principal surgeon performing the operation. This was the case for over 90 percent, or 7,328 patients, of these patients. These patients were treated by 553 surgeons. In table 8.1 we present the results of three ANOVAs based on our adjusted measure of postsurgical outcome. Rows 1 and 2 present the results of an ANOVA for differences in adjusted surgical outcomes among hospitals. Among the fifteen study hospitals, there were highly significant differences ($p \leq .001$). This finding parallels our results in chapter 6 and suggests (*a*) that the hospitals differed significantly in the quality of care delivered and that such differences remained even after taking into account differences that might be due to patient mix (measured by our variables); and (*b*) that it is important to pursue the identity of the specific factors associated with these differences.

The one-way analysis presented in rows 1 and 2, however, ignored an alternative potential source for these observed differences, namely, variations in performance among surgeons treating the patients. Rows 3 and 4 tested for differences in adjusted outcome among surgeons. These results, significant at the .004 level, ignored any effect of the hospital and its associated surgical staff organization on differences in outcome.

A more appropriate model for testing for differences among hospitals and surgeons would evaluate both sources of variation simultaneously. We used a hierarchical analysis of variance to perform a two-way ANOVA in order to take into account the grouping of surgeons by hospital (Kempthorne 1952). The hierarchical, two-way ANOVA is presented in rows 5–7 and can be viewed as decomposing the differences found among surgeons (row 3) into a component for variation among surgeons within a hospital and a component for variation among hospitals, after taking the surgeons into consideration. This resulted in a more valid test for variation among surgeons,[12] since hospital-level effects

12. We tested for variation among surgeons within hospitals. To the extent that surgeons were not randomly distributed in hospitals with regard to quality, we could not distinguish the net difference in outcome at the hospital level using the first approach.

Table 8.1. ANOVAs of adjusted surgical outcome among hospitals and among surgeons

Source	Degrees of Freedom	Sum of Squares	Mean Squares	F Ratio	Significance Level for F	Expected Value for Mean Squares
One-way ANOVA—among hospitals						
(1) Among hospitals, ignoring surgeons	14	82.2113	5.8722	6.646	.001	
(2) Residual, for hospitals	7,313	6,461.9961	0.8836			
One-way ANOVA—among surgeons						
(3) Among surgeons, ignoring hospitals	552	568.8127	1.0305	1.168	.004	
(4) Residual, for surgeons	6,775	5,975.3555	0.8820			
Hierarchical ANOVA:[a] surgeons within hospitals						
(5) Among hospitals, considering surgeons	14	82.2113	5.8722	6.493	.001	$\sigma^2 + \kappa_2\sigma_P^2 + \kappa_3\sigma_H^2$
(6) Among surgeons, within hospitals	538	486.6014	0.9045	1.025	.348	$\sigma^2 + \kappa_1\sigma_P^2$
(7) Residual, for surgeons	6,775	5,975.3555	0.8820			σ^2
Total, for patients	7,327	6,544.1680				

Estimated variances[a]

Variance due to hospitals: $\sigma_H^2 = .0102$
Variance due to surgeons: $\sigma_P^2 = .0018$

[a]The method for performing hierarchical analysis of variance and for estimating the amount of explained variance is based on methods described in Kempthorne 1952. The estimated variances are obtained by setting the expected value of the mean squares to the observed value of the mean squares and solving for σ_H^2 and σ_P^2. The values of the constants were as follows: $\kappa_1 = 12.83$; $\kappa_2 = 28.16$; $\kappa_3 = 484.28$.

were removed. It also provided a better test for hospital-level effects than the one-way ANOVA presented in rows 1 and 2 by removing the effects attributable to differences among surgeons within hospitals. The first of these hierarchical tests (row 5) revealed significant differences among hospitals in the adjusted outcomes of patients, even after removing the variation in outcomes explained by surgeon differences within hospitals. By contrast, in the second hierarchical test (row 6), we observed no significant effects on surgical outcome attributable to individual surgeons within the hospitals.[13]

Although the "hospital effect," taking into account variance among surgeons within hospitals, was significant, while the "surgeon effect," taking into account variance among hospitals, was not, it would be inappropriate to conclude from these tests that surgeon characteristics have no effect on surgical outcomes. The differences attributed to hospitals may be due to the possibility that surgeons are grouped systematically by hospital and thus collectively account for variations observable at the hospital level only. Further, such effects may result either from the operation of the corporate structure created by surgeons within each hospital or from the activities of individual surgeons aggregated across patients at the hospital level. These alternative explanations can be explored in the second approach.

In the next set of analyses, we examined the possibility that what appeared to be differences in hospitals were in reality differences attributable to the professional staff and its organization. We therefore turned to an exploration of the causes of these differences through a series of regression analyses utilizing the measures of hospital context, surgical staff organization, and individual surgeons previously described.

The Effect of the Hospital Context and the Surgical Staff Organization

We first examined the effects on adjusted outcomes of the measures of surgical staff organization. Three measures of the hospital context—size, expenditures, and teaching—were also included but were used as control variables whose effects were taken into account before the measures of surgical staff organization were evaluated. Specifically, a stepwise regression format was employed in which, at step 1, all the measures of hospital context were

---

13. The analyses were complicated by the imbalance in the data: the number of patients per surgeon was not constant for all surgeons, and each hospital did not have the same number of surgeons. We note, too, that in table 8.1, although there were significant differences in adjusted surgical outcomes among hospitals, the amount of variance in adjusted outcomes explained was small. The variance in patient outcomes attributable to hospitals was about five times the estimated variance attributable to surgeons. While the amount of variance in outcomes for a given patient attributable to hospitals and surgeons was small, when expressed relative to total variation in patient outcomes, these differences among hospitals were by no means trivial. (See below; and chap. 5 in this volume.)

forced into the equation and at step 2, the surgical staff organization variables are allowed to enter in a stepwise fashion, the order of inclusion determined by the contribution of each variable to explained variance.

Table 8.2 reports a regression analysis with adjusted surgical outcomes as the dependent variable and three measures of hospital context and five measures of surgical staff organization as independent variables. Among the three measures of hospital context, only expenditures were significantly related to the quality of surgical care. The relationship was in the predicted direction: higher expense per patient-day was associated with better-quality care and was significant at the .001 level.

This finding is in apparent contradiction to the results reported by others, such as Shortell, Becker, and Neuhauser (1976), who found that lower average costs were associated with higher average quality of care in a study of forty-two hospitals in Massachusetts. Their measures for both costs and outcomes differed significantly from ours. They reported average costs per case rather than per patient-day and used a different measure and method of adjusting outcome for case-mix differences. Moreover, their associations were based on aggregate data only and were subject to biases when they tried to interpret the impact of hospital efficiency on an individual outcome. The conclusions reached by their study may be in conflict with ours, but the methodology and kind of analysis make direct comparisons inappropriate. In a more detailed analysis of costs per case measured in terms of amounts of services delivered (chapter 7), we found strong evidence corroborating our finding that a higher level of service intensity was associated with better outcomes when each of these measures had been adjusted to take patient health status into account.

Shortell, Becker, and Neuhauser (1976) argued that their aggregate measures of high costs per use reflected "inefficiencies." It is not always appropriate to equate high costs with inefficiencies, as the many proponents of cost-benefit analyses correctly point out. Our data, while finding that higher costs (per patient) were associated with outcomes better than would be expected given the patient's health, do not imply that inefficiency is good; they imply that providing more and better services than the "typical" hospital offers may actually benefit the patients. More refined conceptualization and research are needed to resolve these apparent contradictions and to understand the full impact of reductions in costs on health care outcome (see the rebuttal in Shortell 1982).

Turning to the measures of surgical staff organization, only two—the proportion of contract physicians and the number of surgical specialties— were found to be significantly associated ($p \leq .05$) with the quality of care. Both relationships were in the expected direction: the higher the level of coordination as reflected in the proportion of contract physicians, and the higher the average degree of specialization among surgeons on the staff, the better the quality of care.

Table 8.2. The effect of hospital context and organization of the surgical staff on adjusted surgical outcome

Independent Variable[a]	Regression Coefficients		Standard Error B	F Ratio	In the Predicted Direction[b]
	Standardized (β)	Unstandardized (B)			
Hospital context					
Size	.012	.000	.000	.551	
Expenditures	−.076	−.004	.001	17.181*	yes
Teaching	.030	.058	.049	1.420	
Surgical staff organization					
Proportion of contract physicians	−.052	−1.205	.407	8.762**	yes
Number of surgical specialties	−.042	−.016	.007	5.254**	yes
Average percentage of practice conducted at the study hospital	.012	.051	.065	.628	
Proportion of board-certified surgeons	.003	.026	.122	.044	
Admission requirements for new members	−.003	−.002	.014	.026	

Multiple *R* of .082
  R² of .007
Overall *F* at final step of 6.724*
F for incremental change in sum of squares from hospital context variables to final step of 7.101*

[a]The hospital-context variables have all been forced into the regression step 1; the surgical staff organization variables are listed in the stepwise order in which they entered the regression.
[b]Since a higher score for adjusted outcome reflects a more severe outcome than expected, a negative coefficient connotes an association with better-quality care.
*Significant at the .001 level.   **Significant at the .05 level.

The measure of the surgical staff's power based on stricter admission requirements for new staff members, was associated significantly with better-quality care in the simple correlation but did not remain significantly associated with quality in the regression. The structural variable most likely to affect the relation between power and outcome quality in this regression was hospital expenditures. The simple *r* between hospital expenditures and power was .47. (A more detailed examination of the relation between power and quality of care is presented in chap. 9.)

The remaining two measures were not significant in this regression or in the simple correlations with quality. We shall return to a discussion of these measures after first exploring the importance of the characteristics of the individual surgeon for explaining the quality of surgical outcomes.[14]

The Effect of the Hospital Context and the Characteristics of the Individual Surgeon

We turn last to an analysis of the importance of the qualifications and training of the individual surgeon for the quality of surgical outcomes. In this approach, we examined the impact of the individual surgeon while taking into account the hospital by first introducing three context variables into the regression and then allowing individual-surgeon measures to enter in the order of their explained variance. Table 8.3 summarizes the results of this regression analysis.

The same relation between hospital-context measures and the quality of care observed in table 8.2 can be observed in table 8.3: expenditures per patient-day had a significant effect on the quality of care; size and teaching were not significantly related to surgical outcomes. Among the five measures of surgeon characteristics, only two—the percentage of each surgeon's practice conducted at the study hospital (a measure of commitment) and the number of residencies completed (a measure of qualifications)—were significantly associated ($p \leq .05$) with the quality of care. In each case the association was in the predicted direction: greater commitment and more residencies were associated with better care. Two other measures of qualification—board certification and the number of years of practice—as well as a measure of surgical specialization were not related to adjusted surgical outcomes.[15]

The second approach to examining the structural correlates of the quality of surgical outcomes, represented by tables 8.2 and 8.3, permitted us to address two additional questions of particular interest in this chapter: (1) Which units of the professional organization contribute to differences in its effectiveness? and (2) Do professionals having similar qualifications and training tend to group together into organizations such that the aggregate levels of qualifications and training could account for effectiveness?

To answer the first question, we needed to compare the overall impact of hospital context, surgical staff organization, and individual surgeons. Here, unlike in the two-way ANOVA, we could distinguish between the hospital structure and the professional staff structure. In these analyses, when the hospital-context variables were entered alone in the first step, the overall regression

14. The total variance explained by the variables in table 8.2 was also quite small: the amount of explained patient variance was 0.7 percent (see n. 13).
15. The total variance explained by all the variables in table 8.3 was again small: the amount of explained patient variance was 0.3 percent (see nn. 11 and 13).

Table 8.3. The effect of hospital context and characteristics of the responsible surgeon on adjusted surgical outcome

Independent Variable[a]	Regression Coefficients		Standard Error B	F Ratio	In the Predicted Direction[b]
	Standardized (β)	Unstandardized (B)			
Hospital context					
Size	−.007	−.000	.000	0.225	
Expenditures	−.054	−.003	.001	19.325*	yes
Teaching	.019	.036	.028	1.651	
Surgeon characteristics					
Percentage of practice conducted at the study hospital	−.026	−.096	.046	4.421**	yes
Number of residencies	−.026	−.027	.013	4.417**	yes
Number of years in practice	−.018	−.002	.001	2.243	
Board certification	.002	.005	.026	0.036	
Surgical specialization	−.002	−.001	.005	0.017	

Multiple R of .058
R^2 of .003
Overall F at final step of 3.328*
F for incremental change in sum of squares from hospital context variables to final step of 1.680***

[a]The hospital-context variables have all been forced into the regression in the first step; characteristics describing surgeons are listed in the stepwise order in which they entered the regression.

[b]Since a higher score for adjusted surgical outcome reflects a more severe outcome than expected, a negative coefficient reflects an association with better-quality care.

*Significant at the .001 level.   **Significant at the .05 level.   ***Not significant at the .05 level.

was significant at the .001 level (Flood 1976). In tables 8.2 and 8.3, we present an F ratio for the incremental increase in variance in the quality of outcome represented by surgical staff measures as a set (table 8.2) and by individual-surgeon qualifications as a set (table 8.3). This incremental F ratio was significant at the .001 level for surgical staff organization but not for the set of measures for the individual surgeon. These tests of significance were consistent with the two-way ANOVA but suggested that both hospital context and professional staff structure account for differences in the effectiveness of the organization.

We next examined the possibility that individual professional qualifications might still account for differences in effectiveness but be masked because the surgeons in each professional staff tended to have similar qualifications. Two results argued against this hypothesis. First, when the qualifications of surgeons within a hospital were examined, considerable variation in each measure was observed (Flood 1976). Second, when the aggregate measures of qualifications were examined for their impact on the quality of care, in table 8.2, only the average level of specialization showed any relation to the quality of care. Neither the proportion of board-certified surgeons nor the average commitment was significantly related to outcome. It would appear that the qualifications of individual professionals were not related to effectiveness at either the aggregate or the individual level.

SUMMARY

We attempted to determine the organizational units responsible for the level of performance observed. Three types of units were identified as possibly accounting for the performance of the organization: the larger organizational context, the corporate structure of organized professionals, and the individual practitioners. For our study of hospitals and surgeons in the IS, we found that characteristics of the hospital organization and the corporate structure of the professional group were more strongly associated with differences in the quality of care than were differences among individual surgeons within the hospital studied.[16]

In our analyses, we explored the effects of different structural dimensions within each organizational unit: the hospital context, the surgical staff organization, and the individual surgeons. For the hospital context, expenditures, measured in terms of expense per patient-day, were found to be associated with better-quality patient care. (See chap. 10 for further analyses of the relation between costs and the quality of care.) For the surgical staff, higher levels of differentiation and coordination were found to relate to better-quality surgical care. Related analyses reported in chapter 9 suggested that greater power of the surgical staff over its own members was also associated with better-quality care. Our measures of surgical staff organization were found to relate significantly to the quality of surgical care beyond any effects attributable to hospital measures of the hospital context. At the same time that these results were statistically significant, the amount of explained variance was low. A question often raised is whether a low R^2 in these analyses indicates that the explaining variables are of no practical importance. We believe not. In other analyses of these data, we concluded that this level of variation among hospitals resulted in

16. Several authors have commented on the implications of the work reported in this chapter (Ross 1982; Rutkow 1982; Shortell 1982; May 1983; Neuhauser 1983; and Rundall 1983). See Conclusions and Implications, following chap. 12, for more details.

a two- to threefold increase in death and morbidity rates for the poorer hospitals relative to the better hospitals (chap. 6).

As we discuss in more detail in chapter 5, Gordon, Kannel, and Halperin (1979) presented an excellent discussion and illustration of the potential for misinterpretation of a small R^2 in regression analyses such as ours, with a noncontinuous, skewed dependent variable. In one example, using a dependent variable analogous to mortality, they presented a statistical argument that the upper limit of R^2 is 1.96 percent. Applying similar assumptions to our data in which the overall, average death rate across hospitals is 3 percent, a hospital characteristic whose presence accounts for a twofold increase in deaths would have a theoretical upper limit for R^2 of .0034 or $(.06)^2$. We agree with these authors' conclusion that "the hazards of arguing analogically from the multivariate case were never more clearly illustrated than in this instance" (433).

Even though the association between individual surgeons within hospitals and measures of the quality of care proved to be quite weak, we attempted to determine which characteristics of surgeons were more strongly predictive of care differences. Better qualifications of surgeons, reflected by the number of residencies, and greater commitment to the hospital, reflected by the percentage of a surgeon's practice conducted at the study hospital, were found to relate to better surgical outcomes. However, the amount of variance explained by surgeon characteristics did not add significantly to that attributable to hospital-context measures.

In sum, differences in the quality of surgical care seemed to be more closely associated with features of the hospital setting in which care was delivered and features of the surgical staff as a corporate body than with the characteristics of individual surgeons. Whether or not these results hold for other types of professional organizations and across other types of effectiveness indicators must be determined by future studies.[17]

17. Rhee and colleagues (Rhee 1977; Rhee, Luke, and Culverwell 1980) reported similar findings using a process measure of the quality of care.

9 · Professional Power and Professional Effectiveness: The Power of the Surgical Staff and the Quality of Care

Ann Barry Flood and W. Richard Scott

A critical survey of the literature conducted by the Committee on Professional Organization and Control of the Medical Sociology Section of the American Sociological Association concluded that after more than two decades of research on professional work in medical settings, we still know very little about "the effect of variations in the organization (including financial arrangements) of physicians and their work setting on the technical and social quality of the medical care provided" (Goss et al. 1977). This chapter deals with this neglected area. We examine the effect of selected structural characteristics of hospitals—in particular the distribution of power among professional role groups and the power exercised by the surgical staff over its own members—on medical outcomes experienced by patients undergoing surgery. We relate detailed measures of hospital characteristics to equally detailed measures of the quality of care. Unlike most other studies of the quality of care, we rely on outcome rather than process measures of quality in the belief that it is important to attempt to focus on results achieved rather than effort expended or conformity to standards of unknown efficacy. Great effort is expended to adjust measures of medical outcome—morbidity and mortality—to take into account medically relevant differences among patients.

THE THEORETICAL APPROACH

In his influential paper on the professions, Goode (1957) argued that professional communities are able to secure a measure of autonomy from the

For an earlier version of this chapter see Flood and Scott 1978.

larger society by organizing themselves to exercise control over their own members. Such controls are often presumed to be exercised by professional associations which set certification standards, promulgate codes of ethics, and administer sanctions to deviate members. The evidence attesting to the efficacy of these control attempts is at best mixed (*Yale Law J.* 1954; Cohen 1973). Perhaps in response to these deficiencies, the locus of control appears to be shifting from the professional community to the professional organization, as Etzioni (1964) and Freidson (1970) noted.

To assert that organizational controls are exercised over professional work is not necessarily to suggest that the organizational control mechanisms are of the conventional hierarchical type. Indeed, a number of descriptive studies have shown that professional organizations tend to develop somewhat distinctive control arrangements that offer considerable autonomy to individual workers and place heavy reliance on collegial processes of control (see Goss 1961; Hind, Dornbusch, and Scott 1974; and Freidson 1975). The extent to which such distinctive arrangements develop depends largely on the power exercised by professional participants in the organization (Scott 1972). These groups organize themselves—as a medical staff in hospitals, as a senate or assembly within universities—in order (1) to secure and protect an arena of professional decision making and activity and (2) to promote fidelity to professional standards by careful selection, control, and continuing education of staff members. Professional groups strongly contend that the performance of these functions—the securing of autonomy for the group, coupled with the regulation of the individual practitioner—is conducive to effective performance.

Our approach can be clarified by briefly describing four classes of variables: the two sets of independent variables measuring professional power, the dependent variables measuring the effectiveness of performance, and a set of control variables whose effects must be considered.

The Power of Professionals in Hospitals

Under the assumption that professionals in organizations need to be able to define and defend an arena of professional autonomy, we chose as our first class of variables those relating to the relative power of physicians, nurses, and hospital administrators in hospitals. We defined *power* as the ability of members of an organization to affect the outcome of organizational decisions. We expected such power to vary depending on the type of decision at issue; such differentiation is the hallmark of organizations and is especially characteristic of professional organizations, where there is likely to be a clear demarcation between the professional sphere and the administrative sphere (Smith 1955; Goss 1961). Further, we viewed power in nonzero sum terms, so that high power for some role groups on an issue did not preclude the possibility of high power for other groups on the same issue.

In general, we argued that for optimal functioning, professional groups must be in a position to exercise a large amount of power, relative to other groups, over decisions within their sphere of competence. Conversely, effectiveness will not be served if professionals exercise a large amount of power over decisions outside their sphere of competence. We distinguished, therefore, between *within-domain power* and *encroachment*. We expected effectiveness to relate positively to the exercise of power by a role group within its domain and negatively to encroachment by one role group on another's territory.

The Power of the Surgical Staff over the Surgeon

We expected the professional staff, having held claim to a sphere of autonomous functioning, to police the conduct of its own members within that realm. Generally speaking, we did not expect professional groups to exercise detailed control over the activities of their members. Such practices are inconsistent with professional norms (Goss 1961). Freidson's studies of control processes among physicians in a group-practice clinic (Freidson and Rhea 1963; Freidson 1975) concluded that colleagues' attempts to regulate performance were rare and usually ineffectual. However, hospital settings may be more conducive than ambulatory settings to the exercise of control. Hospitals tend to be larger and more formalized. Accreditation requirements mandate the operation of a number of quality-review committees under the auspices of the medical staff. In particular, surgical performance is more subject to colleagues' surveillance and regulation. Among the most fateful tasks of every hospital staff is the setting of conditions under which additions to the staff are made and membership privileges withdrawn. Roemer and Friedman (1971) argued that hospitals vary significantly in the amount of power the medical/surgical staff exercises over its own members and that the greater this power, the more effective the hospital is in its delivery of quality medical care. Neuhauser (1971), Shortell, Becker, and Neuhauser (1976), and Rhee (1977) reported some supporting evidence. We expected greater surgical staff power over individual surgeon-practitioners to be associated with more effective performance.

The Effectiveness of Performance

It is widely recognized that the assessment of professional performance is at best a complex and hazardous business. The complexity of the work, the incompleteness of the knowledge, and the variety of individual cases all converge to prevent consistent success. Because "good" performances can sometimes result in "poor" outcomes, professionals emphasize process measures of effectiveness (Were the proper procedures correctly performed?) rather than outcome measures (Did the desired effect occur?) However, process measures evaluate conformity to a given standard of performance; they do not evaluate the adequacy of the standards themselves, and they assume that the activities required to ensure effectiveness are known. Such assumptions are always problematic when the work involved is complex and uncertain, as is the case with surgical care. As argued in greater depth in chapters 4 and 5, we prefer outcome measures of effectiveness for testing hypotheses such as ours. In the analyses reported here we employed measures of patient mortality and morbidity, adjusted for differences in patient characteristics, as indicators of the quality of surgical care.

Control Variables

Clearly, a great many other factors may potentially influence the outcomes experienced by patients following surgery. The factors selected as control variables—We use *control* in the statistical sense—included various characteristics of patients, surgeons, and hospitals.[1] We focused on those factors that may influence patient outcomes and are believed to vary systematically by hospital.

PROCEDURES

Data Sources and the Size of the Samples

The data were collected as part of the Intensive Study (IS) of factors affecting the quality of surgical care in hospitals. Seventeen hospitals were surveyed for the original study, but due to missing data on surgeon characteristics in two hospitals, only fifteen were included in the major portions of this analysis. Organizational characteristics relating both to the hospital context and to the organization of the medical/surgical staff are described in chapter 1 and reviewed in chapter 8. The primary focus of the analyses reported here was the effect of organizational power on patient outcomes. First, however, it was important to take into account other major factors that could influence the outcomes of patient care. To accomplish this, we performed the analyses at the level of the individual patient, matching the patient's outcome with the data describing his or her health at the time of surgery, the characteristics of his or her specific surgeon, and features of the larger hospital structure in which the treatment occurred. Consistent with this patient-level approach, the characteristics for each physician and hospital were associated with each patient, which had the effect of weighting them according to the number of patients

---

1. The question of how much variance in outcome is due to the characteristics of patients or surgeons or to hospitals, after taking into account variance attributed to the first two sources, is addressed in chapter 8.

treated. All means and correlations reported were based on these weighted observations.

Measuring and Adjusting Surgical Outcomes

Surgical outcomes were measured in terms of both the mortality experience—obtained at the fortieth postoperative day—and the extent of morbidity assessed at the seventh postoperative day or at the date of patient discharge, if earlier. Using the Intermediate Scaled Outcome, we employed an indirect standardization procedure to take into account differences attributable to patient characteristics. In effect, measures of care quality were constructed to reflect the difference between a patient's observed outcome score and his or her expected score calculated on the basis of that patient's characteristics. A more detailed discussion of the outcome measures and adjustment procedures used appears in chapters 5 and 6.

Measuring the Relative Power of Professional Groups and the Power of the Surgical Staff over Surgeons

In order to determine the relative power of the medical staff in influencing various types of decisions in hospitals, following the approach of Tannenbaum (1968), we asked a set of informants in each hospital to rate, on a five-point scale, the amount of influence exercised by a given position on a specified type of decision. Responses were obtained by interview or questionnaire from the following types of informants: hospital administrators, chiefs of surgery, chiefs of anesthesia, directors of nursing, ward supervisors, head nurses, and ward nurses. The positions rated included those of the hospital administrator, the chief of surgery, the director of nursing services, and physicians as a group. Eight decisions were selected as representing differing types of issues as well as differing levels, ranging from routine administration to policy determination (see table 9.1). Because we could not presume that all organizational respondents were equally knowledgeable (Aiken and Hage 1968; Scott 1972), we gave greater weight to information from respondents occupying positions higher in the hierarchical structure. Thus, responses for each occupant of a position were combined into a single "position" score, and then scores for all positions were combined to provide an average score for each hospital. The effect was to give greater weight to the judgments of those persons in positions with no or few other occupants. While theoretically justified, this procedure had little effect on the results because of the high level of agreement exhibited by informants on the distribution of influence.

Combining the data from all hospitals, we observed that the distribution of influence by position varied greatly by type of issue, as expected (Comstock 1980). Based on these profiles as well as on the content of the decision items,

Table 9.1. Indices of the relative power of professional groups

Type of Decision[a]	Power Within Domain		
	Hospital Administration	Nursing Administration	Surgical Administration[b]
1. To hire a replacement staff nurse for a patient-care unit.		X	
2. To increase the size of a ward staff by adding a new staff nurse position.		X	
3. How best to discipline a nurse for committing a serious medication error.		X	
4. To purchase contract services, e.g., laundry.	X		
5. To change the nursing care system, e.g., to adopt team nursing throughout the hospital.		X	
6. To add a clinical service, e.g., an intensive-care unit.			X
7. To add an ear-nose-throat specialty room in the operating suite.			X
8. To terminate a major department head, e.g., the nursing director of the operating suite.			X

[a]These decision items were employed in constructing the six measures of power.
[b]Chief of surgery.   [c]As a group.

we distinguished between the within-domain influence of a role group and its encroachment into the decision terrain of other role groups. Table 9.1 indicates the questions used for determining each of these conditions for the role groups of interest. As already noted, our expectations were that higher-quality care would be associated with the exercise of greater influence by role groups within their respective domains and, conversely, with less encroachment by one role group on another's turf.

The second set of power measures was designed to indicate the extent of power exercised by the surgical staff as a corporate body over individual

	Encroachment on Power	
By Physicians[c] on Hospital Administration	By Physicians[c] on Nursing Administration	By Hospital Administration on Surgical Administration[b]
X		
	X	
		X
		X
		X

surgeons. Three measures were developed. The first measured the degree of centralization of decision making within the surgical staff by comparing the perceived influence of the chief of surgery with that of physicians as a group on the decisions to add a clinical service and a specialty room in the operating suite (decision items 6 and 7). The two other measures were based on interview responses by the chief of surgery regarding the strictness of admission requirements for new members of the surgical staff. One measure was based on information on the length of the probationary period, differentiation by specialty, and the number of review bodies; the other considered the extent of restrictions on surgical privileges, the use of written procedures in reviewing surgical privileges, the number of years for which privileges were granted, and the rules defining who could serve as first assistant during surgery. Items were standardized using a Z-score and combined into an index for each measure. While not all forms of control by the surgical staff over its members would be expected to increase the quality of medical care, this was our prediction for the three measures just described.

Table 9.2 reports the intercorrelations among the nine measures of power and with the hospital context. Note that for the hospitals surveyed, less within-domain influence of the surgical administration was related to more encroachment by hospital administrators on surgical administration ($-.85$); but more within-domain influence of the hospital administration was associated with the encroachment on their decision terrain by the surgical administration (.60). Such patterns are consistent with a nonzero-sum view of power. Note also that the two measures of surgical staff control over individual surgeons were uncorrelated and that each related differently to the distribution of influence measures. More stringent admissions requirements for new surgeons were associated with greater encroachment by the surgical administration on the domain of the hospital administration; but greater surgical staff control over tenured surgeons was related to less encroachment on this same measure and to greater influence of hospital administrators within their own domain.

Measuring the Control Variables

As already discussed, additional factors were thought likely to have some effect on the quality of surgical care. These factors were not of primary interest for this analysis; we introduce them here in order to determine whether they needed to be controlled.

Patient Variables

In addition to the patient characteristics employed to adjust surgical outcomes, we measured five other characteristics: ethnicity and marital status were treated as dichotomous variables, while education and income were each coded into seven levels. Finally, we employed a measure of social stress based on selected items from the Holmes and Rahe (1967) instrument.[2]

Physician Variables

Using information from PAS records reflecting all the surgery performed by each surgeon in the study hospital during 1973, we constructed a measure of

2. The application of the Holmes and Rahe instrument to these data, as well as an analysis of the effect of social stress on recovery from surgery for selected surgical categories, is described in Rundall 1978.

Table 9.2. Correlations among the power measures and with the hospital context

			Interitem Correlations							Hospital Context		
	1	2	3	4	5	6	7	8	9	Size	Expenditure	Teaching
1. Within-domain influence of the surgical administration		.342	−.311	.192	.327	−.852*	.119	.065	.161	.377*	.129	.648*
2. Within-domain influence of the hospital administration			.353	.600*	.419*	.076	−.054	−.035	.425*	.319	−.640*	.385*
3. Within-domain influence of the nursing administration				.056	.236	.580*	−.422*	−.336	−.076	−.361*	−.360*	.090
4. Encroachment by physicians on the hospital administration					−.108	.035	.208	.442*	−.682*	−.451*	−.159	.364*
5. Encroachment by physicians on the nursing administration						.026	−.315	−.419*	−.215	.027	−.441*	.192
6. Encroachment by the hospital administration on the surgical administration[a]							−.140	−.197	−.046	.358*	−.453*	−.602*
7. Centralization of decision making within the surgical staff								.287	.284	.160	.247	−.049
8. Admission requirements for new members of the surgical staff									−.066	.095	.473*	.037
9. Power of the surgical staff over tenured surgeons										−.125	−.238	.101

Note: Correlations are Pearson product-moment correlations on per-patient data for 15 organizations and 14 medical staffs.

[a]Chief of surgery.

*Significant at the .1 level or less.

each surgeon's specialization based on the distribution of operations across twelve categories. Three different measures of surgeons' qualifications were employed: board certification, the number of residencies, and the number of years of practice after completion of any residency training. To assess the extent of each surgeon's commitment to the study hospital, we noted the percentage of each surgeon's practice conducted at the study hospital. A higher percentage of practice was associated with less surgical specialization ($-.14$) and with fewer residencies completed ($-.24$). Greater surgical specialization was related to a shorter length of practice ($-.17$) and to fewer residencies ($-.15$). All of these intercorrelations were significant at the .001 level.

Hospital Variables

As in the research reported in chapter 8, three measures were employed to assess the hospital context: size was measured as a product of the number of beds and the average occupancy rate for each hospital; expenditures on patient care were measured by dividing the total annual hospital expenditures by the number of patient-days; and the teaching status was assessed on the basis of the presence or absence of an active residency program. Of these three hospital-context variables, only teaching status and expenses per patient-day were significantly correlated (.53). Table 9.2 reports the intercorrelations among the nine measures of power and the three variables assessing hospital context.

RESULTS

In examining the effect of surgical power on adjusted patient outcomes, we wished first to take into account the impact of any control variables affecting these outcomes. Therefore, we regressed outcomes on each set of control variables to determine the presence of any significant relationships. Among the patient control variables, only income was significantly related to adjusted patient outcomes: patients with higher incomes tended to experience better surgical outcomes. The other patient measures—ethnicity, marital status, education, and social stress—were not significantly related to the quality of care. Among the three hospital control variables, only expenditures were found to be significantly associated with surgical outcomes: greater expenditures per patient-day were associated with better outcomes. Neither size nor teaching status was significantly related to the quality of care. And among the five physician variables, the only measure significantly related to adjusted surgical outcomes was the percentage of each surgeon's practice conducted at the study hospital. The greater the percentage of the surgeon's practice conducted at the study hospital, the better the quality of care experienced by patients. To our surprise, the other measures of surgeons' characteristics—the extent of specialization, board certification, the number of residencies, and the number of years of experience—were not related significantly to the quality of care (see Flood 1976; and Flood et al. 1982 [see also chap. 8 in this volume]).

Given these preliminary results, we retained only the three control variables revealed to have a significant effect on surgical outcomes: patient income, hospital expenditures, and the percentage of the surgeon's practice conducted at the study hospital. These three control variables were forced into the regression equation at step 1; then the measures of professional power were introduced. This approach was conservative in the sense that it permitted the measures of patient, hospital, and surgeon characteristics to account for all of the possible variance in surgical outcomes before examining the impact of the professional power measures on patient outcome.

Table 9.3 reports the results of a regression analysis of the effects of the distribution of power among role groups within hospitals on the quality of surgical care, after taking into account the effects of selected control variables. Of the three control variables forced into the equation at step 1, only two—hospital expenditures and patient income—retained a significant impact on surgical outcomes. Turning to the three measures of the influence of role groups within their own domain, we noted that two were significantly related to the quality of surgical care. The power of hospital administrators to influence decisions within their domain was related to surgical outcomes in the expected direction: the greater their power, the better the quality of care. The power of nursing administrators to influence decisions within their domain was also significantly related to surgical outcomes, but not in the predicted direction: the greater their influence on decisions within their own domain, the poorer was the quality of care observed. The influence of surgical administrators on decisions within their own domain was not significantly related to the quality of surgical care. None of the three encroachment measures was significantly related to the quality of surgical care. The overall F ratio was significant at the .001 level; the F representing the change in the sum of squares for the power measures beyond that attributed to the three control variables was also significant at the .001 level. The total amount of explained variance was quite small, largely due to our methodological approach (see chap. 5).

In summary, these analyses suggest that among the various measures of the power of role groups considered, the perceived ability of the hospital administrators to influence decisions within their own domain was the factor most strongly and consistently related to better-quality surgical care. The relative power of the surgical administration to influence decisions within its own domain showed no effect on the quality of care; and the relative power of the nursing administration within its own domain was seen to relate to poorer-quality care when the standardized Intermediate Scaled Outcomes were used.

Table 9.4 shows the effect of the power of the surgical staff over its own members on adjusted surgical outcome. As in the previous analyses, we first introduced the three control variables and then allowed the surgical staff vari-

Table 9.3. The effect of within-domain and encroaching influence on adjusted surgical outcome (using Intermediate Scale and selected control variables)

Variable[a]	Standardized Regression Coefficient (β)	Unstandardized Regression Coefficient (B)	Standardized Error B	F Ratio	In the Predicted Direction[b]
Control variables					
Percentage of surgeon's practice conducted at the study hospital	−.010	−.036	.047	.577	
Hospital expenditures	−.085	−.004	.001	16.970**	yes
Patient's income	−.028	−.013	.005	5.901	yes
Power variables					
Within-domain influence of the hospital administration	−.133	−.224	.048	23.417**	yes
Encroachment by physicians on the nursing administration	.034	.063	.036	3.110	
Within-domain influence of the nursing administration	.307	.173	.083	4.307*	no
Encroachment by physicians on the hospital administration	.028	.054	.038	1.987	
Within-domain influence of the surgical administration	.082	.187	.109	2.929	
Encroachment by the hospital administration on the surgical administration	.051	.099	.098	1.028	

Multiple $R = .090$; $R^2 = .008$
Overall F at final step $= 7.115$**; F or incremental change from control variables to final step $= 6.654$**

[a]The three control variables were forced into the regression at step 1; the power variables are listed in the stepwise order in which they entered the regression.

[b]Since a higher score for adjusted surgical outcomes reflected a more severe outcome than expected, a negative coefficient connotes an association with better-quality care.

*Significant at the .05 level.   **Significant at the .001 level.

Table 9.4. The effect of the power of the surgical staff over its own members on adjusted surgical outcome (using Intermediate Scale and selected control variables)

Variable[a]	Standardized Regression Coefficient (β)	Unstandardized Regression Coefficient (B)	Standardized Error B	F Ratio	In the Predicted Direction[b]
Control variables					
Percentage of surgeon's practice conducted at the study hospital	−.016	−.061	.046	1.784	
Hospital expenditures	−.032	−.002	.001	5.408*	yes
Patient's income	−.023	−.011	.005	4.238*	yes
Surgical staff power over members					
Power of the surgical staff over tenured surgeons	−.047	−.026	.077	13.654***	yes
Admission requirements for new members of the surgical staff	−.042	−.033	.010	10.469**	yes
Centralization of decision making within the surgical staff	−.010	−.022	.029	.553	

Multiple $R = .085$; $R^2 = .007$
Overall F at final step $= 9.641$***; F for increment from control variables to final step $= 11.249$***

[a]The three control variables were forced into the regression at step 1; the power variables are listed in the stepwise order in which they entered the regression.
[b]Since a higher score for adjusted surgical outcomes reflected a more severe outcome than expected, a negative coefficient conotes an association with better-quality care.
*Significant at the .05 level. **Significant at the .01 level. ***Significant at the .001 level.

ables to enter in a stepwise fashion. Two of the three control variables—hospital expenditures and the patient's income—were significantly related to better-quality care. The percentage of a surgeon's practice conducted at the study hospital was not significantly associated with surgical outcome. Two of the three measures of surgical staff control over surgeons were significantly associated with the quality of care. Both were in the predicted direction: the stricter the admissions requirements for new members of the surgical staff and the greater the power of the surgical staff over tenured surgeons, the higher the quality of surgical care. Centralization of decision making within the surgical staff was not significantly associated with the quality of care. The overall F was significant at the .001 level, as was the incremental F measuring the change in the sum of squares from the control variables to the final step. Thus, these analyses showed strong support for our expectation that greater regulation of the work of individual surgeons by the surgical staff organization would be associated with higher-quality surgical care in hospitals.

SUMMARY

In this chapter we examine the relation between professional power and professional effectiveness as reflected in the organization and work of surgeons in a sample of short-term, acute-care hospitals. The power of surgeons and hospital and nursing administrators was assessed by asking respondents to describe their perceptions of the influence of each role group on a set of hypothetical decisions. In addition, the power of the surgical staff to regulate the work of individual surgeons was examined by determining the degree of centralization of influence within the surgical staff and the stringency of requirements governing admission to the staff and the awarding of surgical privileges to staff physicians. Patient outcomes—the actual effects of the surgical treatments as reflected in the health status of patients following surgery—were used as indicators of professional effectiveness. For such measures to be valid indicators of the quality of care received, they must be adjusted to take into account differences in patient condition prior to treatment. Such an adjusted outcome measure was developed using linear regression techniques. Factors (other than the power measures) thought likely to affect the quality of outcomes were also identified and measured and taken into account. Those observed to have an effect on patient outcomes and, hence, controlled in this analysis were patient's income, hospital expenditures per patient-day, and the percent of all the surgeon's practice conducted at the study hospital. Surprisingly, several measures of the extent of specialized training and experience of surgeons were not significantly associated with the quality of surgical care (see chap. 8).

Among the various measures of the relative power of the three role groups to influence organizational decisions, the strongest and most consistent factor related to the quality of care was the power of the hospital administrators to influence decisions within their own domain. While in general we expected the influence of each role group within its own domain to be associated with better-quality care, we expected the most important factor to be the power of the surgical group to influence decisions within its own domain. However, no significant effects on the quality of surgical care were observed for our indicator of surgical power. The influence of the nursing administration on nursing decisions was observed to be associated with poorer-quality care, although this unexpected relationship was not consistently observed across the three outcome scales. While the strong association of the power of the hospital administration with the quality of surgical care was somewhat unexpected, it is consistent with the arguments of both Perrow (1961) and Georgopoulos and Mann (1962), who viewed the administrator as providing coherence and coordination in a work situation fraught with fragmentation and overspecialization. Encroachment— the exercise of power by one role group in the domain of another—was not related significantly to the quality of care.

The power of the surgical staff over its own members was found to relate to the quality of surgical care: the more extensive the regulations imposed on individual surgeons by the surgical staff, the higher the quality of surgical care. This finding is consistent with the arguments and results of Roemer and Friedman (1971), who placed great emphasis on the importance of the medical/surgical staff organization and the quality of medical services. It is important to recognize that these are controls exercised by professionals over professionals. It does not follow from the findings that any and all attempts to regulate the performance of individual practitioners will result in greater effectiveness. We recognize that the causal processes that link the relative decision-making power in the organization, or even the extensiveness of staff regulations over practitioners, to the morbidity and mortality of individual patients are complex, and we should not expect our measures to explain all the variations in the quality of care. To have discovered some consistent and statistically significant relationships under these circumstances is encouraging.

PART IV

Effects of Hospital Structures and Processes on Hospital Performance

10 · Organizational Determinants of Services, Quality, and the Cost of Care in Hospitals

W. Richard Scott, Ann Barry Flood, and Wayne Ewy

After more than a decade of research on the structural features of organizations (Pugh et al. 1968, 1969; Blau and Schoenherr 1971), researchers are turning their attention from the determinants to the consequences of organizational structure. In particular, attention has recently been focused on the effects of structure on organizational effectiveness and efficiency (Price 1972; Child 1974, 1975; Goodman and Pennings 1977; Steers 1977). Good examples are provided by the quality (effectiveness) and the cost (efficiency) of health care in hospitals. These variables are also of great interest to policy makers because of the recent rapid increases in hospital costs and the uneven quality of hospital care in this country.

A large number of studies have examined factors associated with the quality or the cost of care in hospitals, but only a small number have examined both simultaneously, and an even smaller number have attempted to relate them to structural features of hospitals (Cohen 1970; Neuhauser 1971; Morse, Gordon, and Moch 1974; Rushing 1974; and Shortell, Becker, and Neuhauser 1976). Results from these and related studies have not been clear or persuasive. Important limitations of previous work include (1) a lack of effective techniques for taking into account differences among patients that affect both the cost and the quality of care observed and (2) a lack of attention to the development of output measures that distinguish the outcome of care received from the quantity or costs of services delivered or from the potential to provide care implied by the elaborateness of facilities and the qualifications of health care personnel.[1]

For an earlier version of this chapter see Scott, Flood, and Ewy 1979.

1. Strengths and limitations of the various classes of measures employed to assess care quality are discussed in Donabedian 1966; Scott 1977; and chaps. 4 and 5 in this volume.

We designed our reserach approach to deal with both of these difficult issues. To handle the first limitation, we adjusted the measures of services (including length of stay) and outcomes for hospital patients to take into account variations due to the health status of the patients being treated. To handle the second limitation we developed independent measures of the quality of care, the quantity of services, the costs of care, and the structural measures of the potential of the organization to provide care and examined their interrelationships. Based on this research, we first examined the relations between measures of the average quantity of services delivered and measures of the average quality of outcomes achieved by patients in a hospital (Flood et al. 1979 [see also chap. 7 in this volume]). In this chapter we focus on a set of structural characteristics of hospitals as predictors of variations in the average intensity and duration of services provided to patients, the average amount of expenditure for patient care, and the average quality of outcomes experienced by patients in the hospital.

METHODS

Data Sources

The SIS data used in this chapter were drawn from the seventeen acute-care hospitals. The patient data for the SIS are described in chapters 5 and 6. All patient data were based on information contained in the PAS abstract record, which was available for each of the approximately 600,000 patients discharged from the study hospitals during the period May 1970–December 1973. Data on the organizational characteristics of the hospital and medical staff came primarily from the IS (see chap. 1). For that study, interviews were conducted during the spring of 1974 with key hospital and medical staff personnel, who acted as expert informants, describing the structure and operation of their units. Questionnaires were also administered to the staffs of the operating room, the recovery room, and the surgical wards and to selected physicians providing primary care and selected ancillary services. Data on surgeons' training and experience were collected from either hospital records or American Medical Association (AMA) records. In addition to these data from the IS, information was assembled on selected hospital characteristics from the American Hospital Association (AHA) annual survey for each of the four years studied.

Measures of Major Variables

The principal measures in this study may be grouped into four categories: (1) the outcome of hospitalization; (2) the amount and type of inhospital services; (3) actual hospital costs; and (4) hospital structure.

The Measure of the Outcome of Hospitalization

The indicator of quality of care was the rate of *inhospital mortality* adjusted for patient characteristics—a measure emphasizing the quality of outcome of care for patients.

Measures of Inhospital Services: Rates of the Service Intensity and the Length of Stay

We developed indicators to estimate the number or amount of services of varying types received by a patient during a hospital stay. Although it was not feasible to assess all of the many types of services provided by hospitals, we measured seven types of important diagnostic and therapeutic services provided to inpatients. For purposes of this analysis, we limited our attention to a composite measure of these seven services. An *index of service intensity* reflects the amount and variety of diagnostic and therapeutic services provided to patients, as well as the relative cost of each of these different types of services.[2] We also assessed the duration of the services, as measured in terms of the length of stay (LOS).

General features of the standardizing approach are described in chapters 5 and 6. Briefly, using a combination of classification by diagnosis (with 332 diagnostic groupings) and linear regression, and using indicators that characterized each patient's condition and treatment record, including diagnoses, operations, admission-test findings, and sociodemographic characteristics, we computed the expected levels of service intensity, LOS, and outcome for each patient, conditional on the patient's specific characteristics and physical condition at admission. For each of the three types of measures based on patients, the expected levels reflected the pattern of utilization or outcome obtained on the average in the set of study hospitals by patients with the same type of disease and physical condition. We then calculated difference scores for each patient, which reflected the difference, whether positive or negative, between the expected level of service intensity, LOS, and outcome for a patient of that type and the actual level observed for that patient. To obtain a measure for a hospital, we then averaged these difference scores for the set of all patients treated in the

2. Categories of diagnostic and therapeutic services measured are reported in table 7.1. The costliness of services was reflected in a weight assigned to each individual category before combining them into the composite measure. These weights were based on the average proportion of total charges for a hospitalization episode associated with each category of service. The weights were obtained from data on hospital charges supplied by a nonstudy hospital. Thus, they were not intended to reflect the actual variations in charges among study hospitals but were uniformly applied to all hospitals. The intent was only to reflect differences in *relative* costliness among the various categories of services provided by hospitals. Since we were able to assess not only whether a given category of services was used by a given patient but, often, the amount or number of such services consumed as well, the actual weights applied to each service used by a patient took into account these frequencies.

hospital during the study period. Thus, our measures of service intensity, LOS, and outcome for each hospital were summary measures of observed departures in the experience of individual patients from expected scores based on the typical experience of similar patients treated in all of the hospitals in our sample.

The Measure of Cost Based on Actual Hospital Charges

Unlike the measures of services and outcomes, the measure of cost was not based on data obtained on individual patients and then aggregated to the hospital level, nor was it adjusted for differences in patient mix among hospitals. Data on actual expenditures on, or charges to, each patient were not available; instead, the cost measure was based on data obtained from the AHA's annual survey of 1973 and consisted of the total annual expenditures of each hospital divided by the number of patients treated during that year, which provided the *average expenditures per patient episode*. We attempted to correct this measure for regional differences in cost by dividing each hospital's score by the Medicare reimbursement index for the county in which the study hospital was located. Clearly, however, because our measure of cost did not take into account differences in patient mix, its usefulness was compromised, and it will not receive much attention in our subsequent analyses.

Measures of Hospital Structure

Measures of the structural characteristics of hospitals were grouped into two categories, capacity and control. *Hospital capacity* refers to those aspects of the hospital that represent its potential to supply services. Six types of measures were used. One obviously important measure was that of hospital size or scale. Since hospitals are organizations heavily dependent on personal services, we used as our indicator of size the *total number of personnel employed*. (This indicator was strongly correlated (.93) with the average daily patient census.) Second, to measure the elaborateness of the therapeutic and diagnostic facilities available, we assessed the *number of different types of facilities* and *the proportion of hospital beds devoted to intensive care*. The third set of measures examined the intensity of the staffing, indicated by the *ratio of the total number of staff members to the average daily census* and by the *ratio of direct-care nurses to the average daily census*. Fourth, the teaching status of the hospital was measured in terms of the *presence of residents in approved programs*. Fifth, the qualifications of the staff were determined by several types of measures indicating training, certification, and experience. These included the *ratio of registered nurses (RNs) to other types of nurses,* such as licensed vocational nurses (LVNs); the *average number of years in nursing* for staff nurses; the *proportion of the surgical staff that was board-certified;* and the *average number of years in practice since residency* for surgeons. A final measure assessed the unused capacity or slack resources of the institution as measured by the *occupancy rate*, the ratio of occupied beds to total bed capacity. It should be noted that occupancy rate measured capacity used.

All of the above measures of the hospital's capacity to supply services were based on data supplied by the hospital administrator for each study hospital, with the following exceptions: information on facilities and intensive-care beds was obtained from the AHA annual survey, and information on the average years of nursing experience was compiled from a questionnaire distributed to all ward staff nurses in the study hospitals (average return rate, 75 percent).

Hospital control encompassed several features of the organization, including the distribution of power or influence over decisions and mechanisms for the control and coordination of work activities. We assessed the distribution of influence among two major sets of actors within the hospital, administrators and staff physicians; coordination at several organizational levels; and controls exercised by the surgical staff over its own members. Brief descriptions of the variables used to assess these control features follow; more detailed information on the measures employed is provided in chapter 9.

Three measures of influence were developed based on responses by key hospital informants to a set of hypothetical decision questions. One measure focused on the *hospital administrator's influence on decisions in the administrative area;* a second focused on the *chief of surgery's influence on decisions within his jurisdiction;* and a third examined the extent of *encroachment by physicians on administrative decisions.*

Coordination and control activities were assessed using measures of administrative intensity, clerical support, formalization, and frequency of communication with quality-assurance personnel. Specifically, for the hospital as a whole, we assessed the *ratio of supervisory to direct-care personnel.* At the level of the nursing ward, we measured the *average number of ward clerks and secretaries* present and, based on questionnaire responses from staff nurses, the *explicitness of general nursing policies.* To assess coordination by special professional units, we determined the *frequency of case discussions between physicians and pathologists* as reported by pathologists.

Finally, to assess the control exercised by the medical staff over its own members, we measured the extent of formalized *control exercised by the surgical staff over new members,* as well as the *control exercised over tenured members.* These measures of formalized control were based on the rigorousness of the initial and continuing review of credentials, length of probation, and/or gradations of privileges. A third measure assessed the *proportion of contract (salaried) physicians* on the medical staff, an indicator favored by Roemer and Friedman (1971) as the best single measure of the control of the medical staff.

PREDICTIONS

In general, we expected organizational capacity to be positively associated with greater average service intensity and, hence, higher average costs per patient episode. It should be noted that since service intensity was adjusted to take into account differences in patient mix, the argument was not the conventional one that patients with more severe illnesses were more likely to be treated in larger and more elaborate facilities, where they receive more services. Rather, we argued that patients served in more elaborate and more professionalized facilities were more likely to receive more services than expected, taking into account their specific condition. Such services were expected to be provided both because they were "more available" and because they contributed to other valued organizational and staff goals, such as teaching and research. There is no clear rationale for linking organizational capacity in general to average LOS (ALOS), so no predictions were made.

Hypotheses relating organizational capacity to the quality of care are also somewhat problematic. Since the indicators of care quality vary considerably from one study to another, and since measures of structure, process, and outcome tend to be poorly correlated with one another (Brook 1973; chap. 12 in this volume), we restricted our attention to outcome indicators of quality. There was some evidence to suggest that quality of outcomes is higher in larger hospitals (Kohl 1955; Lipworth, Lee, and Morris 1963; CPHA 1969). The relation between the average level of staff qualifications and surgical outcomes was investigated in the IS data by Flood (1976) and is reported in chapters 8 and 9. In her analysis of these data, Flood reported that better surgical outcomes were associated with hospitals whose surgical staff had completed a greater average number of residencies (e.g., more varied postgraduate training), but, unexpectedly, poorer outcomes were associated with staffs having longer average residencies. Also unexpected was the finding that greater average specialization on the part of surgeons—measured by the types of operations actually performed—produced poorer outcomes, while the proportion of board-certified surgeons on the staff was not associated with the quality of outcomes. The same study showed that better outcomes were associated with hospitals whose nursing staff had longer nursing experience, on the average.[3] Whether one should expect the average length of nurse and physician experience to be positively associated with better-quality outcomes is unclear: a staff with a higher average level of experience signifies, on the one hand, more practice and

---

3. It should be emphasized that these results were observed at the aggregate level of analysis, i.e., using the average level of training and experience as the independent variables. Different results may be expected—and have been observed when the level of analysis is shifted to the individual physician (chap. 4; Flood 1976; Flood et al. 1979 [see also chap. 7 in this volume]).

exposure to varied medical problems but, on the other hand, increasing age and remoteness from training and, perhaps, from contemporary methods of care. Turning to predictions involving control and coordination systems, we expected to see greater controls exercised by administrators and physicians associated with reduced services to patients. Such an expectation for hospitals in a fee-for-service reimbursement setting (all of our hospitals at the time of our study) was probably somewhat utopian, since it was not at all clear that given high influence, hospital administrators or the medical staff had much incentive to curb the services provided to patients and thus to contain the costs of medical care (Fuchs 1974; Enthoven 1980). Also, we should not expect both service intensity and LOS to be affected in the same manner by administrative and professional controls. Thus, our predictions with respect to hospital coordination and control systems and services were unsure, and we hoped to learn from an examination of the empirical relations observed. By contrast, our research in the IS and other studies suggested that better-quality medical care was positively related to administrators' influence over decisions within their own domain (Flood and Scott 1978 [see also chap. 9 in this volume]), to coordination of work at the overall hospital and ward levels (Georgopoulos and Mann 1962; Neuhauser 1971; Longest 1974), and to the ability of the physician staff to regulate its members (Roemer and Friedman 1971; Shortell, Becker, and Neuhauser 1976; Flood and Scott 1978 [see also chap. 9 in this volume]).

Strengths and Limitations of the Data Base and the Approach

Considerable confidence can be placed in our estimates of differences among hospitals in services and the quality of care, since they were based on a very large number of observations per hospital. Also, detailed measures of patient characteristics were used to standardize service and quality measures for differences among hospitals in patient mix. Further, unusually varied and detailed measures of the organizational characteristics of the hospitals and their medical staffs were available. These strengths were offset somewhat by several serious limitations. First, our indicator of the quality of care—death inhospital—while highly reliable, was severely limited in reflecting only mortality experience. Had the data sources permitted, it would have been greatly preferable to include other outcome measures, such as morbidity or return to function,[4] as well as information on patient condition after discharge. Second, although detailed measures of hospital and physician staff characteristics were available, there was some discrepancy in the time at which they were measured in relation to the patient data. As noted, patient information covered the period 1970–73, while on-site collection of organizational data occurred in the spring of 1974.

---

4. An attempt to include inhospital complications as another indicator of care quality had to be abandoned due to the poor quality of data in this area.

One must allow for the possibility that basic structural changes occurred within one or more hospitals during the period under study. A further limitation was that since the original data were collected for a study of surgical care, most of the measures of medical staff were based on the characteristics of surgeons and the organization of the surgical staff. Surgeons constitute, of course, only a subset of the full medical staff. Third, although the measures of services and outcomes were based on the experience of a large number of patients, we had only a small number of hospitals on which to test predictions relating hospital characteristics to these dependent variables. Clearly, in presenting these results, our mode must be exploratory, and the results must be regarded as suggestive rather than definitive.

RESULTS

Interrelations between Service Intensity, Quality, and Cost

Before presenting the data relating to our predictions regarding organizational factors affecting services, quality, and the cost of care, we note briefly the interrelationships between these aggregated dependent variables. In all cases except that of cost, results were based on the standardized measures. There was little or no association between service intensity and ALOS ($-.24$):[5] if anything, hospitals delivering more services to patients than expected tended to exhibit shorter average stays than expected. A longer ALOS was slightly associated with higher average costs per patient episode ($.37$), while the average level of service intensity showed no association with average costs per patient episode ($.07$). What is most important, a higher than expected level of services within a hospital was significantly associated with a lower than expected mortality rate ($-.43$), while a longer than expected ALOS was significantly associated with a higher than expected mortality rate ($.64$). These last two relationships and their implications are discussed in more detail in chapter 7.

The Effects of Organizational Capacity on LOS, Service Intensity, Quality, and the Cost of Care: Zero-Order Correlations

Table 10.1 presents the zero-order correlations among the several measures of organizational capacity and the measures of service intensity and

5. All correlations were Pearson product-moment correlations. The significance level adopted for these analyses was $p \leq .10$. For an N of seventeen and a two-tailed test, an $|r| \geq .412$ was significant at this level.

Table 10.1. The effects of organizational capacity on average levels
of LOS, service intensity, quality, and cost of care: Zero-order correlations

Organizational Capacity[a]	Services		Quality (Inhospital Mortality)[b]	Costs (Expenses Per Hospitalization)[c]
	LOS	Intensity		
Size				
Total number of staff	.35*	.45**	−.04	.55***
Facilities				
Number of different facilities	−.04	.44**	−.15	.54***
ICU beds as percentage of total beds	−.16	.66***	−.15	−.22
Labor intensity				
Ratio of total staff to ADC[d]	−.38*	.56***	−.43**	.15
Ratio of direct-care nurses to ADC[d]	−.12	.09	−.18	−.48**
Teaching				
Active residency program	.38*	.13	−.05	.42**
Qualifications of the professional staff				
Ratio of RNs to LVNs[e]	−.31	.29	.05	.12
Average experience of nurses	−.29	−.32	.30	−.28
Percentage of surgeons with board certification	.05	−.08	−.29	.44**
Average years since residency	.57***	−.58***	.60***	.20
Extent of capacity used				
Occupancy rate	.45**	.29	.26	−.01

Note: The measures of services and quality were based on all patients treated during 1970–73 in the study hospitals. These three measures were standardized to take into account patient diagnosis, surgical procedures, and physical condition (see chaps. 5 and 6 for details).

[a]The measures reported here were based on staff, admissions, expenditures, facilities, and occupancy rates as reported for 1973 in the AHA *Guide.* For this reason, some correlations differed slightly from those previously published, which were based on the IS interview data.

[b]A negative correlation with mortality reflected better-quality outcomes.

[c]Costs were based on average expenditures during 1973 and have been adjusted for regional differences in the cost of living.

[d]Average daily census.

[e]RN = registered nurse; LVN = licensed vocational nurse.

*Significant at the .1 level.   **Significant at the .05 level.   ***Significant at the .01 level.

duration (i.e., LOS), quality,[6] and the cost of care. The pattern for larger hospitals suggests that they were associated with less efficient clinical production of services; that is, they tended to have a longer than expected ALOS, higher average service intensity, and higher average expenditures per hospital episode. Moreover, "excess services" in larger hospitals were apparently unrelated to the quality of outcomes produced. This pattern was fairly consistently observed for all the hospital-capacity measures except those involving staffing levels and qualifications. Note, however, that we had predicted that lower occupancy rates—greater unused capacity—would be associated with higher levels of services and costs, but the data tended to be in the opposite direction: higher occupancy rates were associated with higher service intensity.

The measures related to staff bore more inconsistent relationships to the measures of hospital performance. Hospitals with more staff per patient tended to provide more services and a shorter hospitalization, with a net difference that showed no effect on average costs but did appear to predict better outcomes. When the measure was restricted to nursing staff intensity, however, these relationships generally were not significant.

The measures of qualifications generally were not related to services or to the quality of care. In particular, training levels for both nurses (proportion of RNs) and physicians (proportion of board-certified surgeons) revealed little association with average services and outcomes; average costs tended to be higher in hospitals served by more board-certified surgeons. No significant relation between nursing experience and average services and outcomes was revealed, but a longer average length of practice for surgeons was strongly associated with a longer ALOS, lower average service intensity, and poorer than expected average outcomes.

The Effects of Organizational Control on LOS, Service Intensity, Quality, and the Cost of Care: Zero-Order Correlations

The zero-order correlations among the indicators of influence, coordination, and control within the hospital and physician staff on the measures of services, quality, and the cost of care are presented in table 10.2. Beginning with the measures of the influence of administrators, the surgical chief, and the medical staff, we note that higher influence of both groups tended to be associated with a longer ALOS and with greater average expenses per patient episode (which was significant only for the surgical staff influence). This pattern was observed both for influence measures within each role group's domain of decision making and for the measure indicating physicians' encroachment on

---

6. Since the indicator of the quality of care used is the hospital's mortality rate adjusted for differences in patient mix, a negative correlation is indicative of better outcomes, hence, higher-quality care.

Table 10.2. The effect of hospital control factors on average levels of LOS, service intensity, quality, and cost of care: Zero-order correlations

Hospital Control Factors	Services		Quality (Inhospital Mortality)[a]	Costs (Expenses Per Hospitalization)[b]
	LOS	Intensity		
Influence				
Administrative influence in own area	.66***	−.27	.54**	.21
Surgical staff's influence in own area	.33*	−.02	.28	.54**
Encroachment by medical staff	.39*	.26	.17	.23
Coordination within the hospital				
Ratio of supervisors to direct-care personnel	−.19	.51**	−.38*	−.26
Coordination within wards				
Number of clerks on wards	−.29	.57***	−.58***	.00
Explicitness of nursing policies	−.28	.19	−.05	.03
Coordination by professional units				
Frequency of case discussions with pathologists	−.64***	.36*	−.33*	−.28
Physician staff controls				
Control over tenured supports	.32	−.61***	.42**	−.14
Proportion of contract physicians	.28	.03	.15	.60***
Control over new surgeons	.42**	.13	.07	.20

Note: The measures of services and quality were based on all patients treated during 1970–73 in the study hospitals. These three measures have been standardized to take into account patient diagnosis, surgical procedures, and physical conditions (see chaps. 5 and 6 for details).

[a]A negative correlation with mortality reflects better-quality outcomes.

[b]Costs are based on average expenditures during 1973 and have been adjusted for regional differences in the cost of living.

*Significant at the .1 level.   **Significant at the .05 level.   ***Significant at the .01 level.

administrative decisions. Greater administrative influence was also associated with poorer-quality outcomes.

The several indices of coordination also revealed a rather consistent though not very strong general pattern. Higher levels of coordination within the hospital as a whole and in the patient-care wards and professional staff tended to have little association with ALOS and average expenses per patient episode, but they were related to higher average levels of service intensity and better care outcomes. By contrast, the measures of physician staff control revealed little consistency in their association with the measures of hospital performance.

Combination Effects of Selected Measures of Hospital Capacity and Control on LOS, Service Intensity, Quality, and the Cost of Care: Multiple Regressions

Multiple regression analysis was employed to examine the combined hospital-level effects of selected variables assessing both organizational capacity and control. Variables were selected on the basis of their theoretical interest and the magnitude of their association with the dependent variable and to provide breadth of coverage of the various types of factors considered. The results of one set of regressions are summarized in table 10.3; each was significant overall at a .05 level or lower except as noted for the quality of outcomes. These results were representative of other regressions examined employing various combinations of factors and alternative indicators.

Part A of table 10.3 summarizes the results using the average-adjusted ALOS as the dependent variable. The presence of residents was predictive of longer ALOS, even when other hospital control and coordination measures were taken into account. Among the control measures, greater influence on the part of administrators in their own area acted to increase the ALOS (during an era in which hospitals were reimbursed on a fee-for-service basis almost exclusively), while strong professional coordination acted to decrease it.

Part B reports a multiple regression with the average adjusted service intensity as the dependent variable. Unlike in the case of ALOS, the presence of residents was not significantly predictive of differences in the service intensity provided to patients. By and large, the capacity measures were not very or consistently strongly predictive of service intensity, although there was a tendency for a greater number of facilities to be related to higher average service intensity. The control over tenured surgeons, when adjusted to take into account other hospital characteristics, tended to decrease the services provided.

Part C reports the regression of the measure of quality—the standardized mortality rate—on selected measures of hospital capacity and control. Although some of the variables related to capacity and control were strongly associated with average mortality at a zero-order level, the overall regressions seldom, if ever, reached significance. It would appear that these variables (which in many cases were based on surgical-care facilities and staff) were not significantly related to the overall quality of outcomes for medical and surgical patients.

Finally, part D reports results of the regression of average expenditures per patient episode on selected measures of hospital capacity and control. While the overall regressions reached significance, few individual measures of control and coordination ever reached significance. The major exception was that greater administrative influence was predictive of greater expenditures.

Table 10.3. Summary of associations of selected organizational capacity and control variables with average levels of LOS, service intensity, quality, and cost of care, based on linear regressions

Dependent Variable	Direction	
	Observed[a]	Predicted
A. ALOS		
Presence of residents	Increased	Increased
Administrative influence in own area	Increased	None
Encroachment of medical staff	None	Increased
Frequency of case discussions with pathologists	Decreased	Decreased
B. Average service intensity		
Presence of residents	None	Increased
Number of different facilities	Increased	Increased
ICU beds as percentage of total beds	None	Increased
Control over tenured surgeons	Decreased*	Decreased
C. Average quality of outcomes		
Frequency of case discussions with pathologists	None	Increased
Control over tenured surgeons	None	Increased
Administrative influence in own area	None	Increased
D. Average expenditures per episode, region adjusted		
Presence of residents	None	Increased
Number of different facilities	None	Increased
Administrative influence in own area	Increased	None

Note: The organizational capacity and control measures reported here were those identified in the zero-order correlations as being significantly associated with the dependent variables.

[a]"None" indicates that no significant relationship was observed in the linear regressions. All others except one were significant at .05 or less.

*Significant at the .01 level.

SUMMARY

It is not easy to summarize the results relating hospital characteristics to measures of average services, outcomes, and costs. The small number of hospitals studied—only seventeen—severely limits the confidence to be placed in any generalizations relating hospital characteristics to these dependent variables. Nevertheless, the opportunity to study structure (hospital characteristics), process (service intensity and duration), outputs (patient-care outcomes), and costs in a single study encouraged us to carry out this exploratory analysis.

The prediction that hospitals characterized by greater capacity would tend to provide more services than expected received some empirical support in our analysis. However, measures of capacity to deliver services showed only a slight association with the quality of hospital care as measured by standardized mortality rates. Measures of labor intensity tended to be slightly associated with better average outcomes as assessed by zero-order correlations. Measures of qualifications were not associated with the quality of care, with the exception of average years since residency for surgeons; unexpectedly, this indicator was associated with hospitals having poorer-quality care.

Measures of greater service capacity were positively associated with higher average costs of patient care in zero-order analyses; that is, larger staff size, more facilities, residents, and a higher proportion of board-certified surgeons were all associated with higher costs per patient episode. The only measure of capacity related to lower average costs was an indicator of labor intensity. When examined in multiple regressions, however, none of these measures remained significantly associated with costs.

Turning to measures of coordination and control, for most of the measures, greater coordination was associated with better-quality care, as predicted. When the effect of other variables was controlled, however, few of these measures exhibited partials large enough to be significant. Contrary to expectation, some of the measures of physician staff controls—e.g., control over tenured staff—tended to be associated with poorer-quality care in the zero-order correlations, but this relationship was not sustained in the regression analysis.

No predictions were developed relating coordination and control to measures of average service intensity and ALOS. In general, greater coordination was related to shorter ALOS but higher average service intensity. The two measures of physician staff control discussed above showed just the opposite pattern. Finally, higher administrators' within-domain influence tended to be found in hospitals whose patients typically stayed longer and had higher costs and who received poorer-quality care.

The associations between more control over tenured physicians and poorer-quality care, and between more administrative influence and poorer-quality care, were not only unexpected but contrary to the results of our study using these same organizational measures but studying surgical outcomes in the IS (Flood and Scott 1978 [see also chap. 9 in this volume]). Even though the hospitals and the measures of these independent variables were the same in these two studies, discrepant results were quite possible given differences in the patient populations, methodologies, and outcome measures employed. Nevertheless, we were surprised by the inconsistent results in these two related studies.

Although the specific associations revealed in these analyses were not as clear and consistent as we would have preferred, the general research approach employed—combining measures of organizational structure, processes, and outcomes into a single design and attempting to adjust process and outcome measures for differences in the types of clients served—seems to us promising. Indeed, the low and/or inconsistent associations observed among these three types of measures indicate the dangers entailed in using one type of measure as a surrogate for the others—a practice all too common in health services research specifically and, more generally, in research on organizational effectiveness.

We recommend that analyses of the type explored here be carried out in a larger sample of hospitals. Increased sample size would greatly assist in sorting out the complexities of associations that seem to characterize the relationships between the types of variables considered. Of course, improved measures of costs that take into account differences in patient mix are essential. Finally, we hope that others will explore the uses of patient abstract data as a potential source of information on that most elusive of all measures in service organizations—the outcome experienced by clients.

11 · Does Practice Make Perfect? The Relation between Hospital Volume and Outcomes

Ann Barry Flood, W. Richard Scott, and Wayne Ewy

Quality care and cost containment in hospitals are well-recognized goals shared by policy makers, professionals, administrators, and patients alike. Deciding how best to achieve them produces more divergence of opinion. One explanation for producing better outcomes investigated recently had to do with the importance of a hospital's experience in treating patients of a given type. It has long been suspected, but only recently demonstrated, that hospitals performing more treatments of a given type exhibit better patient outcomes than do hospitals processing fewer patients (Luft, Bunker, and Enthoven 1979; Shortell and LoGerfo 1981). Earlier research based on specific and usually new surgical technologies, such as open-heart surgery, generally found that the survival rate of patients was related to increased experience of the surgical team. Policy makers and professional groups have recommended that a minimum patient volume be required for certain selected procedures, and some have even promoted efforts to concentrate caseloads in the hands of a few surgeons (Graham and Paloucek 1963). However, in a recent study, Studnicki, Stevens, and Knisely (1985) questioned whether high volume for a specific surgeon or surgical team was an appropriate policy goal. In their study of Maryland surgeons, they found that surgeons with a heavy caseload of hospitalized patients also tended to have more inappropriate days of care, as assessed by a peer review organization. The more recent larger-scale and more broadly based studies raise a different issue: organizations themselves may gain from increased volume (for example, increased volume may result in better coordination and a more experienced nursing staff). This so-called volume-outcome relationship, if supported by broadly based additional research, has important

For earlier versions of this chapter see Flood, Scott, and Ewy 1984a, 1984b, and 1984c.

policy implications for the "regionalization" of hospital services, suggesting that important health advantages may be attained by promoting a more explicit division of labor among hospitals in terms of the types of treatments they provide.[1] Data from the ES allowed us to evaluate the volume-outcome hypothesis for a large sample of hospitals and for a different set of patient categories than those previously investigated.[2]

Briefly, in the first section of this chapter we describe our approach combining data on hospitals and patients from the ES data sources. The quality of care was assessed using a single outcome—death inhospital—adjusted to take into account differences in patient condition at the time of admission. A variety of diagnostic categories and patients undergoing both surgical and medical treatment were included. We assessed volume in two ways, one based simply on hospital experience with patients in the same diagnostic category and the second based on experience with patients at a similar risk level within the same diagnostic category. In the second section, using cross tabulations and graphs for several diagnostic groupings, we show the effects of volume or hospital experience on adjusted patient outcomes. In the third section, we control for hospital characteristics in examining this relationship. And in the final section, we discuss the evidence supporting assumptions about causal direction in this relationship.

PROCEDURES AND MEASURES FOR VOLUME-OUTCOME HYPOTHESES

The Selection of Hospitals and Patients

This study was based on the approximately 330,000 patients in one of fifteen diagnostic surgical categories and 227,000 patients in one of two diagnostic nonsurgical categories who were treated in one of the 1,224 ES hospitals. The procedures for selecting ES hospitals and patients and the methods for producing standardized measures of hospital performance based on outcomes (in this case inhospital death) are detailed in chapter 5 and briefly reviewed in chapter 6. Chapter 6 also presents the tests for differences in hospital performance for each category and for various groups of patient categories.

In the present analysis, attention is focused on three classes of study

1. See also comments on the work reported here by Donabedian (1984).
2. The study by Luft, Bunker, and Enthoven (1979) was restricted to surgical patients but investigated a broader set of surgical categories than those covered in the present study. Breadth is an advantage for generalization; however, it makes less tenable the assumption that patients within a given category may be regarded as comparable to one another. That is, it interferes with attempts to adjust outcome measures for patient differences. See new studies by Sloan, Perrin, and Valvona (1985) and Kelly and Hellinger (1985) for further evidence.

patients: (1) *selected surgical categories*, comprising patients who underwent one of nine relatively purer study procedures (that is, the majority of the patients shared the same diagnosis, and the majority of those in the diagnostic group who underwent any related, nondiagnostic procedure underwent the study procedure); (2) *all surgical categories* (the nine selected surgical categories plus six other study surgeries); and (3) *medical categories*, including patients who were hospitalized for one of two study diagnostic groups (biliary tract disease and ulcer disease) but were treated medically rather than surgically. The study patient categories are listed in table 11.1 together with the number of patients, the number of deaths, and the death rate for each category. The order of presentation of the categories of selected surgery and of additional surgery reflects the relative difficulty of each type of surgery as evaluated by a panel of surgeons (Schoonhoven et al. 1980).[3]

The Outcome Measure: Death Inhospital

The outcome measure employed was death inhospital. This indicator was not ideal: it did not take into account many health status outcomes of interest (e.g., morbidity, return to function, quality of life); a sizable proportion of deaths following a hospitalization period do occur, not within the hospital, but following discharge;[4] and death is a relatively rare event, a circumstance reducing the power of statistical attempts to estimate its probability of occurrence. Moreover, Luft (1981b) argued that death rates may exhibit spurious variation by region due to differences in length of stay. Since the ALOS varies significantly by region (the shortest ALOS being in the West and the longest in the Northeast), the number of deaths occurring outside the hospital and thus unrecorded in the data base is likely to be higher in areas with the shortest ALOS. Luft also found that rehospitalization was higher in areas with the shortest ALOS. Since each hospitalization was treated as an independent episode in our analyses, areas with significantly higher rehospitalization could appear to have lower death rates due to the same patient's counting for multiple "survivals" of hospitalization. In chapter 7 we examine the impact of the region of the country

3. In a related study, 550 surgeons were asked to rate the difficulty in terms of the complexity and uncertainty of a set of seventy-one surgical procedures, using a scale of 1 (easy) to 9 (difficult). Using these ratings, the study categories would be ranked: abdominal aorta surgery (7.86 involving renal vessels and 7.16 without renal vessels), arthroplasty of the hip (6.81 for total hip), biliary tract surgery (5.71 involving common duct exploration and 4.11 without), gastric surgery (5.45), repair of the fractured shaft of the femur (5.02), large bowel operations (5.00), and amputation of the lower limb (3.74) (Schoonhoven et al. 1980).

4. For example, in chap. 5, in the IS, we focused on the outcome measure of death within forty days following surgery whether or not the death occurred within the hospital. We obsered that 25 percent of the deaths in our sample of 8,592 study patients occurred within the forty-day period but after the patient had been discharged from the hospital.

Table 11.1. Basic patient and hospital statistics, by patient category

Patient Category	Patient Statistics			Hospital Statistics	
	Number of Patients	Number of Deaths	Death Rate (%)	Number of Hospitals	Average Number of Patients
Selected surgical categories[a]					
1. Intraabdominal artery operations	9,532	1,476[b]	15.5	645	14.78
2. Arthroplasty of the hip	13,424	199	1.5	702	19.12
3. Biliary tract operations	130,749	1,444[b]	1.1	1,196	109.32
4. Stomach operations with ulcer diagnosis	26,688	1,138	4.3	1,100	24.26
5. Large bowel operations with specified diagnosis[c]	16,110	517	3.2	984	16.37
6. Hip fracture diagnosis with other trauma diagnoses	6,925	554	8.0	886	7.82
7. Hip fracture diagnosis with no other trauma diagnoses	52,368	4,774[b]	9.1	1,169	44.80
8. Amputation of the lower limb with no current trauma diagnosis	10,267	1,476[b]	14.4	973	10.55
9. Amputation of the lower limb with current trauma diagnosis	881	75	8.5	217	4.06
All selected surgical categories	266,944	11,653[b]	4.4	1,209	220.80
Additional surgical categories					
10. Stomach operations with cancer diagnoses[d]	1,500	161	10.7	377	3.98
11. Stomach operations with other diagnoses[d]	7,148	578	8.1	875	8.17
12. Large bowel operations with cancer diagnoses	17,872	1,160[b]	6.5	1,040	17.18
13. Large bowel operations with other diagnoses	6,575	817	12.4	858	7.66
14. Fracture of the pelvis	18,033	687	3.8	1,113	16.20
15. Fracture of the shaft of the femur	13,677	562	4.1	976	14.01
All surgical categories	331,749	15,618[b]	4.7	1,216	272.82
Medical categories					
16. Biliary tract diagnosis— nonsurgical	88,839	2,477[b]	2.8	1,210	73.42
17. Ulcer diagnosis— nonsurgical	138,268	3,299[b]	2.4	1,214	113.89
All medical categories	227,107	5,776[b]	2.5	1,215	186.92

[a]Categories are arranged in order of their relative difficulty from greatest to lowest (see Schoonhoven et al., 1980).
[b]The significance level of the test for differences was .0005 (see chap. 6).
[c]Includes benign tumor, enteritis, colitis, and diverticulosis.
[d]Excludes secondary or unspecified malignancies.

on our measures of outcome for the SIS, and find that region explains the differences in ALOS but does not account for the differences in death rates among hospitals. Finally death within a specified number of days is generally regarded as a more appropriate indicator for surgery than for medical treatment. On the positive side, death can be reliably measured and is unarguably a valid indicator of an adverse health outcome.

It is well known that patient mix varies greatly among hospitals (Berry 1970; Lave and Lave 1971; Horn and Schumacher 1982; Young, Swinkola, and Zorn 1982). If outcome measures such as death are to be regarded as valid indicators of the quality of care, they must be adjusted (standardized) to take into account differences among patients in type of illness and general health status.

Since comparison of hospital performance was a major goal of our study, we developed a methodology to predict the probability of dying for each patient, given his or her particular health-related characteristics. (Our standardizing method is described in chaps. 5 and 6.) Thus, we have two measures for each patient: (1) whether they were discharged alive or dead (i.e., "inhospital death") and (2) the probability of their dying inhospital. When we aggregate these measures for a group of patients, the ratio of actual deaths to the expected number of deaths (the standardized mortality ratio, or SMR) is a measure of performance that takes into account the number of deaths that could be expected on the basis of detailed information about patient mix.

Risk Levels of Patients

The expected outcome—the probability of dying inhospital—was also used to rank each patient within each category to provide a measure of risk level. Patients were then partitioned into three risk levels—reflecting a low, a medium, and a high probability of dying—in such a way as to ensure that each level would contain approximately one-third of the patients who died inhospital within each category. The partition of risk into levels was based upon the number of deaths in order to increase the statistical power of our tests for variation in rates per hospital. As already noted, for one of the two measures of volume, hospitals were differentiated according to whether they treated more or fewer than the average number of patients at each risk level within a given category.

Volume Measures

We developed two measures of case volume. Both were based on CPHA data and assessed the extent to which the hospital treating a given patient was experienced in cases of the type represented by the patient. Both measures were dichotomous, indicating whether or not the patient was treated in a hospital that had treated more than the average number of patients of each type—the average based on the combined year-long experience of all study hospitals with at least two patients in the study category.

The first volume measure, *volume within category,* was positive only if for each study patient, the hospital treated more than the average number of patients in the same category. (The categories used are those listed in table 11.1.) The second volume measure, *volume within category and risk level,* was more stringent in its definition of relevant experience: it was positive only if for each patient, the hospital treated more than the average number of patients in the same category and at the same risk level as the patient's. Risk level (already defined) was a measure of the severity of illness (estimated probability of death) and so represented a more refined measure of patient similarity.

Levels of Analysis

For our present purposes, the data analysis was carried out at the level of the individual patient. The effect of this decision was to treat each patient as a separate case and to characterize him or her in terms of the specific volume and other structural measures describing the hospital in which care was received. One important consequence of this approach was to weight these structural variables according to the number of patients receiving care in each hospital. A second consequence of this decision was to place a limitation on the amount of explained variance possible in our analyses. (These points are addressed more fully in chap. 5.)

The patient level was most appropriate for the analyses reported here, since not only were the outcomes and their adjusting variables measured at the patient level but the measures of volume were assessed in terms of the experience of a given hospital with patient subgroups highly similar to the patient of interest in both diagnosis and risk level. Nevertheless, it can be argued that using the patient level leads to overestimates of the significance of differences observed, since it uses as the number of "independent" observations the number of patients rather than the number of hospitals. To compensate for this bias, we employed fairly stringent tests of significance throughout these analyses.

RESULTS: THE RELATION BETWEEN VOLUME AND OUTCOMES FOR SELECTED DIAGNOSTIC CATEGORIES

Volume and Crude Rates of Outcome for Surgical and Nonsurgical Patients

The two diagnoses for which both nonsurgical and surgical cases were studied were ulcer and biliary tract disease. As can be seen readily in our data (table 11.1), biliary tract disease was treated more frequently by surgery than medically (60 percent of all patients with biliary tract diagnosis received surgery). In contrast, ulcers were more commonly treated medically (84 percent were treated medically). The crude death rate was lower in each diagnostic category for the more common treatment; that is, for biliary tract disease, the death rate was lower for surgical patients (1.1 percent versus 2.8 percent), and for ulcers, it was lower for medical patients (2.4 percent versus 4.3 percent). This finding is consistent with the argument that greater experience with a given treatment leads to better outcomes. However, it is also consistent with the argument that the "usual" form of treatment is preferred for routine cases, while more difficult cases receive the "unusual" treatment. To be able to distinguish whether experience is important in explaining variation in outcomes, for both surgical and medical patients, it is necessary to take patient condition into account.

Volume and Standardized Outcomes

In the analyses whose results are presented in table 11.2, we examine the impact of volume, or hospital experience with patients in the same diagnostic-procedure category, on patient outcomes as measured by SMRs. We turn first to the results for each of the five individual diagnostic categories exhibiting more than 1,000 deaths in the set of study hospitals.[5] As expected, there were more patients and, hence, more observed deaths in the high-volume hospitals. For each of the surgical categories, the observed death rate was higher for low-volume hospitals. However, in all cases except that of biliary tract operations, the expected death rate was also higher in low-volume hospitals. This finding was unexpected in that it implies that the low-volume hospitals were more likely to treat more difficult patients. It also underscores the importance of taking patient mix into account before comparing death rates. These same overall patterns were observed for the two groupings of surgical categories— all selected surgical and all surgical categories. Turning to the two medical categories, ulcer diagnosis patients displayed a pattern like those of patients in the individual surgical categories. Biliary tract patients, however, also exhibited a lower death rate in low-volume hospitals that tended to treat more difficult patients.

The SMRs and the results of a statistical test for differences between outcome performances in low- and high-volume hospitals are displayed in the

5. As reported in table 11.1, one of these categories—stomach operations with ulcer diagnosis—revealed significant differences among hospitals at only the .017 level. It was retained in this analysis to permit comparisons with ulcer patients treated medically.

last two columns of table 11.2.[6] The SMRs for patients treated in low- and high-volume hospitals can vary above 1, indicating more deaths than expected, or below 1, indicating fewer deaths. Because of the model used to estimate deaths, the overall number of observed deaths equals the overall expected deaths in each category, and the SMR for all hospitals combined is 1.0.

In each of the six surgical categories, the SMR indicated better outcomes (i.e., fewer deaths than expected) in more experienced hospitals. For four of the six comparisons, the differences were statistically significant at the .05 level or less. (One nonsignificant category, ulcer surgery, was also not significant in the test for hospital differences.) For the two groupings of surgical categories, the more experienced hospitals were more likely to have better outcomes, with a significance level of less than .001.

The last column of table 11.2 reports the ratio of high- and low-volume SMRs, providing an indication of the percentage increase of deaths over what would be expected on the basis of patient condition. Among the significant categories, they range from a 32 percent increase in death rates for less experienced hospitals for intraabdominal aorta operations to an 18 percent increase for amputation of a lower limb with no current trauma. The percentage increase in death rates in the less experienced hospitals for all selected surgical categories combined was 13 percent.

For the medical categories, biliary tract patients unexpectedly had a better SMR (i.e., fewer deaths) in the low-volume hospitals, a finding significant at the .05 level. Neither ulcer diagnosis nor the combined medical categories was statistically different for the two types of hospitals.

In summary, for surgical categories, we found strong evidence that treating a larger volume of patients in the same category was associated with better outcomes than would be expected on the basis of patient health characteristics.

6. The computation of χ^2 utilized the number of expected deaths from the logistic regression analyses. Since the computation of the expected number of deaths was not based on cell margins, there is no loss of degrees of freedom over the number of cells (4). Using the selected surgical categories as an example, we computed $\chi^2 = \sum_{i=1}^{4} \frac{(O - E)^2}{E_i}$, where $(O - E)^2 = (\pm\ 300.2)^2$ and the expected number of patients in each category, E_i, is displayed below.

Hospitals	Expected Number of Survivors	Expected Number of Deaths
Low-volume	66,257.2	3,357.8
High-volume	189,033.8	8,295.2

$\chi^2 = 39.54$ with four degrees of freedom.

Table 11.2. The effects of volume on adjusted and crude outcome: Nonparametric analyses

Hospital Volume[a]	Number of Patients (N)	Number of Observed Deaths (D)	Number of Expected Deaths (E)[b]	Observed Death Rate (D/N)	Expected Death Rate (E/N)	Standardized Mortality Ratio (SMR) (D/E)	Ratio of SMRs, χ^2, p value
Selected surgical categories							
1. Intraabdominal artery operations							
Low volume	2,459	539	448.9	.219	.183	1.201	1.32
High volume	7,073	937	1,027.1	.132	.145	.913	$\chi^2 = 31.38$
Total	9,532	1,476	1,476.0	.155	.155	1.000	$p < .001$
3. Biliary tract operations							
Low volume	33,818	456	384.4	.013	.011	1.190	1.27
High volume	96,931	988	1,059.6	.010	.011	.930	$\chi^2 = 18.38$
Total	130,749	1,444	1,444.0	.011	.011	1.000	$p < .005$
4. Stomach operations with ulcer diagnosis							
Low volume	7,418	353	334.1	.048	.045	1.057	1.08
High volume	19,270	785	803.0	.041	.042	.977	$\chi^2 = .08$
Total	26,688	1,138	1,138.0	.043	.043	1.000	$p > .05$
7. Hip fracture diagnosis with no other trauma diagnoses							
Low volume	13,627	1,411	1,357.0	.104	.100	1.040	1.06
High volume	38,741	3,362	3,416.0	.087	.088	.984	$\chi^2 = 3.3$
Total	52,368	4,773	4,773.0	.091	.091	1.000	$p > .05$
8. Amputation of the lower limb with no current trauma diagnosis							
Low volume	3,001	504	451.6	.168	.151	1.116	1.18
High volume	7,266	972	1,024.4	.134	.141	.949	$\chi^2 = 10.2$
Total	10,267	1,476	1,476.0	.144	.144	1.000	$p < .05$

All selected surgical categories (9 categories)							
Low volume	69,615	3,658	3,357.8	.052	.048	1.089	1.13
High volume	197,329	7,995	8,295.2	.041	.042	.964	X = 39.54
Total	266,944	11,653	11,653.0	.044	.044	1.000	p < .001
Additional surgical categories							
12. Large bowel operations with cancer diagnoses							
Low volume	4,492	344	299.7	.077	.067	1.1484	1.21
High volume	13,380	816	860.3	.061	.064	.9487	$\chi^2 = 9.48$
Total	17,872	1,160	1,160.0	.065	.065	1.000	p < .05
All surgical categories (15 categories)							
Low volume	87,676	4,879	4,519.1	.056	.052	1.080	1.12
High volume	244,076	10,739	11,098.9	.044	.046	.968	$\chi^2 = 55.96$
Total	331,152	15,618	15,618.0	.047	.047	1.000	p < .001
Medical categories							
16. Biliary tract diagnosis—nonsurgical							
Low volume	28,036	759	834.9	.027	.030	.909	0.121
High volume	60,803	1,718	1,642.1	.028	.027	1.046	$\chi^2 = 10.7$
Total	88,839	2,477	2,477.0	.028	.028	1.000	p < .05
17. Ulcer diagnosis—nonsurgical							
Low volume	42,932	1,169	1,145.0	.027	.027	1.021	1.03
High volume	95,336	2,130	2,154.0	.022	.023	.989	$\chi^2 = .03$
Total	138,268	3,299	3,299.0	.024	.024	1.000	p > .05
All medical categories (2 categories)							
Low volume	70,968	1,728	1,979.9	.027	.028	.974	0.96
High volume	156,139	3,848	3,796.1	.025	.024	1.014	$\chi^2 = 2.10$
Total	227,107	5,776	5,776.0	.025	.025	1.000	p > .05

[a] High-volume hospitals are those that treated above the average number of patients in the same category as the patient.
[b] The sum of the individual patient's probabilities of dying.

These results characterized both groupings of surgical categories as well as all six individual surgical categories, although they were significant for only four. According to our data, the importance of the experience of the hospital for improving surgical outcomes was not dependent upon the relative difficulty of the procedure. Medical outcomes presented a mixed story: greater experience was not significant for explaining different outcomes in ulcer patients or in the combined medical categories but was weakly related to poorer outcomes for biliary tract patients.

Volume, Risk Level, and Outcomes

We turn next to the effect of volume on outcomes when patients' risk level is taken into account. Two approaches were pursued. First, we sought to determine whether a hospital's overall experience in treating patients in a given category revealed differential benefits to patients at varying risk levels. Up to this point volume had been assessed for the patient category as a whole, while outcomes had also taken into account the patient's risk level. We began by examining the relation between volume and outcome for each risk level separately. Second, we defined our measure of volume to include experience in treating the patient's risk level as well as his or her diagnostic category. Experience counted only when a hospital treated patients in the same category and at the same risk level. We focused first on the surgical categories.

Our first question was whether experience in treating patients in a given category was more or less beneficial for high-, medium-, or low-risk patient groupings. Figures 11.1 through 11.6 present the results of our tests for the six surgical categories exhibiting more than 1,000 deaths. Each figure graphs the SMR for each of the three risk groupings in high- and low-volume hospitals, *volume* being defined as experience in treating patients in the same surgical category. Also reported is the SMR for all risk groupings combined. Recall that an SMR greater than 1 indicates that more deaths were observed than were expected, and an SMR less than 1, fewer deaths. Significance tests for each comparison indicate whether or not the differences observed between high- and low-volume hospitals were larger than could be expected by chance.

The findings for the six categories revealed both similarities and differences. It appears that high-volume hospitals did exhibit fairly consistent effects on patient outcomes regardless of risk level (note the relative flatness of their graph line)—a possible exception was for the amputation of a lower limb (fig. 11.6)—while low-volume hospitals exhibited effects that interacted with risk level. Focusing on the patterns in low-volume hospitals, we observed that low- or medium-risk groupings generally seemed to fare worse, while high-risk patients experienced better outcomes (lower SMRs). It appears that for patients in low-volume hospitals, those undergoing surgery for intraabdominal aorta, hip fracture, and amputation of a lower limb (figs. 11.1, 11.5, and 11.6)

Figure 11.1. Standardized mortality ratios for high- and low-volume hospitals, by risk level of patients: Intraabdominal aorta surgery

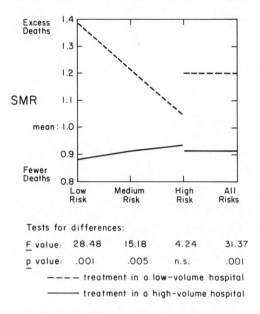

Tests for differences:

F value:	28.48	15.18	4.24	31.37
p value:	.001	.005	n.s.	.001

- - - - treatment in a low-volume hospital

———— treatment in a high-volume hospital

Figure 11.2. Standardized mortality ratios for high- and low-volume hospitals, by risk level of patients: Gall bladder surgery

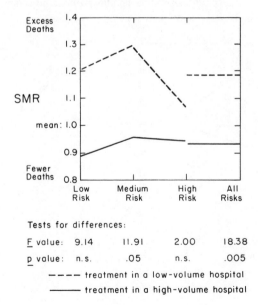

Tests for differences:

F value:	9.14	11.91	2.00	18.38
p value:	n.s.	.05	n.s.	.005

- - - - treatment in a low-volume hospital

———— treatment in a high-volume hospital

Figure 11.3. Standardized mortality ratios for high- and low-volume hospitals, by risk level of patients: Stomach operations with ulcer diagnosis

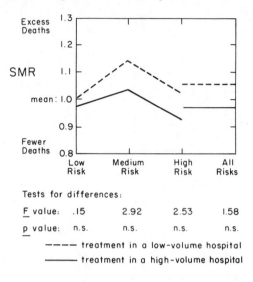

Tests for differences:

	Low Risk	Medium Risk	High Risk	All Risks
F value:	.15	2.92	2.53	1.58
p value:	n.s.	n.s.	n.s.	n.s.

– – – – treatment in a low-volume hospital

——— treatment in a high-volume hospital

Figure 11.4. Standardized mortality ratios for high- and low-volume hospitals, by risk level of patients: Large bowel operations with cancer diagnosis

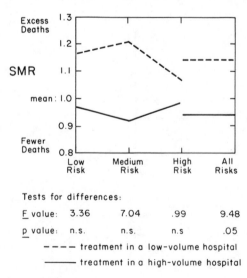

Tests for differences:

	Low Risk	Medium Risk	High Risk	All Risks
F value:	3.36	7.04	.99	9.48
p value:	n.s.	n.s.	n.s	.05

– – – – treatment in a low-volume hospital

——— treatment in a high-volume hospital

Figure 11.5. Standardized mortality ratios for high- and low-volume hospitals, by risk level of patients: Hip fracture diagnosis with no other trauma diagnosis

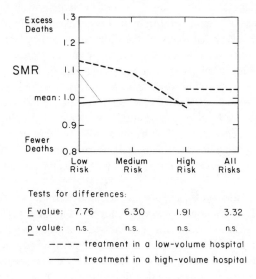

Figure 11.6. Standardized mortality ratios for high- and low-volume hospitals, by risk level of patients: Amputation of the lower limb with no current trauma

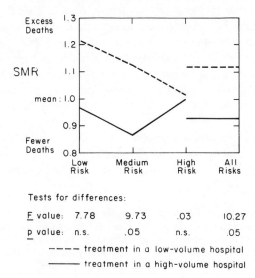

experienced somewhat worse outcomes in the low-risk level as compared with other risk levels. On the other hand, for patients in low-volume hospitals undergoing surgery for biliary tract, ulcer, and cancer of the large bowel (figs. 11.2, 11.3, and 11.4), those at the medium-risk level experienced somewhat better outcomes. Note, however, that many of the differences between high- and low-volume hospitals associated with risk groupings were not significant, in part because of the smaller number of deaths in each subgroup. In no instance was the difference between high- and low-volume hospitals significant for high-risk patients. The greater fluxuation of SMRs by risk level for the individual categories (figs. 11.1–11.6) for low-volume hospitals as compared with high-volume hospitals could have been due in part to the smaller number of cases being analyzed in the low-volume hospitals. We shall return to an examination of the interaction between risk level and volume when we look at the combined study categories.

Before commenting further on these patterns, let us determine whether they held when the second volume measure was employed. Is hospital performance improved by experience in treating *any* patient within a given category or by treating only patients at the *same risk* level? If experience depends importantly on risk level as well as category, we would expect to see stronger results in each of the risk levels for the second volume measure; in particular, we would expect to see an effect of experience on high-risk patients.[7] Figure 11.7 reports the relation between volume and outcome for patients undergoing intraabdominal aorta surgery by risk level for high- and low-volume hospitals, using two measures of volume: greater than average experience in treating any patient in the category (i.e., the same measure reported in fig. 11.1–11.6) and greater than average experience in treating patients at the same risk level in the category. It appears that the effects of volume on outcome for each of the three risk groupings were very similar for the two measures of volume. To the extent that there were any differences between the measures, the use of the more refined volume measure tended to be associated with smaller, not greater, differences between the two types of hospitals. These results held for all the other surgical categories studied except that of biliary tract surgery, where differences between types of hospitals were slightly greater using the more refined volume measure.

To combat the problem of reduced numbers, we examined the relation between volume, risk level, and outcomes for all selected surgical categories combined. The findings revealed by inspection of the individual categories

---

7. If risk level is an important qualifier of experience, then ignoring risk could be particularly misleading for high-risk patients, since they represented such a small percentage of all patients. For example, over 90 percent of all biliary tract patients undergoing surgery were in the low-risk category. Recall that patients were distributed among risk-level groupings to equalize the numbers of observed deaths, not the numbers of patients treated.

Figure 11.7. Standardized mortality ratios for high- and low-volume hospitals, by risk level of patients, comparing two measures of volume

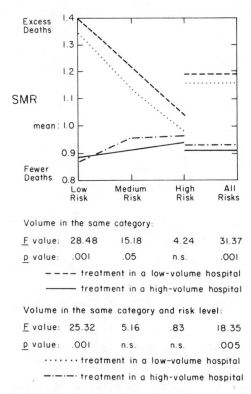

Volume in the same category:

F value: 28.48   15.18   4.24   31.37

p value: .001   .05   n.s.   .001

  – – – – treatment in a low-volume hospital

  ———— treatment in a high-volume hospital

Volume in the same category and risk level:

F value: 25.32   5.16   .83   18.35

p value: .001   n.s.   n.s.   .005

  • • • • • • treatment in a low-volume hospital

  —•—•—• treatment in a high-volume hospital

were sufficiently similar to suggest the appropriateness of examining them in combination. Results for all selected surgical categories combined for both volume measures are reported in figure 11.8. The general pattern for patients to have better outcomes in high-volume hospitals at each risk level was consistent with the results already noted, but differences in SMRs between high- and low-volume hospitals were significant at the .001 level for both low- and medium-risk patient groupings as well as overall.

We concluded first that hospitals having more experience in conducting a given type of surgery produced better outcomes for their patients, particularly those at low or medium risk levels, than did hospitals having less experience. Figure 11.8 also reveals an interactive relation between risk level and volume. As before, SMRs for high-volume hospitals varied little by risk level. SMRs in low-volume hospitals, however, varied greatly by risk level. The poorest outcomes were observed for low-risk patients in low-volume hospitals. Moreover, the discrepancy in performance between low- and high-volume hospitals was

Figure 11.8. Standardized mortality ratios for high- and low-volume hospitals, by risk level of patients: All selected surgical categories combined

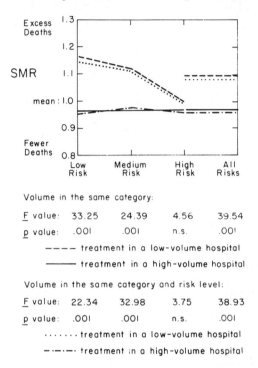

Volume in the same category:

F value:	33.25	24.39	4.56	39.54
p value:	.001	.001	n.s.	.001

–––– treatment in a low-volume hospital

——— treatment in a high-volume hospital

Volume in the same category and risk level:

F value:	22.34	32.98	3.75	38.93
p value:	.001	.001	n.s.	.001

······· treatment in a low-volume hospital

–·–·–· treatment in a high-volume hospital

greatest for this group of patients—a difference significant at .001. Medium-risk patients in low-volume hospitals fared relatively better but were still significantly worse off than their counterparts in high-volume hospitals. High-risk patients in low-volume hospitals were relatively better off than either medium- or low-risk patients, and they did not differ significantly from their counterparts in high-volume hospitals. Thus we concluded, second, that there was support for the overall relation between volume and surgical outcomes to be mitigated by the risk level of the patient (fig. 11.8) and the type of diagnostic procedure involved (figs. 11.1–11.6). Last, since the results in figure 11.8 demonstrated no difference between the two measures of volume, we concluded that there was no support for the effect of experience, or volume in treating patients, to depend upon treating surgical patients in the same category *and* at the same risk level.

We turn now, more briefly, to the two medical categories: biliary tract and ulcer patients treated medically rather than surgically. As reported in figures 11.9 and 11.10, there were no significant differences in outcomes associated with differences in patient risk level. As already noted, higher-volume hospitals

Figure 11.9. Standardized mortality ratios for high- and low-volume hospitals, by risk level of patients: Nonsurgical gall bladder diagnoses

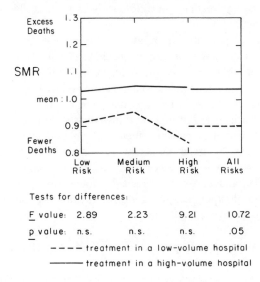

Tests for differences:

F value: 2.89   2.23   9.21   10.72

p value: n.s.   n.s.   n.s.   .05

— — — treatment in a low-volume hospital

——— treatment in a high-volume hospital

Figure 11.10. Standardized mortality ratios for high- and low-volume hospitals, by risk level of patients: Nonsurgical ulcer diagnoses

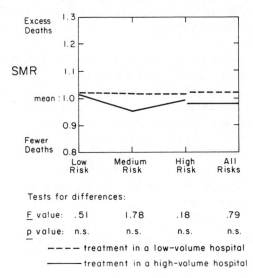

Tests for differences:

F value: .51   1.78   .18   .79

p value: n.s.   n.s.   n.s.   n.s.

— — — treatment in a low-volume hospital

——— treatment in a high-volume hospital

performed no better than low-volume hospitals on ulcer patients, and contrary to prediction, high-volume hospitals experienced poorer outcomes than low-volume hospitals for biliary tract patients, a difference significant at the .05 level for all risk levels combined.

For biliary tract medical patients, the relation between risk level and volume paralleled the pattern observed for surgical patients. That is, there was no evidence of an interaction between risk and outcome in the high-volume hospitals. For low-volume hospitals, on the other hand, high-risk patients appeared to fare better than either low- or medium-risk patients. As before, in no instance were the differences between high- and low-volume hospitals significant for any risk level. For ulcer patients, there was no evidence of an interactive effect between risk level and outcomes. In analyses not reported here, we examined the impact of using the second volume measure and found the same pattern as reported above. We concluded that there was little consistent support for the effect of experience, or volume in treating patients, for producing better outcomes for medical patients.

Volume and Outcomes: Alternative Explanations for Their Relationship

We can only speculate on the bases of these patterns. The tendency for high-risk surgical patients to fare somewhat better than low- or medium-risk surgical patients in low-volume hospitals may indicate that these hospitals treat high-risk surgical patients differently, perhaps by providing special facilities or arrangements, such as intensive care, that help to overcome the limitations of the hospital's general lack of experience. Alternatively, high-risk patients may not be randomly distributed among hospitals performing these procedures but may be concentrated in certain types of hospitals—for example, teaching hospitals or larger hospitals—that have arrangements that compensate for their low volume.

Many other factors may enter into these results to obscure any connection between volume, risk level, and outcomes for surgical patients. Surgical procedures vary greatly in complexity (see n. 3), and the benefits of experience may vary accordingly, although our data provide little support for this argument. Our measures of volume were crude, allowing us to assess only whether a hospital had more or less experience than the average study hospital. For some procedures, this led us to designate some hospitals as low-volume even though they treated, in absolute terms, a large number of patients.[8] Finally, as already noted, death is not a sensitive measure of surgical outcome, particularly for patients in low- and medium-risk groupings.

8. We were not able to redefine our measures of volume to test for this possibility because precautionary steps taken to protect the anonymity of the study hospitals, required by our contract with CPHA, precluded the redefinition of any measure.

The absence of strong outcome effects associated with volume and/or risk level for medical patients is consistent with several varying explanations. Experience in dealing with medical patients may not have the same positive impact on performance that it appears to have in the case of surgical patients. Or it may be that inhospital death is not a valid indicator of medical performance either in general or in the case of these two diagnostic categories. Alternatively, it is possible that the medical categories chosen are in evidence frequently enough that even those hospitals with below-average volume see sufficient numbers of patients to be experienced in their care. Finally, it is possible that volume is highly intercorrelated with other structural characteristics of hospitals affecting outcomes, so that the true effect of volume is masked in our results. This final explanation is one that we evaluate for both surgical and medical patients in the next section using other data from the ES.

RESULTS: THE RELATION BETWEEN VOLUME AND OUTCOMES AND OTHER HOSPITAL CHARACTERISTICS

Volume measures constitute the principal independent measures for explaining differences in quality in the current analyses. However, hospitals as a type of organization vary along several major structural dimensions that have been found to be associated with quality. Some researchers have found teaching to be associated with better care, particularly for process measures (Lee, Morrison, and Morris 1957; Lipworth, Lee, and Morris 1963; Goss 1970; Palmer and Reilly, 1979; Shortell and LoGerfo 1981); others have found greater expenditures associated with better care (Flood et al. 1982 [see also chap. 8 in this volume]) or worse care (Shortell, Becker, and Neuhauser 1976); and still others have reported evidence that surgery is safer in larger hospitals (Roemer 1959; Rhee 1976). Many of these studies did not take multiple structural variables into account at the same time; moreover, patient mix often was ignored or was estimated at the hospital level only in these studies. Each of these dimensions can, in turn, be expected to be related to volume. Other researchers have suggested that the relation between structure and outcome is more complex: the impact depends upon the difficulty of the cases being treated (Schoonhoven et al. 1980). For example, experience may be more critical for high-risk patients. In the previous section we found little evidence to support this hypothesis; indeed we found no significant differences between low- and high-volume hospitals for high-risk patients. We also observed some evidence that high-risk patients were grouped by type of hospital rather than distributed randomly. It is possible that the true relation between volume and outcome and the difficulty of the patients being treated was masked in our previous analyses. For all these reasons, it was important to control for these hospital contextual measures, as well as patient mix, when examining the impact of volume on outcome.

In the previous section we examined the volume-outcome hypothesis for each study category of patients and for classes of surgical patients and for medical patients; in these analyses we use only classes of patients: selected surgical patients (nine categories) and medical patients (two categories). Because the effect of experience can be argued to be more critical for more difficult cases, we also examined patients grouped as low-, medium-, or high-risk based upon their probability of dying.[9] The major analyses in the previous section were based on nonparametric techniques; here we used linear regression to examine the impact of multiple independent variables on outcomes. We turn next to a definition of these additional hospital characteristics.

Measures of Hospital Structure

Hospital *size* was measured by the average daily patient census, calculated by multiplying the total (short-term) bed size by the average occupancy rate. The log base 10 of this figure was used as a correction for nonlinearity. Data for this measure were available from the American Hospital Association (AHA) annual survey. Size was highly correlated with the volume of selected surgical patients ($r = .656$).[10]

Teaching status was assessed using a measure that combined information regarding both the existence of residency programs (advanced post-M.D. training for specialized practice) and their current activation. AHA annual survey data pertaining to the existence of one or more residency training programs were supplemented by information obtained from the American Medical Association (AMA) *Consolidated List* of approved residencies indicating whether residency positions were vacant or filled. For this chapter, a hospital was regarded as a teaching hospital if (1) both AHA and AMA sources reported it to be conducting one or more residency training programs and (2) the AMA source reported that there were at least two residents actually present in the hospital.[11] Teaching was correlated strongly and positively with size ($r = .531$) and with volume ($r = .301$).

Hospital *expenditures* were measured so as to focus attention not on re-

---

9. The probability of dying for each patient was obtained using a logistic regression to estimate the impact of patient health variables at the time of admission on inhospital death. This procedure is described more fully in chap. 5.

10. The Pearson correlations involving volume reported throughout the description of hospital contextual measures were based upon the selected surgical categories, all risk levels combined. All correlations reported were those used in the linear regression analyses and so were weighted by the number of patients at the hospital. The number of hospitals was 1,196 (some hospitals were dropped due to insufficient cases in these categories); the number of patients, 266,944.

11. See chap. 12 for a more refined definition and analysis of teaching and the quality of care in the ES.

source holdings (e.g., capital equipment) but on resources actually expended on patient care. The measure used was the total annual expenditure reported by the hospital divided by the total number of patient-days of care. Data for this measure were available from the AHA annual survey. Expenditures were correlated positively with size ($r = .233$), teaching status ($r = .331$), and volume ($r = .169$).

Throughout the overall research design and analyses of the determinants of hospital performance from which these data derive, these three structural dimensions were expected to have an important impact on hospital performance. For this reason and because the three measures were interrelated, we report on all three dimensions in the work described here even though expenditures were not strongly related to volume.

Hospital Size, Volume, and Outcomes of Surgery

We begin with analyses comparing the impact of size and volume on the death rate. Size, not unexpectedly, was the hospital variable most highly correlated with volume. Since the size of a hospital is likely to be indicative of a more differentiated and complex organization, involving multiple departments and subunits as well as more specialized facilities and staff, the question of *how* organizational features affect performance depends very much on whether experience with similar cases or size is the primary determinant of differences in performance.

In table 11.3 we report the impact of volume alone and size alone on deaths before examining their impact conditional on each other. In all cases we include as an independent variable the probability of dying for each patient based upon the patient's health status. Two statistics are reported for each independent variable: the standardized regression coefficient (β) and the F ratio and its associated significance level. The β is a partial correlation coefficient representing the slope of the regression with all other independent variables held constant, and the standardized version permits the direct comparison of one coefficient with another. The F statistic provides a test of significance for each β by beginning with that portion of the total sum of squares that is unexplained by earlier variables and comparing the ratio of the remainder that is explained to that which remains unexplained. Significance levels are also provided for reference. Finally, with each equation the F ratio at the final step and the R^2 are reported. Because the dependent variable is mortality, a negative relation indicates that the variable is associated with a lower death rate, that is, better outcomes.

In each test reported in table 11.3, the strongest predictor of death was each patient's probability of dying, which summarized the information on the patient's health condition. In the first test, volume was the only hospital characteristic included. This information reproduced in another form the findings for

Table 11.3. The effect of volume on surgical death, adjusting for patient mix and hospital size (selected surgical patients)

	Death in Hospital					
	All Patients Combined (N = 266,944)			High Risk Patients Only[a] (N = 13,956)		
Test	β^b	F	p	β^b	F	p
1. *Patient Variable*						
Probability of dying[c]	.397	49,838	.0001	.314	1,531	.0001
Hospital variable						
Volume	−.013	51	.0001	−.010	1.5	.221
Overall statistics						
R^2			.158			.099
Overall F (p)			24,994 (.0001)			768 (.0001)
2. *Patient variable*						
Probability of dying[c]	.397	49,989	.0001	.314	1,527	.0001
Hospital variable						
Size	−.001	0	.600	.018	5.1	.024
Overall statistics						
R^2			.158			.099
Overall F (p)			49,700 (.0001)			770 (.0001)
3. *Patient variable*						
Probability of dying[c]	.396	49,697	.0001	.312	1,501	.0001
Hospital variables						
Volume	−.021	82	.0001	.038	13.0	.0001
Size	.017	31	.0001	.043	16.6	.0001
Overall statistics						
R^2			.158			.100
Overall F (p)			16,695 (.0001)			518 (.0001)

[a]Parallel analyses were also performed for low- and medium-risk patients. The results for both of these subsets closely resemble those reported for all patients combined, with no difference in the direction and the magnitude of the level of significance for volume. Size did not reach statistical significance for medium-risk patients (p = .08) and was less significant for low-risk patients (.001) in test level 1 regressions.

[b]β = the standardized coefficient from the linear regression.

[c]The probability of dying for an individual patient is the result of applying the logistic regression coefficients to predict death on the basis of the patient's actual age, physical status, stage of disease, type of procedure, and so on, as detailed in the previous section.

selected surgical patients reported in table 11.2 and figure 11.8 and showed that volume significantly reduced the likelihood of dying even after patient health condition was taken into account for all selected surgical categories combined but not for high-risk patients only. In the second test, size was the only hospital variable included. Size alone was not significantly predictive of differences in deaths for all selected surgical patients but was weakly related to more deaths than would be expected for high-risk patients. In the third test, both volume and size were entered simultaneously. For selected surgical categories combined, volume significantly reduced the likelihood of death even when size was taken into account. Size, on the other hand, was significantly related to an increased likelihood of death when volume was taken into account. For high-risk patients, when size was taken into account, volume for the first time was significantly related to a reduced likelihood of death. For the high-risk patients, increased volume evidently was highly interrelated with being treated in larger hospitals. As observed for all patients combined, larger hospitals were significantly related to more deaths after both patient mix and volume were taken into account. Similar analyses were performed for the low- and medium-risk patients as well, although they are not reported in table 11.3. For these subgroups the findings resembled those reported for all patients combined, except that size was not as significantly related to higher death rates when both volume and size were included.

The R^2 statistic in this and related tables was low (.158) compared with those observed in analyses involving linear regressions on dependent variables that are continuous and have normal distributions. The small R^2 was primarily an artifact of the type of dependent variable employed—death is dichotomous and highly skewed (the overall death rate for the selected surgery categories is 4.4 percent)—and our use of patient-level analyses. As detailed in the previous section, we believed that the adjustment for patient mix was most appropriately performed at the patient level, taking into account the patient's age, sex, type of disease, procedure, and so on. Volume was also defined at the patient level and represented experience with cases similar to the patient's. When this model was employed for our tests, the R^2 was constrained to be small. (We have adapted the arguments of Gordon, Kannel, and Halperin 1979; see also above, chap. 5, for details.) For example, if we take a death rate of 4.5 percent (approximately that of selected surgical patients) and expect deaths to be doubled due to the low volume of patients treated (3 percent versus 6 percent), an estimated R^2 due to the hospital characteristic would be only .005. Thus, applying the usual criteria for evaluating the magnitude of our R^2 is inappropriate.

Hospital Control Variables, Volume, and Outcomes of Surgery

In analyses reported in table 11.4 the full set of hospital variables was introduced into the regression of volume on death with essentially no change from the regression with size and volume only. That is, neither teaching nor expenditures was significantly related to death when conditioned on the other variables; size continued to be significantly related to an increase in deaths, and volume to a decrease, when all variables were in the equation. Although we do

Table 11.4. The effect of volume on surgical death, adjusting for patient mix and hospital size, teaching status, and expenditures (selected surgical patients)

	B	Standard Error of B	β	F	p
		Death Inhospital[a] (N = 266,944)			
Patient Variable					
Probability of dying	.984	.004	.396	49,700	.0001
Hospital Variables[b]					
Volume	−.010	.001	−.021	80	.0001
Size	.012	.002	.017	32	.0001
Teaching status	−.001	.001	−.002	1	.387
Expenditures	−.001	.000	−.005	5.7	.017
Overall Statistics					
R^2	.158				
Overall F (p)	10,019 (.0001)				

Change in F for all three hospital control variables beyond volume: 12.32
Change in F for teaching and expenditures beyond volume and size: 3.04

[a]Parallel analyses were performed for each of the three subsets of patients by risk level. The direction and magnitude of the results for each subset were the same as those reported here, although size was less significant for low- and medium-risk patients (.002 and .03, respectively).

[b]In addition to analyses reported here, interaction and squared terms for the hospital control variables were also entered. There was no change in direction nor significance level for the impact of volume on death for any subset or for the combined patients. The change in F for these additional variables as a set was 8.50 for all patients.

not report them in table 11.4, we performed parallel regressions for the three risk groupings of patients. As was the case when size and volume were entered, high-risk patients revealed the same pattern and significance levels as the entire set of patients. Although low- and medium-risk patients showed the same pattern, size was not significantly related to increased deaths. When interaction terms and squared terms for the hospital control variables were entered, there was no change in the direction and magnitude of the impact of volume on outcome.

Hospital Structure, Volume, and Outcomes for Medical Patients

Similar analyses were conducted to examine the effect of volume on outcomes for medical patients, taking into account patient condition and the size, teaching status, and expenditures per patient of the hospital treating the patient. The results are reported in table 11.5 in a form parallel to that of table 11.4. Here for the first time, by taking into account the effects of size, teaching status, and expenditures, we found a highly significant association between volume and outcome for medical patients in the predicted direction. Higher-volume hospitals were observed to have significantly better patient outcomes for the two types of medical patients combined. And as was the case for selected surgical patients, larger hospital size was significantly associated with poorer outcomes. Further, both teaching status and expenditures exhibited a significant relationship with outcomes: medical patients in teaching hospitals were more likely to experience poorer outcomes, while patients in hospitals with higher expenditures per patient were somewhat more likely to experience better outcomes. Contrary to earlier results in which volume was observed to have no effect or a weak adverse affect on patient outcomes for medically treated cases, when various measures of hospital structure were introduced, volume was significantly associated with better patient outcomes.

Hospital Structure, Volume, and Outcomes: Policy Implications

This study based on 266,944 selected surgical patients and 227,107 medical patients treated in over 1,200 hospitals examined the effect of a hospital's

Table 11.5. The effect of volume on medical death, adjusting for patient mix and hospital size, teaching status, and expenditures (medical categories)

	B	Standard Error of B	β	F	Level of Significance
		Death Inhospital[a] (N = 227,107)			
Patient Variable					
Probability of dying	.978	.005	.362	34,330	.0001
Hospital Variables[b]					
Volume	−.006	.001	−.017	48.6	.0001
Size	.016	.002	.033	90.1	.0001
Teaching status	.004	.001	.011	26.5	.0001
Expenditures	−.000	.000	−.005	3.7	.053
Overall statistics					
R^2	.133				
Overall F (p)	6,967 (.0001)				
Change in F for all three hospital control variables beyond volume: 87.0 (.0001)					

[a]Parallel analyses were performed for each of the three subsets of patients by risk level. The direction and magnitude of the results for each subset were the same as those reported here except that expenditures were not significant for medium- or high-risk patients (p = .83 and .74, respectively), and the effect of all hospital variables was reduced for high-risk patients (significance levels: volume [.068], teaching [.070], and size [.002]).

experience in treating patients similar to those studied on the outcomes experienced—death inhospital—by these patients, taking into account their condition at the time of treatment. When only hospital experience was considered, better than expected patient outcomes were observed in the more experienced hospitals for most categories of surgery examined but not for medical patients. Indeed, for one category of medical treatment—biliary tract disease—patients in high-volume hospitals were somewhat more likely to have poorer outcomes than expected. When related hospital characteristics were taken into account, however, both surgical and medical patients treated in more experienced hospitals exhibited outcomes significantly better than expected. Moreover, the effect of experience on outcomes was significant for all three levels of risk when other hospital characteristics were included. Among the three hospital characteristics examined, hospital size, although positively associated with experience, was consistently associated with poorer than expected outcomes for patients.

Although the differences in death rates among hospitals due to volume may appear to be small, they were in fact rather substantial if projected to a national context. Using the unstandardized coefficient (.010) and its standard error (.001) for volume, we estimated the number of deaths among selected surgical patients in our study hospitals that might have been prevented if the surgeries had been performed in high-volume hospitals to be between 627 and 766. As detailed in the previous section, the entire patient population from the study hospitals represented about one-fifth of all patients discharged from nonfederal acute-care hospitals during the study year. Our sample of hospitals was not a random sample of all nonfederal acute-care hospitals. (See chap. 5 for details.) It is also probable that our sample was biased in including a disproportionate number of patients treated in high-volume hospitals. Nevertheless, we used the proportion one-fifth to generalize our results to the national experience. We estimated that between 3,100 and 3,800 excess deaths—representing about 5 percent of the patients in our study hospitals—were attributable to treatment in a low-volume hospital during the study year in the nine study surgical categories alone.

We have argued that our results have important implications for regionalizing health care. Does this estimate of excess deaths justify trying to influence where people go for surgery? Many factors influence whether people are willing to take additional risks in receiving health treatment. The convenience of the hospital location to the patient's home and family may be perceived by the patient to be more important than decreasing the probability of dying. For example, for low-risk biliary tract surgery (90 percent of all biliary tract surgeries), a patient's probability of dying would be reduced from .404 percent to .400 percent if he or she went to a high-volume hospital. At the other extreme, the probability of dying for average high-risk patients receiving abdominal surgery would decrease from 61.9 percent to 61.3 percent if they received surgery in a high-volume hospital. For the patient as well as for the physician, larger changes and higher probabilities are more likely to be convincing. A general expectation that greater experience is more important for more difficult cases, coupled with the belief that larger hospitals are more likely to be experienced, may account for the observation in our data that high-risk patients were more often found in larger hospitals.

Federal or state health policies could be implemented to encourage use of high-volume hospitals in several ways. A system to monitor and disseminate information about the volume of cases at each hospital could provide information to influence the patient's or the physician's decision on where the patient should be hospitalized. Regulations or reimbursement incentives could be used to encourage use of high-volume hospitals (such as by restricting the facilities to perform certain types of surgical procedures, coupled with minimum volume standards necessary to maintain facilities, or by selecting preferred provider organizations on the basis of volume). Our data suggest that such policies should try to encourage use of hospitals with high volume in the same diagnosis and procedure rather than simply larger hospitals. We found evidence that after volume was taken into account, larger hospitals did worse than expected.

Before contemplating enacting such recommendations, it is important to try to assess the potential magnitude of the benefits and risks involved. Is our finding limited to low volume's being implicated in increased numbers of deaths, or are other indicators of outcomes worse too?

Using Length of Stay to Estimate the Cost of Volume-Outcome Effects

We have argued that adjusted death rate is an indicator for the quality of care provided and that other adverse postsurgical outcomes such as infections and morbidity would also be more prevalent than expected in hospitals with greater death rates than expected. In additional analysis using the IS, we found some evidence that the poor quality of outcomes, measured by death, was indeed correlated with increased postsurgical morbidity, even after patient health variables were taken into account (chap. 6). Thus, to the extent that the quality of surgical care is poorer in low-volume hospitals, patients may also have an increased likelihood of morbidity and infections, an increased length of stay or other hospital services, and days lost from work—factors that contribute to the increased cost of care as well.

Although we were unable to measure morbidity and days lost from work in the ES, we could measure the length of stay (LOS) of patients. LOS is not a particularly good surrogate for the quality of care as measured by health outcomes (Ro, 1969; Rhee, Lyons, and Payne 1978; chap. 4 in this volume). It is subject to the same needs as death to take patient health variables into account before comparing hospital rates. It also varies by region, type of insurance, and utilization-review mechanisms. Last, there are potential pitfalls in assuming that shorter stays imply a proportional reduction in costs (Jönsson and Lindgren

1980). Nevertheless, we examined the relation of volume to LOS in order to assess the potential costs of surgery in low-volume hospitals beyond its impact on deaths.

Although these analyses are not detailed here, the pattern observed for the LOS of hospitalized patients closely resembled the relationships for death inhospital. That is, after patient mix was taken into account, high-volume hospitals were significantly more likely to have a reduced LOS.[12] When the three major structural variables were also included, size was consistently associated with increased LOS; volume remained predictive of reduced LOS. The pattern for LOS for high-risk patients paralleled that observed for death also. Volume was not significantly related to shortened LOS for this group until hospital size was taken into account. One explanation consistent with our findings is that care is better in experienced organizations, and the subsequently lowered postsurgical morbidity permits earlier discharge. When we used the estimated impact of volume on LOS (-3.004) and its standard error ($.077$), the selected surgical patients in low-volume hospitals in our study stayed an excess number of days totaling between 781,345 and 822,454 days. Projecting to a national level, we estimated that patients undergoing one of the nine study procedures stayed 3.9 million to 4.1 million extra days during the study year because they were treated in low-volume hospitals. In addition to the direct daily costs of extra hospital days, these patients probably incurred greater postsurgical morbidity and days lost from work on normal activity. We concluded from these estimates that there is a substantial impact on care of great policy importance associated with treating patients in low-volume hospitals— an impact measurable in terms of increased deaths and increased LOS.

The results of this analysis support earlier studies linking better outcomes with greater volume of patient care. It is important to emphasize that it was not just volume of patients per se that improved performance but volume of patients of a type highly similar to those whose care was being evaluated. While we found some support for the importance of volume for both medical and surgical categories of patients, the evidence was more consistent and stronger for selected surgical patients. Having more experience with similar types of patients might be associated with improved performance for a number of reasons. Individual staff members may become more highly qualified because of their increased experience in dealing with such patients; organizational routines are more likely to be devised, and their regular use may enhance the performance of all participants; and specialized facilities and equipment may be more likely to

---

12. Analyses for LOS paralleled those reported in tables 11.1–11.3, except that two additional patient-level variables were included to control for the effects of censoring of LOS; the discharge status, including discharge with incomplete recovery or transfer, and death within forty days of admission.

be on hand to support diagnosis and therapy as the flow of patients requiring such facilities become larger. More specific causal linkages need to be determined in future research, but our results do provide encouragement to those who argue that health care services should be regionalized so that to the extent possible, patients can be treated within facilities and by staff who have ample experience in dealing with similar problems.

DOES PRACTICE MAKE PERFECT, OR VICE VERSA?

An objection has been raised—not to our findings but to our imputation of causal direction—that on the average, more volume (experience) in treating a particular disease at a hospital leads to better outcomes (Dranove 1984). The counterargument is that good providers attract more patients, so that volume follows the quality of care, not vice versa (Luft, Hunt, and Mearki 1985). We agree that causal direction was not established in the analyses we presented. However, we do not find the alternative explanation—namely, that the association between volume and outcomes arises from patients' and doctors' selecting hospitals where care of a particular disease is good—to be as plausible as ours, for several reasons.

Choosing a Hospital on the Basis of a Disease-specific Indication of Quality

First, there is little evidence that patients or doctors select hospitals on the basis of their reputation for care of a specific disease or surgical procedure, particularly in the case of common benign diseases. With the possible exception of intraabdominal artery operations (1.2 percent of our study patients), all of our study categories involved common, benign disease and well-established procedures. Thus, for our evidence to reflect greater overall volume due to the general reputation of the hospital, the hospital would have to have greater volume and consistent quality for each category. Further, the hospital's reputation among patients would have to be consistent with the quality of care as assessed by standardized outcomes. As we argue in our review of the quality of care (chap. 3), there is considerable evidence that quality-of-care measures at the hospital level do not uniformly tap the same dimension of care; that is, a good reputation or patient satisfaction may or may not coincide with the best standardized outcomes (see Neuhauser 1971).

Patient Choice and Hospital Performance

Second, there is little evidence that patients participate actively in choosing hospitals. The modern movement of consumerism in medicine was relatively new at the time of the ES (1972), though demands for increased participation by patients in their treatment decisions and by consumers in the setting of local health policy were being made. Nevertheless, the actual influence of patients in choosing a hospital, then or now, has seldom been studied. Wolinsky and Kurz (1984) provided a rare attempt to examine patient attitudes about choosing a hospital. In their survey, conducted in 1981, they asked a random sample of adults in one metropolitan area about their attitudes in choosing a hospital, whether or not they had in fact been hospitalized recently. They found that (1) 50 percent of people believed that they, rather than their doctors, chose the hospital; (2) the quality of care was the most important criterion for selecting a hospital; and (3) people generally were not happy with hospitals. These results, assuming they can be generalized to earlier years as well as other areas of the country, would suggest that our critics may be right. People do care about quality and do attempt to choose on that basis. However, the question remains, How do people evaluate the quality of a hospital? How well should a global reputation for quality predict standardized outcomes for a specific category of patients?

Indeed, how do patients assess quality and choose a hospital? As we argued in the previous section, we do not believe that the variation in death rates by disease is sufficiently high to alter patient choice even if patients know the standardized death rates. Work on patient risk-taking behavior supports our view (see Eraker and Sox 1981). What is more important, the assessments of the quality of care in hospitals that patients make are not closely linked with either the clinical process or outcomes (see Lebow 1974; Nelson-Wernick et al. 1981; and chap. 4 in this volume). We believe that patients are more likely to select hospitals on the basis of global characteristics such as proximity to their home, religious affiliation, and amenities or on surrogates for quality like size, teaching status, or reputation. Still, especially in large metropolitan areas, there will be many nearby hospitals from which to choose. If volume truly follows quality, we might expect to see in our data that hospitals with the largest number of patients—controlling for community size—were associated with better quality. Recall that when we controlled for three global characteristics— size, teaching status, and expenditures per patient-day—we found that our results were, if anything, strengthened, not weakened as would be more consistent with the alternative explanation. Adding community size (measured in terms of the SMSA) did not alter our findings.

Physician Choice and Hospital Performance

Third, a slightly different version of the alternative explanation would argue that patients can influence the choice of the hospital indirectly by choosing more often to go to physicians who have a good reputation for care of the type they need. Physicians, in turn, are more likely to influence where hospital care will occur, though, we would argue, on the basis of hospital-level criteria such as the physician's having admitting and surgical privileges there; convenience to the physician, for example, having most of his or her hospitalized patients at the hospital; and, to some extent, cost, convenience, or the personal preferences of the patient. If such choice factors were the true explanation for our findings that volume is related to outcome, one might expect to see that better physicians are found at better hospitals. Recall that in chapter 8, using the IS data base, we examined whether variation in outcomes was explained by surgeon characteristics or hospital characteristics. In three different types of analyses we found no evidence that surgeon characteristics—including the surgeon's qualifications, such as board certification and years in residency, and the surgeon's experience, such as total number of patients operated on or the extent to which the surgeon specialized in operations within a specific specialty—predicted outcomes. Though hospitals differed significantly in the quality of outcomes for their patients, we found no evidence that physicians with better qualifications or greater overall experience were grouped into hospitals providing better care. (See Sharp 1986 for further support for this finding using biliary tract surgical patients.)

In addition to the more straightforward examination possible in the IS, we had available some indirect measures of the experience of individual surgeons in the ES. Using these, we found some limited evidence that greater volume per surgeon predicted better outcomes, but adding these measures to the linear regressions reported in the previous section did not alter the direction or the significance of the observed relation between volume and outcome. Kelly and Hellinger (1985), in their study of four surgical procedures in 373 nonfederal hospitals, were able to examine this question more directly and found no evidence to support that the volume-outcome relationship occurred at the surgeon level, but they did find evidence of the effect at the hospital level.

The Direction of Causality in the Volume-Outcome Hypothesis

Our finding regarding surgeon experience may help to shed light on why smaller hospitals were observed to give better care. In the selected surgical categories, our measure of greater volume per surgeon was associated with smaller, nonteaching hospitals and those that had a low volume. When we controlled for these relationships, we found that the extent to which a greater proportion of surgeons were experienced, the better the care; this relationship may be especially important in smaller nonteaching hospitals. Since the experience of the surgical staff was not consistently important for predicting better care, one interpretation of our findings would be that we were observing a threshold or minimal level of experience necessary for surgeons to maintain skills and quality outcomes. That is, once each surgeon exceeds a minimal level of current experience, the outcomes of patients are not discernibly different—at least with respect to the current level of experience of the surgeon. Other reasons for a surgeon's low level of current experience may account for the association with poorer quality: he or she may (*a*) be a newly trained physician setting up a private practice; (*b*) not receive many referrals due to a poor professional standing; or (*c*) conduct most of his or her practice in a different hospital, leading to less staff familiarity with the doctor's procedures and less time for the surgeon to devote to follow-up visits on the ward. Further research is needed to verify the importance of and the explanation for the observed association between the greater experience of the surgical staff as a whole and better outcomes.

We concluded that there was little evidence in our work to support the explanation that greater volume was associated with better outcomes due to patients' and/or surgeons' selecting hospitals known to provide good care for the specific disease of the patient, with the potential result that hospitals that provided better care for the disease had more volume. We also found little evidence that the relation between volume and outcome was explained by greater experience on the part of the surgical staff rather than by hospital-level variables. Nonetheless, we agree with Luft (1980) and Sloan, Perrin, and Valvona (1985), who argued that prior to implementation of a policy to promote regionalization of patients, more research is needed to establish how hospitals can be best organized to establish efficient and adequate provision of care. In particular, our study suggests that a regionalization policy that resulted primarily in increasing the overall size of hospitals would not be desirable; we found evidence that larger hospitals had significantly worse outcomes than expected, after controlling for the volume of patients treated and for other hospital characteristics, including the experience of the surgical staff.

12 · Hospital Characteristics and Hospital Performance

Ann Barry Flood, W. Richard Scott, and Wayne Ewy

INTRODUCTION AND OVERVIEW

In this chapter we present the major tests of hypotheses relating organizational characteristics to hospital performance based on the ES. The major strength of the ES was, of course, the large number of hospitals and patients, which permitted statistically reliable estimates on outcomes and employed a methodology amenable for monitoring the quality of care on a nationwide basis. On the other hand, reliance on already collected data bases for assessing both hospital and patient characteristics has a negative side: it measures only death upon discharge, provides only crude or incomplete measures of patient mix, and permits the development of only limited measures examining hypotheses and providing explanations for why and how hospital arrangements affect patient outcomes.

We begin with a brief restatement of the theoretical overview presented in detail in chapter 1, emphasizing those aspects that are especially relevant for the ES. The general conceptual approach to assessing hospital performance is to view patient outcome as reflecting the health status of the patient upon admission (predicting the expected course of the illness) and the quality of care he or she received during hospitalization for treatment of the disease. Because hospitals differ greatly in the types of patients they treat, it is imperative to take into account the differences in patient outcomes that reflect patient-related characteristics before using outcome as a measure of the quality of care provided by the hospital.

Much effort has been expended to obtain measures of hospital performance based on outcomes of patients that have already taken into account patient diagnoses, other indicators of initial health status, and, when appropriate, the type of surgical procedure undergone. The purpose of this effort has been to make it possible to attribute any remaining differences among hospitals in these outcomes to the operation of the hospitals themselves rather than to differences in the types of patients treated. Chapter 5 presents details of the standardization procedure used to remove patient variation for a set of seventeen categories of study patients, and chapter 6 details results establishing that hospitals did differ significantly in the outcomes achieved by the study patients, even after differences in outcomes expected on the basis of patient characteristics were removed. In the majority of analyses presented here, the fully standardized measures of patient outcomes for combinations of study patients were used because we considered them to be the best measures of hospital performance. In addition to these more fully standardized measures of hospital performance, we had available standardized measures of outcome based on fewer adjustment variables for nonstudy patients, which provided an important comparison with the fully standardized study categories.

The primary goal of this chapter is to identify which structural features of hospitals appear to explain these variations in performance. Predictions relating hospital organizational dimensions and subunits to patient outcomes are based on several theoretical traditions in the social sciences, including the view that there are a number of important structural dimensions that are especially relevant to the quality of work performance; the contingency view that the most effective hospital structure depends upon what kinds of patients it treats—more or less difficult, varied or similar, or some other relevant dimension; and the view of a hospital as a professional work organization highly dependent upon the qualifications of its participants and the use of appropriate types of control and coordination systems.

In the remaining sections, three separate types of issues are addressed using the ES data. Within each section the issue is presented, new indicators are defined, and the results of analyses are presented and discussed. The second section addresses the extent to which outcome, process, and structural measures of the quality of care were intercorrelated at the hospital level. In the third section we focus on three major hospital characteristics that have been widely argued to be related to the quality of care: size, teaching status, and expenditures. These same hospital characteristics are then used as control variables in the fourth section (as they were in chap. 11), as variables whose effects are taken into account prior to examining how and why more specific organizational dimensions of hospitals affect performance, testing hypotheses detailed in chapter 1. Finally, in the fifth section we summarize the findings of the ES regarding organizational characteristics and hospital performance.

In the ES, data for characterizing hospital dimensions came primarily from the annual survey of hospitals conducted by the American Hospital Association (AHA) in the study year 1972. There are many important limitations to these data for characterizing organizational dimensions. First, such data were limited to general descriptive information and to formal structural features. For example, while information on over forty different facilities was reported in this survey, we only knew whether each type of facility was present or absent. Survey data describing staff made only two types of distinctions: (1) whether staff members were full-time or part-time and (2) in which of four occupational groups they were classified: nurses (registered nurses [RNs] or licensed vocational nurses [LVNs]), house staff (residents or interns), hospital salaried physicians (M.D.'s or D.D.S.'s), or "others." Such data did not support more refined occupational distinctions (e.g., whether the "others" provided primarily custodial or hotel services, administration, clerical support, or laboratory and other patient-care support services). Nor did they permit distinctions in organizational position (e.g., whether the nurses provided patient care or occupied administrative positions).

The AHA data also provided no information on the occupational group considered by most to be of vital importance to the outcomes of patients treated—all physician members of the medical staff not directly reimbursed by the hospital, that is, virtually all the physicians involved in direct patient care. In order to help overcome this obviously severe limitation of the AHA data, we obtained some measures concerning the numbers of physicians performing surgery, the numbers of admitting physicians, and so on, from the PAS data. In addition, the PAS data were used to provide measures of experience: hospitals were identified as having treated more or fewer than the 1,224-hospital average number of study patients for each category. In Flood, Scott, and Ewy 1984a, 1984b (see also chap. 11 in this volume), we analyzed the effect on patient outcomes related to hospital experience with a given type of care.

In order to obtain additional information on the numbers of house staff and the level of affiliation, if any, with a medical school, we supplemented the AHA data with information from the AMA *Consolidated List* of approved residency programs. The AMA source was considered superior to AHA sources for two reasons: (1) it allowed the compilation of information for hospitals involved in more than one program of residency or intern training; and (2) it provided more detailed information about teaching status, including the level of affiliation with a medical school and the numbers and types of residency positions—both potential, or "approved," and filled.

In all, almost 100 organizationally related measures were developed. For the full report on their definitions and relationships see Forrest et al. 1978 (54–138). We have chosen a subset to present here, based on their relevance to our theoretical interests and on preliminary analyses presented in the full report.

The Effects of Time on Our Generalizations and Findings

Since the time of our ES study (1972), some important changes and developments have occurred in clinical practice and in the organization and delivery of, as well as the reimbursement for, hospital care. Moreover, in many cases the actual configuration, staffing, and facilities at the individual hospitals in our data bases have undergone significant changes (e.g., hospital systems have merged or individual hospitals have closed down). We argue that some of these changes limit the generalizations that can be made from our data. In particular, the descriptive statistics about the hospitals can be used to make relative comparisons among hospitals at the time of our study (such as comparisons of large, medium, or small hospitals) and between nonfederal, community hospitals then and now; but these descriptive statistics should not be assumed to correspond directly to the current set of hospitals, let alone to the specific hospitals in our sample.

Similarly, for some of the diagnostic categories and surgical procedures in our study, there have been significant improvements in diagnostic tools and changes in therapeutic strategies. Although the death rates and risks estimated in our data may no longer apply, the methodology for using information from medical record abstracts is still relevant. What is most important, the examination of structural determinants of the quality of care based on these data is still very useful for understanding the extent of the organizational arrangements of hospitals and the processes whereby they can have an impact on the type of medical care provided to patients. Thus, we argue that the methods we used and the arguments we advanced and found evidence to support or refute are important bases upon which to continue to study the quality of care and the production of services in the majority of our short-term hospitals. These findings also have practical importance for policy makers who would like to alter our health care delivery system to encourage lower costs but safeguard the quality of care provided in our nation's hospitals.

Use of the Term *Ratio* in Names of Our Measures

Many of the measures developed were expressed as the ratio of the value for the variable for a given hospital to the corresponding mean value of the same variable for all hospitals combined. This procedure was followed for computational convenience and in order to make all variables center around the value 1, independent of their original scale. In this sense they were "standardized" to remove differences in magnitude introduced by the scale of measurement. We denote such types of measures by using the term *ratio* in the name.

THE RELATIONS BETWEEN STRUCTURAL, PROCESS, AND OUTCOME MEASURES OF THE QUALITY OF CARE

In chapters 3–5 we discuss Donabedian's classic distinctions between the measures of the quality of medical care applied to hospitals: structural, process, and outcome indicators. We note that analysts who use process measures or structural measures alone to assess the quality of care must assume that correctly performing the task (appropriate process) or having excellent staff and facilities (appropriate structure) in fact leads to better outcomes for the patient, though there is evidence to suggest that these assumptions are not always correct. In the ES, we had available some indicators from all three types of measures, so that relationships between them at the hospital level may be examined rather than assumed.

Quality Assessed by Patient Outcomes

Measures of Outcome for Study Patients
For each patient in the seventeen categories of study patients, outcome was measured by inhospital death or live discharge. A standardized outcome was produced based on the discrepancy between the patient's actual outcome (dead or alive) and the corrected probability of dying inhospital. In this chapter we focus on the nine selected surgical categories (see also chap. 5).

Measures of Outcome for Nonstudy Patients
All patients not selected for inclusion in any of the original study categories (that is, the thirty-three original analytical categories and the group of qualifying patients with unspecified cancer) were designated "nonstudy patients" and were used in creating the two following types of measures.

Crude outcome ratios for nonstudy patients were obtained by dividing the number of nonstudy patients experiencing inhospital death by the total number of patients at each hospital. Two such measures were available, one based on all nonstudy patients, and the other based only on nonstudy patients who underwent an operation.

Standardized outcome ratios for nonstudy patients were based on all nonstudy patients and were standardized to take into account the patient's age (in one of five ranges of age) and the patient's diagnosis (the final diagnosis explaining admission as classified into one of 349 List A diagnostic categories). (See CPHA 1975 for definitions and listings of both the List A groups and the five groups of ages.) One measure used all nonstudy patients, and the second, only nonstudy patients who were operated on.

Quality Assessed by Process Measures

We developed several traditional but relatively crude indicators of the quality of process care (i.e., activities performed that were indicative of appropriate clinical actions) and an indicator of service intensity (how much and what kinds of services were provided). These process measures were limited to hospital-level summaries of process; they did not include physician-specific measures used in quality assurance or patient-level measures of the quality of the medical care process such as those reported by Rhee (1976) and Payne, Lyons, and Neuhouse (1984). Most of these measures were based on the information for final-study patients; the data base for each measure is indicated in the definitions.

The first three measures were based on the pathology reports for the most important operative procedures undergone by the patient. Thus, they were based on information on only those final-study patients who actually underwent an operation. The pathology report on the PAS abstract for a patient noted three classifications of tissue removed: disease A (the tissue findings supported removal), disease B (the tissue findings alone did not indicate that removal was necessary), and "no disease" (the tissue was without disease). In interpreting any results based on these measures, it is important to note that reports of questionable pathological evidence have the potential of raising serious legal and professional questions about the appropriateness of the surgery. Thus, there are professional pressures, as well as legal and financial incentives, for a hospital to underreport "no disease" and overreport disease A, especially in relatively public data sources. Misreporting could arise either from the pathologist's under- or overreporting of pathological support for tissue removal, especially in borderline or otherwise ambiguous situations, or from poor recording of pathology reports in the PAS data forms. Moreover, we recognize that the connection between a finding of no pathology and the implication of unnecessary surgery is far from perfect, even if all pathologists could agree about the tissue and there were no data recording errors.[1]

Path Report Ratio

In the first measure, *path report ratio*, we recorded the rate of reporting any type of results from a pathology examination, given that the patient had undergone an operation. We interpreted the rate as an indication of the seriousness with which the pathology report was collected for reporting purposes by the hospital. All measures using the path report were standardized on the basis of the risk level and the analytic category of the patient.

---

1. The Study on Surgical Services for the United States (ACASA 1976) identified six categories of surgical procedures that might be labeled unnecessary: (1) operations in which no pathological tissue is removed; (2) operations in which indications are a matter of judgment; (3) operations to alleviate endurable or tolerable symptoms; (4) discretionary operations for asymptomatic, nonpathological, or nonthreatening disorders; (5) operations currently considered outdated, obsolete, or discredited; and (6) operations for which there is little justification by clinical, x-ray, or laboratory study. Not only do we have no measure of most of these categories of unnecessary surgery but there is considerable disagreement among clinicians and patients alike about the necessity of the first four categories of procedures, since psychological comfort, ability to tolerate symptoms, and clinical judgments play an important part in deciding whether such procedures should be performed on a given individual.

Path Report: Disease A Ratio

In the second measure, *path report: disease A ratio,* we recorded the rate at which patients who had been operated on were reported to have disease A, that is, indications of diseased tissue supporting surgery. A higher score indicated that more surgery was substantiated by the pathology results.

Path Report: No Disease Ratio

The third measure, *path report: no disease ratio,* indicated the rate at which patients operated on were reported to have had no disease, that is, to have had no pathological support for the surgical removal of tissue.

Autopsy Ratio

The fourth measure of process care, autopsy, is traditionally interpreted to indicate that the hospital staff performed important diagnostic checks in following up inhospital deaths (Roberts 1978; McPhee and Bottles 1985). In a study comparing autopsy rates in a university teaching hospital in 1960, 1970, and 1980, Goldman et al. (1983, 1004) concluded that even in community hospitals, "the current very low autopsy rate in many hospitals is inappropriate and autopsies (are) vital for ensuring the quality of care." Our measure, *autopsy ratio,* was the percentage of all patients dead upon discharge who were given an autopsy. We standardized the autopsy rate to take into account whether or not the patient had undergone an operation, since having surgery increases the probability of an autopsy. (The mean autopsy rate for all ES hospitals for patients operated on who died was 36 percent; for all not operated on who died it was 25 percent.)

Special-Care Unit Ratio

The importance of intensive-care units (ICUs) for improving the quality of care has long been a matter of dispute (Bloom and Peterson 1973; Scheffler et al. 1982; National Institute of Health, Office of Medical Application of Research 1983; Singer et al. 1983; Madoff et al. 1985). There is general agreement that at least in the short term, use of the ICUs increases the cost of care. Two issues regarding their performance are (1) who is appropriately admitted to such units for care and (2) to what extent does their use predict better outcomes. Our measure, *the special-care unit ratio,* indicated the use of any type of ICU at the hospital. It was based on all study patients and was standardized to take into account the patient's diagnostic-surgical category and overall probability of dying.

Hospital Structures as Indicators of Quality

Three characteristics of hospitals have been widely assumed to indicate institutions where better-quality care is provided: the extensiveness and quality of the facilities and of the staff and the existence of approvals from various professional accreditation bodies (cf. Roemer and Friedman 1971; Donabedian 1980; and Maxwell et al. 1983). We describe measures of facilities and accreditation status here and discuss staffing measures in the fourth section.

Facilities

Based on the AHA list of facilities (which included some patient services, such as home-care programs), the measure of *total facilities* was a simple count of clinical facilities available at the study hospital, after duplications such as a part-time and a full-time pharmacy were removed (the number ranged from zero to thirty-nine with an average of sixteen facilities per hospital). The measure of *surgical facilities* used the same data, but only facilities relevant to surgical care were considered, and those more crucial to surgical care were given extra weight. In particular, a recovery room had a weight of 2; an ICU and a CCU each had a weight of 3; and a pharmacy, a diagnostic radioisotope, a histopathology laboratory, a blood bank, an inhalation therapy department, and an occupational therapy department each had a weight of 1 (the scores ranged from 0 to 11, with a mean of 8.6).

Accreditation Status

JCAH accreditation, or accreditation by the Joint Commission on Accreditation of Hospitals, was reported to the AHA (89.3 percent of the hospitals were accredited). An *approved cancer program* was one that had been reported to the AHA as having the approval of the American College of Surgeons (21.1 percent of the hospitals had such approval).

Comparisons of the Three Types of Measures of the Quality of Care

The primary comparisons we made were based on simple Pearson correlations (r), since the three types of measures were supposed to be tapping the same underlying dimension of the quality of performance. We examined both the apparent consistency among multiple indicators within a given type (intracorrelations) and the extent to which the different types of indicators of quality based on outcome, process, and structure tended to "agree" in their assessment of hospital performance (intercorrelations). Most of the measures were aggregated to produce a single measure for each hospital; thus, there were 1,224 observations. The only exceptions were measures based on outcomes of the selected surgical patients.[2] As explained more fully in chapter 5, we assumed that the "proper" number of cases for determining the level of significance of a

---

2. We also examined these same sets of correlations substituting the study patients in the two medical categories for the selected surgical patients and found essentially no differences from the pattern reported here.

correlation when a hospital-level variable was correlated with a patient-level variable was the smaller number, in this case 1,224.

The intracorrelations are presented in table 12.1. Looking at outcomes first, the indicators based on nonstudy patients were all strongly correlated with each other, as would be expected, since they involved part-whole comparisons in some cases and crude versus standardized versions of measures on exactly the same patients in others. These correlations illustrate (1) that crude outcomes were correlated with, but not identical in their assessment of hospital performance to, outcomes that took patient mix into account and (2) that outcomes of patients operated on were not necessarily consistent with those for medical patients, even after patient mix was taken into account. The outcome measures for nonstudy patients were all essentially unrelated to the crude and standardized outcomes for the selected surgical patients. The reason for no observed relation between outcome measures of nonstudy patients and of study patients is not clear. It could be due to the differences in the standardization procedure (although crude rates were unrelated too). It may also illustrate that not all patients in any given hospital receive the same quality of care, a result that is also suggested by our analyses reported in chapter 11 and by work reported by others (Luft, Bunker, and Enthoven 1979; Sloan, Perrin, and Valvona 1985).

Of ten possible correlations among process measures, 50 percent were significant at .001 or less. These measures were not all independently constructed, however. We found that the three measures based on the pathology report tended to be related. In particular, a hospital with a higher recorded percentage of pathology reports tended to have fewer cases with no disease, that is, with normal tissue removed. Also, a hospital with a high rate of pathology fully justifying surgery was likely to have a low rate of normal tissue removed. (Remember that there was an intermediate report of pathology which by itself did not fully justify surgery.) These relationships may indicate that better-quality peer review (indicated by careful recording of pathology reports) produced a desirable reduction in "unnecessary" surgery (less surgery with no disease). An alternative explanation is that a hospital that diligently recorded its pathology reports in the medical record abstract was likely to underreport surgery as being without any pathological justification. The measures based on pathology reports were essentially unrelated to the other process measures, except that a higher percentage of recorded pathology reports tended to occur in hospitals with a higher percentage of autopsies. Autopsy rates and the use of intensive care were also correlated, perhaps because both occurred in resource-intensive hospitals, which could support such types of care.

The structural indicators of the quality of care were the most strongly interrelated (all of the measures were correlated at the .001 level). The strong correlation of total facilities to surgical facilities was expected, since they form a part-whole relationship. However, facilities also tended to be related to JCAH accreditation and to an approved cancer program. Since such indications of

Table 12.1. Intrameasure correlations for outcome, process, and structural measures of the quality of care

Outcomes

	1	2	3	4	5[a]	6[a]
1		.427	.697	.201	.048	.024
2			.391	.641	.045	.022
3				.496	.043	.038
4					.033	.029
Mean	1.000	1.000	1.009	0.953	0.044	0.000
Standard deviation	0.767	0.789	0.258	0.373	0.204	0.188

Process

	1	2	3	4	5
1		.110	-.213	.134	.069
2			-.328	-.082	-.014
3				.054	.006
4					.208
Mean	0.936	0.984	2.81	0.869	0.873
Standard deviation	0.397	0.295	19.18	0.504	0.907

Structure

	1	2	3	4
1		.759	.264	.470
2			.275	.292
3				.179
Mean	16.27	8.56	0.893	0.211
Standard deviation	7.62	2.60	0.309	0.408

Note: Correlations are Pearson product-moment correlations. $|r| \geq .200$ are significant at $p \leq .001$, $N = 1,224$.
[a]Patient-hospital correlations; an N of 1,224 (hospitals) was used for tests of significance.

Key:

Outcomes (inhospital death)
1 Nonstudy patients, crude ratio, all patients
2 —, patients operated on only
3 —, standardized ratio, all patients
4 —, patients operated on only
5 Study patients, crude ratio, selected surgical patients
6 —, standardized rate, —

Process
1 Path report ratio
2 Disease A ratio
3 No disease ratio
4 Autopsy ratio
5 Special-care unit ratio

Structure
1 Total facilities
2 Surgical facilities
3 JCAH accreditation
4 Approved cancer program

approval follow an examination of the quality of the facilities, this correlation, while not tautological, was not surprising.

Tables 12.2 and 12.3 present the correlations across the different types of measures. The story they tell supports those who would question the interchangeability among the three types of measures of the quality of care. In particular, table 12.2 shows that outcomes were remarkably unrelated to process measures and to structural indicators of quality. None of the fully adjusted outcome measures of study patients was significantly related to any process or structural measure of quality, and the standardized outcome measures based on nonstudy patients were not consistent in their relation to process or structural measures. In all, only eleven out of fifty-four, or twenty percent, of the comparisons were significant at the .001 level, with .224 being the largest *r* value. Indeed, among those structural measures correlated significantly with outcomes, almost all predicted higher death rates, or poorer-quality outcomes. In table 12.3, on the other hand, there was some evidence of an association between process measures and structural indicators of quality—at least for autopsy rate and intensive care. The association between these process measures and the structural measures based on facilities and approvals is probably best explained by the fact that they were all dependent upon or indicative of the availability of intensive clinical resources. However, resource-intensive hospitals did not necessarily produce the best outcomes.

In summary, we concluded that there was little or no consistent association between some of the traditionally used indicators of the quality of care for hospitals based on structure, process, and outcomes of patients. We can offer no comfort to those who would prefer to offer simple assurances to the public that a hospital can be assumed to provide the highest quality of outcomes if it has been approved by a major accrediting group, if it adopts a policy of conducting autopsies, if it has many facilities and the latest medical technologies, or even if it has a good record of surgical treatment for patients when a nonsurgical regimen is indicated. Since we have argued that process indicators are once removed, and structural indicators twice removed, from measuring the impact of care on a patient's health status, we are particularly concerned that outcome measures were essentially unrelated to the process and structural indicators of the quality of care. Given the weak relationships observed, we believe that it is better to measure hospital performance in terms of what happened to the patient's health status—that is, to use outcomes standardized to take into account the patient's initial health status and the diagnoses and treatments undergone.

THE MAJOR STRUCTURAL MEASURES AND HOSPITAL PERFORMANCE

In chapter 3 we review the literature linking hospital performance to three important structural measures: size, teaching status, and expenditures. The

Table 12.2. Intercorrelations of outcome with process and structural measures of the quality of care

Outcomes	Process				
	1	2	3	4	5
1	−.162	.015	−.017	−.171	−.079
2	−.061	.001	−.003	.100	.081
3	−.103	.027	−.039	−.194	−.065
4	.025	−.016	−.018	.047	.070
5[a]	−.003	.005	−.002	−.014	.001
6[a]	−.000	.006	−.002	−.017	−.002

Note: See table 12.1 for note, footnote, and key.

Table 12.3. Intercorrelations of process with structural measures of the quality of care

Process	Structure			
	1	2	3	4
1	.207	.304	.091	.091
2	−.033	.001	−.025	−.006
3	.007	−.003	.031	−.011
4	.488	.380	.176	.322
5	.314	.376	.124	.106

Note: See table 12.1 for note, footnote, and key.

arguments for and against the importance of size and expenditures for explaining hospital performance are developed fully in chapter 3, and selected findings based on the ES are detailed in chapter 11. Here we focus primarily on the relation between teaching status and the quality of care.

Definition of the Three Major Structural Measures

Size

Size was measured as the log base 10 of the average daily census. (The mean average daily census was 170, with a standard deviation of 139.) For nonparametric analyses, we divided size into small (under 100 occupied beds: 40 percent of the ES hospitals), medium (100–250 beds: 37 percent), and large (more than 250 beds: 23 percent).

Structure			
1	2	3	4
−.090	−.119	−.038	−.040
.224	.135	.084	.119
−.012	−.003	.045	−.072
.193	.183	.086	.055
.003	−.004	−.003	−.000
−.007	−.005	−.004	−.008

Expenditures

Expenditures were the expenses per patient-day. For nonparametric analyses, we used three categories of expenditures: low (less than $90 per patient-day: 46 percent of the ES hospitals), medium ($90–$115: 33 percent), and high (more than $115: 22 percent).

Teaching Status and the Quality of Care

There is general agreement that not all teaching hospitals are alike. Before examining the effects of training residents on patient services and outcomes at a hospital, it is important to note that teaching hospitals vary in the extent to which residents are responsible for patient-care decisions. At one end of this continuum, "teaching" indicates that clinical decisions made by residents are closely supervised and reviewed by well-trained, experienced clinicians prior to their implementation. At the other end, it can indicate that decisions are being made by relatively inexperienced M.D.'s who are expected to learn from trial and error.

Two basic definitions of *teaching status* attempt to assess what kind of teaching occurs in a teaching hospital. One is based on the extent to which the hospital is affiliated with a medical school (e.g., whether it is involved as a major teaching site including medical students and residents or as indicated by membership in the Council of Teaching Hospitals). The argument that closer ties with a medical school represent more supervised or better teaching is based on the assumption that faculty more closely involved with a medical school are better trained, have more current knowledge, are more experienced, particularly with difficult cases, and spend more time in "teaching"—that is, in training and supervising the house staff.

The second definition is based on the ratio of the house staff to patients (e.g., Medicare in 1985 paid an additional reimbursement to teaching hospitals based on the number of house staff per patient). Note that this definition depends not on the absolute size of the teaching program at the hospital but on its size relative to the number of patients being treated there. Thus, a small residency program (e.g., five residents) in a small hospital could have an intensity ratio identical to that of a large residency program in a large hospital. The validity of this definition rests on the assumption that the intensity of residents per patient is a reasonably good surrogate for how much patient care is being provided by residents. When residents provide a large proportion of patient care, the teaching program is more likely to resemble the model that involves care being provided to publicly supported or charity patients and by a hierarchy of residents, with supervision of junior residents by senior residents rather than by faculty. In such a teaching program, each resident is typically given major responsibility for patient orders, with little or no review of clinical decisions prior to their implementation. Several studies of clinical orders in teaching programs have found that such programs tend to lead to services' being ordered in excess of what would have been ordered both by community physicians and by residents whose orders were reviewed prior to being carried out (Schroeder and O'Leary 1977; Martz and Ptakowski 1978; Garg et al. 1982; Boice and McGregor 1983). Jones (1984) suggested that the model of teaching in such situations could be best characterized as learning by doing instead of by example. Thus, we argued that when "more teaching" meant that there was a greater intensity of residents, more care was being provided by relatively inexperienced physicians with little close supervision of clinical orders by faculty prior to their implementation. Although most studies have examined effects on the services provided rather than the quality of outcomes, we reasoned that care by relatively inexperienced physicians was likely to be of lower quality.

We will use these two definitions to examine the relation between the quality of outcomes and teaching, recognizing that they are at best indirect measures of the true qualifications of the faculty and the extent of supervision prior to the implementation of clinical orders.

Measures of teaching status. Medical school affiliation was reported in the AMA data by the medical schools and programs.[3] Hospitals were divided according to whether they were listed as affiliated with medical schools (18

---

3. According to the AMA *Consolidated List* of residencies, affiliated hospitals were identified as follows: M = a major affiliate (8.3 percent of the ES hospitals), L = a minor affiliate (8.6 percent), or G = affiliated but having only a graduate-level program (1.6 percent). Unaffiliated teaching programs (7.4 percent) had approved programs but did not fit the above definitions of affiliation. Due to the original analyses linking medical school affiliation with hospital performance, we were unable to separate hospitals that were affiliated into M, L, or G categories.

percent of the ES hospitals), as teaching hospitals but having no formal affiliation (7 percent of hospitals), or as nonteaching (74 percent).[4]

The second measure of teaching was *house staff intensity*. Based on the AMA data for total numbers of house staff and the AHA report of the number of occupied beds, this measure was the ratio of total house staff to occupied beds. For most analyses reported here we divided this variable into (1) hospitals with no house staff (78 percent of the ES hospitals), (2) hospitals with low house staff intensity (13 percent of our hospitals), and (3) hospitals with high house staff intensity (9 percent).

The Major Structural Variables and Their Relation to Outcomes

In table 12.4 we present the intercorrelations, the mean, and the standard deviation for each of the major types of structural variables. As indicated by the Pearson correlations, the major structural variables were strongly correlated, but not to the point that multicolinearity was an important issue. Teaching hospitals, whatever the definition, tended to be larger and to have higher expenditures per patient-day. The measures of teaching were strongly correlated, as would be expected, but obviously tap slightly different definitions of the extent and type of teaching of physicians ongoing in the hospitals. In our data, almost 50 percent of affiliated hospitals had a high intensity of residents, compared with only 25 percent of unaffiliated hospitals.

The remainder of the results presented in this section were based on our nonparametric analyses relating the three major types of structural variables to the standardized outcomes for the selected surgical patients.[5] In tables 12.5 and 12.6 we present the basic results for each structural variable considered individually. In addition to displaying the number of hospitals and patients in each category, we present the total number of deaths, since the power of our tests (a modified chi-square test, described in chap. 11, n. 6) depends upon this number's being at least 1,000. The mean risk, or average probability of dying, can be interpreted as the average difficulty of the case mix in each category. Finally, the standardized mortality ratio (SMR) reflects the quality of the outcomes after adjusting for patient mix. Recall that an SMR of 1 reflects average

4. The results of the parametric analyses parallel those presented here and can be found in Forrest et al. 1978.

5. This measure was chosen as the major control variable to represent teaching. It requires that the data sources AMA and AHA agree that the hospital was teaching and report that there were at least two residents actually at the hospital. A slightly different version was used if osteopathic teaching status was indicated: the sources must agree that the hospital was an osteopathic teaching hospital and that at least one resident and at least three full-time-equivalent interns were in residency at the hospital.

Table 12.4. Basic descriptive statistics for the major structural variables: Size, teaching, and expenses

		Teaching Status		
Variable	Size	Medical School Affiliation	House Staff Intensity	Expenditures
Size (log)[a]	—	.487	.357	.314
Medical school affiliation[b]		—	.610	.361
House staff intensity[a]			—	.395
Expenditures				—
Mean	2.07	19%	2.4	$96.38
Standard deviation	0.406	39%	6.4	$30.81

Note: Correlations are Pearson product-moment correlations, at the hospital level ($N = 1,224$). All are significant at $p \leq .001$.
  [a]A continuous version of the variable was used.
  [b]Dichotomous variable.

care, and an SMR of below 1 indicates fewer deaths than expected, or "better outcomes."

Each major structural variable was strongly associated with the quality of outcomes as measured by SMRs. When only size was taken into account, large hospitals appeared to provide better care; that is, they had fewer deaths than expected ($p \leq .10$). For expenditures too, the more expenditures per patient-day, the lower the standardized death rate ($p \leq .001$).

In table 12.6 we present the results employing the two measures of teaching status. Since there were virtually no teaching hospitals (by either definition) among the smallest hospitals in our sample, we included for comparison only patients in the medium or large hospitals; in this sense, size was partially taken into account. The relation between teaching and SMRs was more complex but consistent with the arguments about the extent to which "teaching" reflects careful supervision by qualified faculty or major involvement in patient care by relatively inexperienced clinicians. Examining affiliation status first, the "best" SMRs occurred among hospitals affiliated with medical schools, and the "poorest" outcomes occurred for teaching hospitals having no affiliation with medical schools. Turning to house staff intensity, the "best" SMRs occurred where there was low house staff intensity (i.e., greater supervision), and the "poorest," where there was a high house staff intensity. Note, too, as would be expected, that the mean risk (representing more ill patients) was higher as the hospital engaged in more intensive or affiliated teaching programs.

Recall from table 12.4 that there was a strong tendency for teaching hospitals to be larger and to spend more per patient. We next analyze these

Table 12.5. Standardized outcomes by size and expenditure level of hospitals (selected surgical categories)

Variable	Number of Hospitals	Number of Patients	Number of Deaths	Mean Risk	SMR
Size[a]					
Small (under 100)	483	32,156	1,415	4.4	1.006
Medium (100–250)	544	135,881	5,841	4.3	1.003
Large (over 250)	197	98,907	4,382	4.7	0.952
Chi-square[b] 10.3					
Significance .10					
Expenditures[c]					
Low (under $90)	559	87,331	4,061	4.3	1.083
Medium ($90–115)	398	105,192	4,344	4.3	0.962
High (over $115)	267	74,421	3,252	4.6	0.956
Chi-square[b] 39					
Significance .001					

[a]Number of occupied beds.
[b]Six degrees of freedom.
[c]Expenses per patient-day.

relationships simultaneously in order to understand the contributions of each type of structural measure. The SMRs are graphed in figures 12.1 and 12.2. Note that the shorter the bar, the lower the SMR and thus the better the outcomes. In each case, a bar depicting a lower than average SMR is solid. In figure 12.1, hospitals affiliated with a medical school had the best overall SMRs. There was also some evidence of an effect of size among these teaching hospitals, with larger hospitals having relatively poorer care than medium-sized hospitals. Teaching hospitals with no affiliation had the poorest overall SMRs, with some indication of a size effect in the reverse direction: larger hospitals showed some tendency to do better than medium-sized hospitals, at least at lower expenditure levels. The relation between size and expenditures was most complex for the nonteaching hospitals. For this category, there appeared to be a strong effect of greater expenditures predicting better care for each size classification of hospitals. For teaching hospitals by either definition, expenditures showed little association with outcomes. There was some evidence that larger hospitals did better than other hospitals at low and medium levels of expenditures but provided poorer care than other hospitals at higher levels of expenditures.

Figure 12.2 presents a similar analysis for the definition of teaching status based on house staff intensity. Again, we observed that hospitals with the

Table 12.6. Standardized outcomes by teaching status (selected surgical categories)

Variable	Number of Hospitals[a]	Number of Patients	Number of Deaths	Mean Risk	SMR
Affiliation status					
No teaching	488	132,496	5,669	4.3	0.998
Teaching but no affiliation	84	25,729	1,208	4.4	1.065
Medical school affiliation	169	76,563	3,359	4.5	0.977
Chi-square[b] 15					
Significance .02					
House staff intensity[c]					
No house staff	488	127,039	5,363	4.2	1.004
Low[d]	157	63,446	2,691	4.5	0.949
High[e]	112	45,256	2,227	4.7	1.052
Chi-square[b] 14					
Significance .05					

[a]Only medium and large hospitals are included, since there were virtually no small teaching hospitals.
[b]Six degrees of freedom.
[c]Residents per occupied bed.
[d]More supervision.
[e]Less supervision.

highest house staff intensity (i.e., with less supervised teaching) had the poorest-quality outcomes. This result was observed irrespective of size. For these hospitals, there was a tendency for greater expenditures to predict better outcomes than did lower or medium expenditures, but only for large hospitals. Among hospitals with a low house staff intensity (i.e., more closely supervised teaching), there was a tendency to provide the same or better care than nonteaching hospitals for low-expenditure hospitals. At medium or high levels of expenditures, teaching hospitals provided care that was better than average but intermediate between that of nonteaching hospitals (with the best SMRs) and hospitals with a high house staff intensity (with the poorest SMRs). The relation between size and expenditures for nonteaching hospitals in figure 12.2 (which involves a slightly different group of hospitals than those identified as nonteaching in fig. 12.1) paralleled those discussed in figure 12.1 but tended to be less pronounced in their trends. (The significance level of all of these comparisons using the chi-square approach was .001 for the simultaneous comparisons.)

Focusing on the selected surgical categories, we have examined the relations between size, expenditures per patient-day, and two definitions of teach-

Figure 12.1. Standardized mortality ratios by hospital size, expenditures, and affiliation status: Selected surgical categories

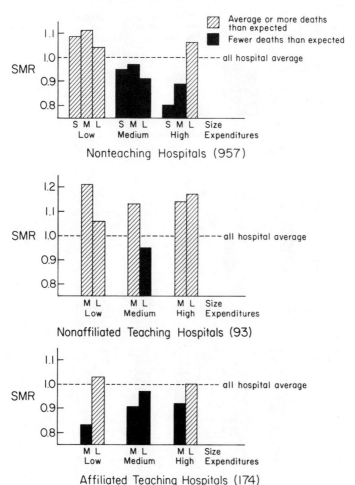

ing status as predictors of differences in the quality of outcomes. We found some support for concluding that greater expenditures per patient-day led to better outcomes than expected, particularly for the 75 percent of hospitals with no teaching programs.

The evidence relating to size was mixed, especially when teaching status and expenditures were considered. There was some weak but inconsistent evidence that greater size was associated with poorer outcomes. These results were similar to those of other recent reports that hospital size does not bear a

Figure 12.2. Standardized mortality ratios by hospital size, expenditures, and house staff intensity: Selected surgical categories

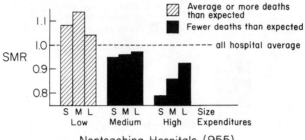

Nonteaching Hospitals (955)

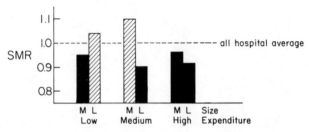

Hospitals With Low House Staff Intensity (157)

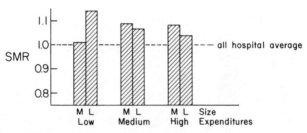

Hospitals With High House Staff Intensity (112)

predictable relationship to either expenditures or outcomes. There are several reasons why this is possible. Larger organizations differ from smaller ones in many ways, so that size cannot be considered in isolation. For example, larger hospitals tend to be located in major metropolitan areas, where there are more opportunities to attract both patients and staff. Larger hospitals tend to have more highly differentiated subunits, leading to more complex coordination requirements. They also tend to have more complex goals and to provide more kinds of services. Finally, the effects of size in a competitive environment may be mitigated somewhat by cooperative arrangements or shared services with other health care organizations.

We found some evidence to support the view that not all teaching hospitals are alike with respect to their quality of care. For both measures of teaching, there was evidence that those hospitals with less supervision by a qualified faculty (i.e., those with a higher house staff intensity or those without an affiliation with a medical school) provided the poorest-quality care. In contrast, teaching hospitals with more supervision by a qualified faculty (i.e., those with a low house staff intensity or affiliated hospitals) provided care better than or equivalent to that in nonteaching hospitals. This evidence is consistent with other findings that newly trained physicians tend to order excess tests and provide less good care during the early years of their career, when they are still learning clinical skills and acquiring experience. When patient care by these residents is supervised more closely by qualified faculty, these potential disadvantages appear to be overcome. Such teaching hospitals provide better care than expected—a consequence that some have argued occurs due to the quality and experience of medical school clinical faculty. Our findings about the importance of close supervision of residents, if verified in additional studies, have important policy implications for federal-level programs that reimburse for patient care by residents (like Medicare's formula based on house staff intensity) or provide direct support for medical education. Our results suggest that in the interests of providing better care, policies encouraging closer supervision of house staff may be most appropriate.

HOSPITAL STRUCTURE AND HOSPITAL PERFORMANCE

In chapter 1 we present the overall theoretical design for both the ES and the IS, review the relevant literature, and describe four major dimensions of structure for which variation is expected to have an impact on hospital performance (differentiation, coordination, power, and staff qualifications). Also in chapter 1 we identify five major organizational units within the hospital that are expected to have major impact on the quality of care delivered to patients, namely, the hospital, the ward, the operating suite, the medical staff, and the individual physicians providing direct patient care. We present hypotheses and causal arguments relating each of these dimensions to performance, featuring the organizational units related to the treatment of surgical care and the types of indicators available in the richer data base of the IS. Throughout our discussions of both the IS and the ES, we treat hospital size, teaching status, and expenditures per patient both as important predictors of variations in hospital performance, and as control variables, in the sense that we expect them to be related to many of the indicators of the structural dimensions of primary interest. As such, if their presence is not taken into account while examining the impact of each dimension on performance, it is possible that misleading conclusions could be drawn about relationships that are better explained by the three-way associations between these major structural variables, the dimension of concern, and the measures of performance. Finally, we present dimensions of technology, referring broadly to the nature of work being performed, and we describe hypotheses relating structural dimensions to effective performance contingent upon the nature of the work. Although we made every effort to develop a set of measures parallel to those available for the IS, the limitations of the organizational data base for the ES were quite severe. For example, relatively few measures of coordination, differentiation, and power were available, and even these few had many limitations.

Measures of Coordination and Power

The types of AHA and AMA data available provided little information about the kinds of power and coordination activities carried out in the hospital. We were limited to formal and indirect measures of the amount of power and coordination present, such as the number of contract physicians as an indicator of the coordination of the medical staff. For the nursing and hospital staff, we were limited to measuring the need for coordination, as evidenced by the presence of a large number of part-time staff, which increases both the need for and the difficulties of coordinating workflow. In addition, part-time staff are less likely to be experienced and well informed about the patient-care activities (i.e., less well qualified). We were unable to distinguish between the effects of these dimensions in testing our hypotheses with the ES data. We argued simply that more reliance on part-time staff was likely to be associated with poorer outcomes. For physicians, we examined the extent to which they had a core of active staff members who provided care for most of the patients. None of these was considered a very good measure of coordination, but there were no other relevant data for this dimension.

Measures of Medical Staff Organization

Control over the medical staff. Roemer and Friedman (1971) argued that the proportion of employed physicians is the single best indicator of the tightness of control over the medical staff—control exercised by the medical staff over individual physicians. We argued that it indicates the potential for coordination and peer review among the members of the medical staff. The employed-physician ratio made use of data from two different sources. From the AHA we learned the total full-time equivalents (FTE) of salaried physicians (M.D.'s and D.D.S.'s) at the hospital. From the PAS abstract, we obtained a count of all the different physicians listed as the attending physician for at least one patient during the year. The *employed physician ratio* was simply the ratio of these two figures, or, roughly, the number of contract physicians per direct-care physicians at the hospital. Note that in operationalizing the measure of contract physicians for the IS, we did not limit the type of contractual obligation to that requiring direct remuneration by the hospital. In the ES, only salaried physicians were included in the definition of contract physicians.

The level of involvement of the medical staff. In the IS, time commitment was obtained by asking physicians participating in the prospective study to estimate the proportion of their practice that they performed at the study hospital. We were, of course, unable to obtain such information for the ES; instead, these measures were based on information available on the PAS abstracts and were intended to measure the degree to which some or all of the direct-care physicians were actively involved in treating patients at the study hospital.

There are several reasons to expect our measures of physician activity at the hospital to be related to the quality of care. A hospital with a large number of physicians relative to the number of patients has a complex set of work demands, which means that much coordination is required in order to provide good care. A high physician-patient ratio at the study hospital could also indicate that there are few medical staff members who have a strong time commitment to the hospital and who therefore may be less likely to serve actively on committees for the medical staff organization or to be responsive to peer-review efforts. A high physician-patient ratio at the study hospital may also reflect an overall low volume of cases treated by each physician. Our measure is not considered an accurate measure of overall volume for individual physicians, because each could have an active practice at a nearby hospital and those patients would not be detected in our data base. As is true for our nursing staff measures, we cannot distinguish among these theoretical explanations in testing hypotheses about the activity of the medical staff and hospital performance. We simply expect that the more diffuse the medical staff, the lower the quality of outcomes.

The measure of the *diffuseness of the medical staff ratio* was the proportion of the attending physicians required to account for 50 percent of all patients treated, obtained from the PAS abstracts. A higher score reflected a more "diffuse" staff, that is, one having more physicians who each treated a smaller number of patients. The average number of patients treated annually in the hospital by a given physician was 83, with a standard deviation of 82 and a range of from 2 to 512. The all-hospital mean proportion of attending physicians required to account for 50 percent of a hospital's patients was 20.5 percent.

The measure of the *diffuseness of the surgical staff ratio* was the proportion of the surgeons required to account for 50 percent of the patients operated on, obtained from the PAS abstracts for all patients operated on. The average annual number of patients for surgeons was 75, with a standard deviation of 70 and a range of from 1 to 512. The all-hospital mean proportion of surgeons accounting for 50 percent of the patients operated on was 13.5 percent.

Measures of Hospital and Nursing Staff Organization

As noted above, we based our measures of coordination for the hospital and nursing staff on the proportion of part-time staff, using the argument that such staff present a greater need for coordination. Registered nurses (RNs) and licensed vocational nurses (LVNs) were combined and referred to jointly as *nurses*. Using AHA data for all employees except physicians and house staff, we also measured the *proportion of part-time employees*.

Staff qualifications have been characterized along four separate subdimensions: training, labor intensity, experience, and time commitment to the hospital. Training and experience and the hypotheses relating them to hospital performance are discussed in detail in chapter 1. The expectations regarding time commitment for physicians and part-time staff are discussed above in this chapter. Here we develop arguments for considering the intensity of labor to be a measure of staff qualifications that can have an important effect on the quality of care.

There are two organizational strategies for assigning staff to perform complex tasks: (1) provide staff with special skills and experience or (2) reduce the workload of each staff member, thereby making the tasks for each staff easier. Hospitals use both strategies; an obvious example is staffing in the intensive-care unit, where nurses are likely to have specialized training in intensive care and to have fewer patients per nurse. We argue that given staff members with equal training and experience, a lighter workload in terms of numbers of patients (i.e., a higher labor intensity) should be associated with better-quality care, due to the availability of more time to provide nursing care to each patient. While more time for care does not necessarily imply better care, we expect that a higher labor intensity is likely to be associated with the provision of a higher intensity of services of the type that were associated with better outcomes (Flood et al. 1979 [see also chap. 7 in this volume]).

In measuring nurses' training, we assumed that the RN had more relevant training than the LVN. Our data included nurses involved in administrative and educational positions, as well as nurses involved in direct patient care. Using AHA data, we measured the *proportion of FTE nurses who were RNs*.

We used AHA data to measure both *nursing staff intensity* and *hospital staff intensity*. We measured the former as the ratio of total FTE nurses (including RNs and LVNs) to the average daily census. We obtained the latter measure by dividing the FTE for all staff except physicians by the average daily census.

Our indicators of the *volume of cases of a particular type* (using the study procedures) provided measures of experience for the hospital patient-care staff. These measures are described in detail in Flood, Scott, and Ewy 1984a, 1984b (see also chap. 11 in this volume).

Relationships between the Measures

We examined first the Pearson correlations between these structural measures, including the three hospital control measures: size, teaching status, and expenditures. For the most part, the various measures were not highly correlated (see table 12.7). Since they were usually intended to tap different dimensions within different subunits of the hospital, this was no surprise. The measures based on all hospital employees were highly correlated with those based on nursing staff alone (.829 and .808), but again, this was due to a part-whole correlation. We focused on the nursing staff measures, since they were more likely to include direct-care personnel. The two measures of diffuseness of the medical staff were strongly correlated too (.443), in part because surgeons were included in the medical staff measure. Because of our interest in the quality of surgical outcomes, we focused on the surgical staff in our subsequent analysis. Only the two diffuseness measures were strongly correlated with the control variables: more diffuse medical staffs were likely to be found in hospitals that were smaller and nonteaching and spent less money per day.

Testing the Relation between Hospital Structure and Performance in the ES

The methods we used to examine the relations between hospital structure and performance paralleled those described in chapter 11. That is, we first adjusted inhospital death for all the patient health characteristics, as detailed in chapter 5. The probability of dying for each patient was estimated using a combination of log and linear regressions; the resultant estimate and its corrective factor were included in our regression in step 1. In this same step we also controlled for the three major structural characteristics identified in the literature as predicting the quality of care (size, teaching status, and expenditures) and therefore potentially confounding the relationships we wished to examine. Then in step 2 we entered all of the hospital structural variables of theoretical interest. For simplicity's sake, we present only the results from step 2 and for the variables of primary interest in this chapter: the measures of control, coordination, and qualifications. Correspondingly, the overall tests of significance we present were based on the change in the sum of squares when this set of regression variables was entered in step 2. (See chap. 11 for the regression coefficients associated with the patient predictors; see the third section of this chapter for analyses focused on the three hospital control variables.)

In addition to analyses based on inhospital death, we present parallel analyses using LOS as the dependent variable. As discussed in chapter 11, LOS may be considered a crude indicator of the efficiency or costs. To adjust for LOS, we used the same estimates of the patient's probability of dying, plus whether the patient actually died or was discharged with a destination or status

Table 12.7. Basic statistics for hospital structural measures

Hospital Structural Measure	Power, Coordination, and Workflow					Staff Qualifications			Control Variables		
	(1)	(2)	(3)	(4)	(5)	(6)	(7)	(8)	Size	Teaching Status	Expenditures
(1) Employed-physician ratio	—	-.067	-.025	-.136	-.105	-.018	-.010	.071	.122	.166	.195
(2) Diffuseness of medical staff ratio		—	.443	.072	.119	-.210	.037	.043	-.524	-.333	-.451
(3) Diffuseness of surgical staff ratio			—	.071	.112	-.096	-.016	-.015	-.430	-.221	-.267
(4) Proportion of part-time nurse				—	.829	.254	-.011	-.060	-.094	-.122	-.040
(5) Proportion of part-time employees					—	.201	.036	-.074	-.188	-.176	-.092
(6) Proportion of FTE nurses who are RNs						—	-.042	.040	.143	.081	.228
(7) Nursing staff intensity							—	.808	-.187	.001	.165
(8) Hospital staff intensity								—	-.151	.104	.201
Mean	1.00[a]	1.00[a]	1.00[a]	0.30	0.24	0.67	0.88	3.20			
Standard deviation		0.45	0.57	0.15	0.12	0.15	0.42	1.44			

Note: Correlations are Pearson product-moment correlations. |r| ≥ .200 are significant at $p \leq .001$, $N = 1{,}224$.
[a] Expressed as a ratio to the all-hospital mean.

indicating less than full recovery. We included these additional variables because they were expected to predict a shorter or "truncated" LOS for such patients compared with patients with the same probability of dying who were discharged with full approval and to home.

Results: Medical and Nursing Staff Structure and Performance

In the first section of table 12.8 we present the results from a regression of our adjusted measures of hospital performance on the medical staff organization variables. In contrast to what we had predicted, a greater proportion of employed physicians was associated with poorer outcomes than expected, and a more diffuse surgical staff was associated with better outcomes, after controlling for hospital size, teaching status, and expenditure levels.

In the second section, we present the measures associated with the nursing staff structure, controlling for hospital size, teaching status, and expenditures. In contrast to our predictions, we found that a higher proportion of part-time nurses was associated with better outcomes than expected and that the proportion of nurses with RN training was unrelated to the quality of outcomes. As predicted, a greater intensity of nurses per patient was related to better outcomes. In the third section, we include all of the above measures in the same regression to examine whether their relationships were altered by inclusion of the remaining variables. They were essentially unchanged from the relationships observed above.

In table 12.8 we also present the results of regressing the same variables on LOS, adjusted for patient characteristics and the three major hospital control variables. Although we did not predict any particular relations between our hospital structural measures and LOS, the relation between shorter LOS and structure were essentially identical to those between better outcomes and structure. The consistency of these relationships involving shorter LOS and fewer inhospital deaths, after adjusting for patient mix and major hospital characteristics, suggests that hospital adaptations to reduce LOS and lower patient-care costs, particularly where they involve changes in hospital characteristics such as the intensity of nurses and the volume of cases, may affect the quality of outcomes achieved by patients as well.

Discussion

We can only speculate about why the two measures of medical staff structure in the ES data base (the proportion of employed physicians and the diffuseness of the surgical staff) were related to the quality of care in a direction opposite to that predicted. In the IS, we found some support for the expectation that a higher proportion of contract physicians would be associated with better outcomes; this measure was also associated with more stringent peer review and

Table 12.8. The effects of regressing death and LOS on the structure of the medical and nursing staff (selected surgical categories)

Set of Measures in Each Regression	Adjusted Death[a]			Adjusted LOS[b]		
	β	F	Significance	β	F	Significance
Medical staff structure[c]						
Employed-physician ratio	.022	144	.000	.072	1,496	.000
Diffuseness of the surgical staff ratio	−.011	35	.000	−.031	253	.000
Nursing staff structure[c]						
Proportion of part-time nurses	−.009	27	.000	−.015	64	.000
Proportion of FTE nurses who are RNs	−.004	4	.04	.001	0	n.s.
Nursing staff intensity	−.015	54	.000	−.048	557	.000
Medical staff structure and nursing staff structure combined[c]						
Employed-physician ratio	.020	117	.000	.068	1,306	.000
Diffuseness of the surgical staff	−.010	26	.000	−.024	149	.000
Proportion of part-time nurses	−.007	14	.000	−.010	27	.000
Proportion of FTE nurses who are RNs	−.002	1	n.s.	.005	7	.011
Nursing staff intensity	−.012	38	.000	−.041	408	.000

[a]Adjusted for patient health characteristics and hospital controls—size, teaching status, and expenditures.

[b]Adjusted for patient health characteristics and hospitals controls, plus whether the patient died or was transferred.

[c]Set was significantly related to both dependent variables at $p \leq .000$, for each set, based on change in the sum of squares after the adjusting variables were entered.

medical staff power. Note, however, that the definition of contract physicians in the IS was broader and included all physicians with a contractual relationship to provide services to the hospital, whether or not they were salaried. Perhaps this difference in defining hospital-based physicians led to identifying different types of hospitals or medical staff organizations in the two studies. For example, suppose that government-run hospitals were more likely than other hospitals to have salaried physicians. Suppose, further, that government-run hospitals tended to have poorer outcomes (both of these correlations in the ES were significant at the .001 level). Such associations with government sponsorship (or other unidentified factors that pick out *salaried* hospital-based physicians) might account for the observation that a higher proportion of salaried physicians was correlated with poorer outcomes. In contrast, suppose that nonprofit community hospitals with stringent peer review were likely to have more hospital-based physicians with contractual arrangements to provide services but were not likely to have such physicians remunerated by salary. In this case, with a different measure of hospital-based physicians, we might have observed that such physicians tended to occur in hospitals with better outcomes (as suggested by our IS results).

Turning to the second medical staff measure, we examined the relation between physician's time commitment and performance at two levels in the IS. At the level of the individual surgeon, we found some evidence that physicians who had a higher time commitment (i.e., conducted relatively more of their practice at the hospital) tended to have patients who had better outcomes than predicted (Flood and Scott 1978 [see also chap. 9 in this volume]). However, when this measure was aggregated to the level of the medical staff (i.e., when the surgeons as a group had most of their patients at the study hospital), the hospital tended to have poorer-quality outcomes than predicted for its patient mix (Flood 1976). This second IS measure at the hospital level corresponds more closely to the measure used in the ES, and both studies provided some evidence that a medical staff made up of surgeons whose practices were concentrated at a single hospital (i.e., a less diffuse surgical staff) was associated with poorer care rather than with better care as we had predicted.

One post hoc explanation for these hospital-level observations is that medical staffs that concentrate their patients at one hospital may be present in a particular set of circumstances that leads to poorer-quality care. For example, such a hospital may be located in a relatively isolated or undesirable community setting, which in turn can offer only relatively poor supporting facilities or staff, can attract only physicians with less rigorous or up-to-date training, or offers little stimulation to maintain or update the medical practice at the hospital, thereby leading to poorer-quality care. In any case, our findings underscore the need to be wary of methodological and theoretical problems introduced by conceptualizing and testing variables at different levels. That is, our measure based on the aggregated qualifications of the staff—a measure that characterizes the medical staff organization or hospital—behaved quite differently in its relation to the quality of care than did the same concept applied to the performance of an individual staff member.

Turning to our findings regarding the structure of the nursing staff, we had argued that a greater proportion of the part-time nurses indicated greater demands on coordination, as well as a greater likelihood of receiving care from less well trained or less informed nurses. We found instead that greater use of part-time nurses was associated with better outcomes than expected. It is possible that any disadvantages of using part-time staff were overcome by increased coordination and management efforts or that the advantages of flexibility in staffing levels that part-time staff permit outweighed the disadvantages. Unfortunately, in the ES we were unable to examine the types and extent of coordination and other management tools used at the hospital.

Greater qualifications of nursing staff tended to be related to better-quality care, but not significantly. A drawback to all of our measures based on nurses was that they included nurses in managerial and educational positions as well as in direct patient care (which also included nonsurgical wards, the surgical suite, and the recovery room). It is possible that the average qualifications for nurses providing direct patient care on the postoperative wards may be related to the quality of outcomes, but our measures may not be sufficiently indicative of the qualifications of nurses providing postsurgical care on the wards to provide a good test. An alternative explanation is that the quality of outcomes of surgical patients (especially for relatively common types of procedures) is not affected by the average qualifications of the nurses at the hospital.

There is one final explanation regarding the processes whereby the nursing staff could affect the quality of care of surgical patients, based on our observations in the ES. Recall two factors—observed to increase the quality of care in our data: a greater intensity of nurses (i.e., a high nurse-to-patient ratio) and a greater volume of similar cases treated at the hospital. These positive relationships to quality, coupled with the observations about nurses' qualifications, suggest that the level of skill and services that nurses are able to provide to patients (and thus their contributions to the quality of outcomes) may be more dependent on the number of patients for whom they must be responsible (fewer is better) and on their greater familiarity with the types of care to be delivered than to their formal training or part-time status. These speculations, if true, suggest that hospital administrators seeking to maximize the quality of care efficiently would be well advised to concentrate on managerial techniques to maximize placement of patients with nurses familiar with their care and in sufficient numbers rather than to rely on greater qualifications of the staff.

SUMMARY

Despite the severe limitations on organizational measures that could be constructed for hospitals in the ES, we were able to examine some hypotheses and models relating hospital structure and performance. In this chapter, we have examined three basic models of these relationships: the consistency of structural, process, and outcome measures of hospital performance; the interrelationships between the three major structural dimensions characterizing nonfederal short-term hospitals (size, teaching status, and expenditures) and their impact on performance; and the medical staff and nursing staff qualifications and structures as predictors of better hospital performance. Our findings and their implications can be briefly summarized.

There was little consistency among the various types of measures of hospital performance. (Measures were adjusted for patient characteristics whenever possible.) There are three major implications of this inconsistency:

1. Hospital performance, even when it is limited to the quality of patient care, is a complex phenomenon, and assumptions about the quality of care received by patients that are based on the capability of the structure or staff to perform well are not warranted.
2. Health policies, incentive systems for reimbursing medical services, or accreditation bodies that rely on only structural or process measures of the quality of care may not be effective in ensuring better or adequate quality of outcomes.
3. More research is needed in order to understand the processes (the how) and circumstances (the when) that lead "good" structures to affect the quality of process decisions and the quality of outcomes. The need to identify effective organizational strategies is especially important under conditions of organizational "belt tightening," which permeate our health care system in the 1980s.

We found that greater average expenditures were strongly associated with better outcomes, especially for nonteaching hospitals; that size was not predictably related to outcomes; and that some teaching hospitals were better than or equal to their nonteaching counterparts, while others appeared to provide poorer care. (These relationships were examined after controlling for patient mix and the other two hospital characteristics.) The policy implications of these findings are as follows:

4. In an era of cost containment, there is a great need for more research and careful examination of the association between expenditures and the quality of outcomes. Our study does not address the reasons for higher average expenditures (but size and teaching status and patient mix were taken into account). There is ample evidence that some production efficiencies and clinical efficiencies need to be introduced into the health care system, but our results would suggest that better-quality outcomes may indeed carry a higher price tag.
5. Policies relating to the reimbursement of inhospital patient care in teaching hospitals and to the funding of graduate medical education should promote more stringent supervision of resident care of hospitalized patients.

The medical staff measures of peer review (based on the proportion of salaried physicians) and time commitment (based on the relative concentration of care by members of the surgical staff at the study hospital) were related to poorer care, contrary to our predictions. Nursing staff measures based on formal qualifications were not related to outcomes, while a greater use of part-time staff and a higher nursing staff intensity were associated with better outcomes. (In each case, patient mix, hospital size, teaching status, and expenditure level were taken into account.)

6. The measures of structural dimensions available in the ES presented severe limitations in testing the organizational structure. Additional research is needed in order to understand the relation between structural dimensions, such as staff qualifications and coordination and power, and hospital performance.

7. One finding in particular bears further study. The importance of formal qualifications and experience for producing better-quality care is apparently more complex than we first hypothesized. Instead of finding that the formal training or average level of qualifications for the staffs as a whole is important for explaining higher-quality outcomes, we found evidence that better hospitals apparently adopt strategies such as using part-time staff or providing a high nursing staff intensity rather than rely on a staff with higher-than-average qualifications.

Conclusions and Implications

The chapters in this volume describe three complex data sets and report a variety of analyses conducted on these data over a period of more than ten years. Here we attempt to provide an overview and an assessment of this work. First, we discuss the major strengths and limitations of the data sets and the work conducted as we (and some commentators on our work) perceive them. Second, we briefly review the principal findings emerging from the research. We do not attempt to summarize all of the results, but emphasize those that seem to us to be both strongly supported and of substantive interest. Finally, we discuss some of the implications of our findings for those concerned with improving the performance of hospitals, as well as for those devoted to improving our knowledge of hospitals as complex professional organizations. In this discussion, we attempt to be sensitive to the changes that have occurred in the organization of hospital services since our data were collected.

STRENGTHS AND LIMITATIONS

A major strength of the research conducted is that it permits comparison of the performance of hospitals as measured by a variety of types of indicators of quality and of costs. Most previous studies have utilized only one or a few types of measures. Our results suggest that conclusions based on limited measures of quality or cost may be misleading. Most studies of the quality of care rely on either structural or process indicators: measures of hospital facilities or personnel qualifications are frequently employed to assess structural quality, and measures of autopsy rates or numbers of tests ordered are often used to measure the quality of care processes. Outcome measures that attempt to assess changes in the state of health of patients are relatively rare; and when they are employed, they frequently do not take sufficiently into account differences in patient mix. The appropriateness of using structural or process indicators as surrogates for outcome measures is severely challenged by our analyses, which show low and inconsistent correlations between structural features and procedures presumed to be associated with better health care and measures of health outcomes (see chap. 12).

A second strength of our research is the use of outcome measures adjusted for differences among patient populations, the adjustments being based on detailed information concerning each patient entering the study. Using a combination of classifications by diagnosis and linear regression, and using indicators that characterize each patient's condition and treatment record, including diagnoses, operations, admission test findings, and sociodemographic characteristics, we computed the expected levels of outcome—and for a subset of patients, the expected levels of service utilization—for each patient conditional on his or her specific characteristics and physical status at admission. For outcomes, the expected levels reflect the average probability of experiencing an adverse event for all similar patients treated in the study hospitals (rather than some theoretically determined ideal standard of care). Measures of expected and observed quality of care for each hospital, adjusted for differences in patient population, were obtained by aggregating individual patient measures within hospitals. We utilized a similar approach to arrive at observed and expected measures of service intensity for some patients (see chaps. 5 and 6).

Careful attention was given to which patient variables should be included in the standardization equation. Selected for inclusion were those items of available patient information for which the hospital (and/or the physician during hospitalization) should not be held responsible. Most of the variables were based on values at the time of admission or on diagnoses explaining the hospitalization. Excluded were data on those events or services that might be responses to poor care received during the hospitalization period itself (see chap. 4).

It is a great advantage to be able to use the individual patient records as a starting point for constructing indices of adjusted quality and/or service intensity rather than to rely on data already condensed or aggregated for some other purpose. Previous researchers studying hospital differences have not provided convincing adjustments for differences in the population of patients in each hospital (see chap. 3). Their conclusions are open to the charge that the observed differences in service intensity and quality are due simply to hospital variations in the condition and prognoses of patients admitted. While our own approach may not take into account all of the differences in patients that may impact on health care outcomes, it represents a considerable advance over previous attempts.

A third strength is that a large portion of the data utilized were obtained from an ongoing patient abstracting service. PAS abstracts, compiled by CPHA, provided the primary data source for several of the studies conducted, supplying information for patient-related measures, including patient characteristics, services received, and outcomes experienced. Since this patient abstracting service is widely used in the United States—as of 1985 over 1,400 nonfederal U.S. hospitals subscribed to it—any serious effort to evaluate its capability to function in some fashion as a system to contain costs and promote the quality of care in hospitals must be of widespread interest. Moreover, almost all short-term hospitals now use some form of computerized medical abstracts containing the same basic types of information utilized in our work.

Yet another strength in the design of the Institutional Differences Study (IDS) is the conjunction of the Extensive Study (ES), based on patient data obtained from the PAS for 1,224 hospitals supplemented by data from other types of secondary sources, with the Intensive Study (IS), based on the prospective collection of more elaborate data from a subset of 17 hospitals. The latter provided us with an opportunity to develop more sensitive measures of the quality of care, measures that took into account patient morbidity within the hospital and mortality up to forty days after discharge. What is more important, it permitted us to collect a variety of more detailed measures assessing hospital structure and physician staff characteristics. The use of the two data sets in combination permitted an independent assessment of both the reliability of data collected by abstract and the procedures developed to standardize outcomes for patient differences. To a lesser extent (because of the relatively poor measures of hospital structure available for the ES), the two data sets allowed us to better test hypotheses relating hospital structure and performance.

All research has limitations, and ours is no exception. Three major limitations affect the confidence to be placed in the results reported in this volume. First, although the techniques developed to adjust patient outcome measures for differences in patient mix constitute a strength, the outcome measures themselves are not very sensitive indicators of health care status. Most of the results reported are based on measures of death inhospital. The definition of mortality as an adverse health event seems unproblematic. One difficulty is that it is a rare event—very rare in the case of some types of diagnostic categories—and thus insensitive to actual variations in the quality of care. In addition, the small number of deaths observed, even in a study involving many patients, reduces the statistical reliability of the comparisons among hospitals. Yet another problem associated with the use of death inhospital is that hospital discharge policies vary; some hospitals are more likely to dismiss dying patients to other facilities, resulting in data that are censored. For the IS, additional outcome data were gathered. Nursing assessments of patient morbidity were collected seven days after surgery; also collected were assessments of all deaths occurring up to forty days postsurgery, including patients discharged alive prior to forty days after surgery. Such measures represent a considerable improvement over death inhospital but were only available for a limited number and type of patients (about 8,500 patients receiving one of fifteen types of surgical procedures) and a small group of hospitals (see chap. 6).

A second limitation is that each of the two major data sets was flawed in important, albeit differing, respects from the standpoint of testing hypotheses relating hospital structure and performance. The IS provided detailed measures of hospital and medical staff structure but contained so few cases—seventeen hospitals—that only limited multivariant analyses could be conducted, and the results must be treated as exploratory. By contrast, the ES contained many cases—1,224 hospitals—but the measures of hospital structure available from the secondary sources were limited and relatively crude. Overlap in the two data sets served to verify differences among patient populations in adjusted mortality rates—the dependent variables—but proved to be less adequate in providing usable data on differences in structural characteristics—the independent variables. Thus the combined analysis of data from the ES and data from the IS served to establish differences in the quality of care among hospitals but was less useful in testing hypotheses developed to explain these differences.

A third limitation in the work carried out concerns the magnitude of the findings reported. Several critics have called attention to the small amount of variance accounted for by the structural variables in differences among hospitals' mortality rates (see May 1983). We view this limitation as more apparent than real, as discussed in chapters 5, 8, and 9. Most of the measures of variance explained referred to variation among individual patient outcomes that could be attributed to the independent variables of interest. Two factors must be considered in interpreting the amount of variance explained. First, because the dependent variables employed were both noncontinuous and skewed, a small R^2 is subject to misinterpretation, as Gordon, Kannel, and Halperin (1979) noted. Second, it is obvious that many factors contribute to patient outcomes and that many of these—e.g., the general health status of the patient, the nature of the disease, or the types of surgical procedures performed—will be much more influential than the types of organizational variables that are the primary focus of our analyses. That a significant portion of variation in patient outcomes was accounted for by organizational features is, we believe, noteworthy.

MAJOR FINDINGS

Quality of Care

The hospitals studied differed significantly in the quality of medical and surgical care delivered as measured by standardized mortality and morbidity rates. This conclusion was verified for every data set containing outcome measures utilized in the research. In the larger data sets and for the best-adjusted surgical outcomes, slightly more than a twofold difference in death rates separated the better from the poorer hospitals (the top 16 percent versus the bottom 16 percent) (see chap. 6). Considerable variation across types of patients and/or procedures was observed; hospitals performing better than average on one set of surgical procedures did not necessarily perform similarly on other sets (see chaps. 6 and 11). This suggests that there is considerable intrahospital variation in the quality of care.

Service Intensity and Outcomes

Hospitals providing more than average specific services to patients exhibited better outcomes than hospitals supplying fewer services (see chap. 7). For these analyses, both outcomes—death inhospital—and specific services—measures of particular therapeutic and diagnostic services consumed, weighted by cost—were adjusted to take into account differences in the characteristics of individual patients at the time of admission. Preliminary analyses also revealed that adjusted length of stay inhospital was associated with the quality of care, shorter stays being correlated with better outcomes, but these differences did not persist when the regional location of hospitals was taken into account.

Structure, Process, and Outcome Measures of Quality

Widely employed measures of the quality of hospitals as assessed by structural, process, and outcome indicators showed weak and inconsistent intercorrelations (see chap. 12). Structural indicators of hospital quality included the elaborateness of facilities, the proportion of board-certified surgeons, and accreditation by the Joint Commission on the Accreditation of Hospitals. Process indicators included the proportion of surgical patients whose pathology report supported removal of the tissue, the proportion of inhospital deaths that were autopsied, and the proportion of patients utilizing an intensive-care unit. Outcome measures utilized were standardized measures of inhospital mortality and the rate of reported complications following surgery. Intercorrelations of these measures across categories revealed at best weak levels of association. In particular, outcome measures were remarkably unrelated to process measures and to structural indicators of quality. Structural, process, and outcome measures of hospital quality appear to be tapping differing dimensions; they should not be regarded as substitutable indicators of quality.

Organizational versus Individual Provider Characteristics

Hospital-wide characteristics and, in particular, the characteristics of medical staff organization had a greater impact on surgical outcomes than did the characteristics of individual surgeons (see chap. 8). Differences in the quality of care were associated with differences at the hospital and/or the medical staff level and were essentially unrelated to differences among individual surgeons in training and experience. These findings are consistent with those reported by Roos, Ross, and Hentelett (1977) and by Rhee (1977). Data from the IS supported the conclusion that better outcomes were to be found in hospitals in which the surgical staff was in a better position to regulate the behavior of its own members, as reflected by the strictness of admission requirements for new staff members and the length of the probationary period. When the effects of such organizational controls were taken into account, the qualifications of individual surgeons—for example, measures of specialization and of qualifications such as board certification—were not associated with differences in the quality of care.

Organizational Characteristics and the Quality of Care

Broadly speaking, hospitals that exhibited a strong medical staff structure, had more experience in treating similar categories of patients, were affiliated with a medical school or had a lower ratio of house staff to patients, or reported higher expenditures per patient episode were more likely to provide better care. These results were the most consistently observed across the various data sets and controlling for the effects of other variables. Each can be briefly summarized:

1. Hospitals with a medical staff exercising more stringent controls on surgeons, as measured by the strictness of admission requirements for new staff members and more extensive restrictions on surgical privileges, were more likely to provide better-quality surgical care (see chap. 9).

2. Hospitals with greater experience in treating similar patients were more likely to exhibit better outcomes. We designated patients as "similar" if (1) they shared the same diagnosis and underwent the same surgical procedure and/or (2) they faced the same risk of dying, that is, the predictive power of the measures of their physical status and stage of disease was similar. While the effects of the volume of diagnostically similar patients on outcomes varied somewhat by type of surgery across six selected categories, greater volume was associated with better outcomes for all, and a significant association was observed for four of the six. The effects on outcomes were more complex when dealing with experience with patients who had not only the same type of diagnosis and procedure but also the same risk of dying, based on their physical status or stage of disease, with some mixed evidence that more specifically defined experience was important for predicting better outcomes. Experience in treating a higher volume of similar medical patients was also positively associated with the quality of care when controls were introduced for hospital size, teaching status, and expenditures per patient episode (see chap. 11).

3. Hospitals that were affiliated with a medical school or had a lower

intensity of house staff officers were more likely to provide better-quality care. There are two different although interrelated definitions of "teaching" hospitals: (1) hospitals with a residency program directly affiliated with a medical school (in contrast to hospitals with an approved residency program but no affiliation); and (2) hospitals with a high or low ratio of residents in training to patients. In the first case, hospitals affiliated with a medical school exhibited outcomes equal to or better than the outcomes of nonteaching hospitals, while those with unaffiliated residency programs exhibited poorer care. In the second case, hospitals with a lower intensity of house staff, that is, a lower proportion of total house staff to occupied beds, provided care better than or equal to that of nonteaching hospitals, while those with a high house staff intensity delivered poorer care. House staff intensity was interpreted as an index of the amount of supervision residents receive from experienced physicians: the greater the intensity, the less the supervision and the poorer the care (see chap. 12).

4. Hospitals reporting higher average expenditures per patient episode experienced better patient outcomes. Expenditure data were available only at the hospital level and consisted of reported total annual expenditures divided by the number of patients treated during that year. Expenditures were corrected for regional differences in cost but did not take into account differences in patient mix among hospitals. In most of our analyses, expenditures were treated as a variable used for statistical control and not of primary interest. Still, it is useful to point out that the relation between greater expenditures and better outcomes was consistently observed (see chaps. 10 and 12).

A number of other features of hospitals bore an unexpected or inconsistent relationship to the quality of care. For example, neither the qualifications of the surgical staff nor those of the nursing staff on surgical wards were correlated with the quality of care. Nor, as reported above, did the qualifications of individual surgeons affect the quality of outcomes. Neither the average level of commitment of surgeons to the hospital as reflected in the proportion of their care provided in the study hospital nor the proportion of contract physicians— both variables assumed to improve coordination of services—was consistently associated with better outcomes. Similarly, controls exercised by hospital and nursing administrators within their own domains were not consistently associated with better-quality care.

The relations between organizational characteristics and outcomes can also be summarized in reference to the general arguments developed in chapter 1, where better outcomes are predicted in hospitals characterized by (1) higher levels of differentiation, (2) more resources devoted to coordination, (3) higher levels of total power, (4) higher levels of professional staff control, and (5) higher levels of staff qualifications. The only hypotheses receiving consistent support across the various data sets and analyses were those pertaining to professional staff controls.

Chapter 1 also describes two models of hospital structure, a bureaucratic model emphasizing differentiation, coordination, and controls exercised by appropriate authorities; and a professional model emphasizing qualifications of individual staff members and collegial control systems operating within the medical staff. Differentiation, coordination, and administrative controls may provide important benefits within complex professional organizations such as hospitals, but there is little in our data to suggest that they have palpable effects on the quality of inpatient care as measured by adjusted patient outcomes.

The professional model fares somewhat better. Although there was little evidence that staff qualifications, whether of individual surgeons or average levels of training for the surgical and the nursing staff, were associated with better than expected outcomes, there was strong evidence linking staff experience with better outcomes—not experience in general, not years of practice or length of training, but experience at the hospital level in dealing with similar types of patients. (As discussed in chap. 11, it is possible to interpret experience as a property of the hospital rather than, or in addition to, as a property of the staff, since hospitals may improve services to high-volume groups by providing specialized facilities, equipment, and procedural routines.)

Strong support for the collegial control model comes from the evidence linking surgical staff controls to the quality of care. In addition, the findings on medical school affiliation and lower house staff intensity may be interpreted as signifying the effects of closer professional supervision on care delivery.

Technology and Structure

Characteristics of the technology employed—the complexity and uncertainty of tasks—were more strongly associated with work arrangements at the subunit (ward) level than at the hospital level. Moreover, it is important at the subunit level to distinguish between individual task demands, which pertain to worker characteristics, and workflow demands, which pertain to ward structures. More unpredictable tasks were associated with higher levels of worker training and professional activities at the individual level. And more unpredictable workflows were associated with reduced standardization and centralization of decision making at the ward level (see chap. 2).

At the hospital level, support was found for the expectation that increased organizational capacity would be associated with higher levels of service intensity and higher costs per patient episode. That is, patients served in more elaborate facilities were more likely to receive more services than expected. It is difficult to know which direction this relationship takes: it is likely that more complex services will give rise to more complex structures, but it seems equally likely that more complex structures, once developed, will generate more complex services, independent of patient requirements (see chap. 10).

At best, only modest support was obtained for the contingency predictions that the quality of outcomes was dependent on an appropriate match between hospital or staff characteristics and patient-care demands. For example, there was evidence that higher qualifications of individual surgeons and ward-level nurses were associated with better outcomes for patients undergoing more complex surgical procedures, but these results were not replicated at the hospitalwide or the surgical staff levels (see chap. 6).

IMPLICATIONS

At a conference designed to take stock of twenty years of health services research, Brook and Lohr (1985) reaffirmed the need to evaluate the relation between health care structures, processes, and outcomes. While much work has been done and some progress has been made, there remain critical gaps in our ability to adequately measure these constructs and understand their interrelationships. Brook and Lohr strongly endorsed the need to include outcome measures, stressing that "our fundamental concern in quality assessment is the end result of care (i.e., the patient's eventual outcome or health status)," and proceeded to suggest that "what is needed might be characterized as an epidemiology of effectiveness: some way of routinely collecting information that describes the outcomes of tests, procedures, drugs, and other services as they are customarily used in everyday practice" (715, 713).

There is little doubt that we remain far from this objective. However, the methodology for adjusting outcomes developed and tested in the Stanford studies moves us along the path toward this desirable goal. We have demonstrated that it is feasible to utilize abstracted, routinely collected patient-level data to standardize outcomes so that variations in effectiveness of care become visible. If there were routine collection of more sensitive and more proximate outcome measures to supplement mortality as an ultimate adverse event, the methodology would be even more useful. The adjustment methods devised can serve as the basis for the development of routine monitoring systems to evaluate the quality of care. These systems could be attached to various rewards and penalties and function to detect and sanction individual practitioners and/or hospitals producing outcomes of either better or poorer quality than expected.

A control system with some of these features was designed and established as a part of the Professional Standards Review Organization (PSRO) program, mandated as a national quality-assurance and utilization-review system in the 1970s. This program ran afoul of many obstacles—professional, medical, and political—and its mission to monitor quality was swamped by the rapid rise in hospital costs and the pressure to contain utilization. Since it was not possible to demonstrate that PSROs were more effective than previously existing mechanisms in reducing hospital utilization, the program was discontinued (see Dobson 1978; and Goran 1979). A replacement program, the Peer Review Organization (PRO), offers a new opportunity to put into place a routine system to monitor the costs and quality of care. Komaroff (1985) suggested that since prospective reimbursement policies already exist to encourage cost-reducing behavior, PROs should be encouraged and may be allowed to address their primary attention to monitoring the quality of care. Whether they will do so and how effective they will be remains to be seen.

Monitoring systems are not only useful as mechanisms for external regulation and control. They are also essential for the systematic improvement of professional practice. Criteria for determining effective practices and procedures must be validated in terms of their effects on outcomes. Clinical trials represent the preferred contemporary methodology for devising and testing new treatments. However, their major use is to evaluate the *efficacy* of some technology or procedure under ideal conditions of use. They are not used to routinely evaluate *effectiveness*, "performance under ordinary conditions by the average practitioner for the typical patient" (Brook and Lohr 1985, 711). Routine monitoring of clinical practice would allow the regular comparisons of existing variations in practice with adjusted outcomes, providing a systematic basis for learning from experience.

In addition, in a cost-containing climate, better measures of quality are necessary to ascertain when and whether reductions in expenditures and services occasion reduced benefits. The findings reported in chapter 7 suggest that higher than average levels of services do not necessarily represent excessive or inappropriate services. Higher than usual levels of specific services resulted in better than expected outcomes. It is unnecessary to take issue with those economists who argue that we may have set too high a standard of medical quality— that we may not be able to afford to provide "Cadillac care" for all. The point to be made is that if trade-offs are required, we need better information not only on the costs we are asked to pay but also on the benefits we are being asked to forgo.

The recent trend toward more corporate forms of medical care and, in particular, the development of multihospital systems has implications for the development of such monitoring systems. On the one hand, it is in the interests of these corporations to develop better control and information systems of all types: uniform patient records, reports, and accounting procedures, uniform records on personnel and performance, and better measures of capital facilities and equipment. Information to compare performance across facilities is essential to rationally guide strategic decisions concerning which units are to be expanded, modified, or closed. Other things being equal, we would expect the chief executive officer of a multihospital system to have more interest in the comparative performance of hospitals and thus to be more likely to invest resources in monitoring systems assessing costs and quality. However, as the health care sector becomes more competitive, executives in hospitals and multihospital systems may regard any information on comparative costs and/or quality as proprietary information—available only for the use of the system that assembles it. Such an attitude would reduce the possibility that the data collected might inform and improve professional practice generally.

Yet another possibility is that because the increased prevalence of multi-hospital systems represents a heightened level of concentration in the hospital industry, future governmental efforts to establish regulatory systems making use of routine monitoring techniques may be both more likely and more effective—more likely because increased regulation is viewed as more necessary since competition no longer occurs between many small independent hospitals, more effective because there are fewer units to police.

The principal substantive results emerging from our research pertain to the important role played by the controls exercised by the medical staff in contributing to the quality of patient care. Whereas the conventional professional model places primary stress on the training and socialization of individual practitioners and only secondary emphasis on the collegial controls that augment these talents and reinforce these internalized controls, our findings stress the significance of the latter. Organizational context—the provision of a supportive and constraining environment within which to engage in state-of-the-art professional practice—may be a more significant contributor to the quality of work than the type of past training or the length of prior experience.

This conclusion is consistent with a stance long held by Freidson, a careful student of professional behavior, who asserted that "far too much attention has been paid to the personal characteristics and attitudes of individual members of occupations and far too little to the work settings. This is particularly the case for the professions. On the whole, students of the professions in general and medicine in particular have adopted the same individualistic value position of the men they study" (Freidson 1970, 88). And within the work setting, the potentially most influential structures are those erected by the professionals themselves, as Roemer and Friedman (1971) observed.

It is important to stress that the control structures at work in the hospitals we surveyed were created by and for the physicians themselves. They were not structures imposed on the practitioners by some external authority, whether in the administrative offices of the hospital, the corporate offices of the hospital system, or some federal regulatory agency. Professionals are highly resistant to externally mandated control systems that attempt to regulate their clinical decision making, and they can be quite ingenious in circumventing their intent. The optimal clinical control systems are those that professionals impose on themselves. Again, Freidson stated the case persuasively:

> Discretion on the part of the health worker . . . may be taken to be the prerequisite for providing a truly human service. It alone is flexible enough to serve as faithfully as possible the needs of varied individual

patients. . . . But discretion has . . . its own dangers. It is more easily subject to abuse than is formally regulated behavior. . . . Discretion must, while remaining the core of service, nonetheless be disciplined by a concern for the quality of work in light of the general public and particular patient interest. It cannot be disciplined by administrative rules because such rules either destroy it in the course of regulating it or drive it under ground where it cannot be controlled. What is needed for optimal service to human beings is thus not more elaborate and constraining administrative schemes but rather some way of getting workers to discipline themselves in the light of public interest. That is the optimal alternative. (Freidson 1975, 225)

The moves toward larger and more comprehensive administrative units within the hospital field are not necessarily contradictory to these professional collegial control systems. There are many levels and layers of decision making within complex organizations, and a great variety of administrative, financial, and marketing decisions may be made that are not inimical to the exercise of clinical discretion. On the other hand, some types of managerial decisions— such as those placing limits on costs—do impose constraints on clinical judgments and require that professional providers and administrative managers work together so that each understands the trade-offs that may result between cost and quality. Such discussions and negotiations are more likely to be productive if the medical staff is organized to accept responsibility and speak for the professional concerns of its members. Conflicting values are more likely to be taken into account in some compromise arrangement if organized groups are present to articulate and defend them (see Scott 1982, 1985).

At present, even in multihospital systems, medical staffs tend to be organized at the level of the individual hospital. A survey conducted in 1983 by the research arm of the American Hospital Association reported that over 80 percent of the hospitals currently operating within a multisystem framework had separate medical staff organizations. The analysts concluded that "overall, the findings reflect organizational structures that favor decentralization, perhaps to deal with operational complexities at the hospital level or as a reflection of the traditional influence of physicians on decisions affecting their professional activities" (Alexander and Cobbs 1984, 6). A second study examined changes in medical staff organization occurring during the decade 1971–82 (Shortell, Morrisey, and Conrad 1985). This research reported sizable increases both in the extent of the organization of the medical staff (e.g., the number of staff committees, the numbers of physicians serving on committees, and the percentage of salaried physicians) and in physicians' involvement in hospital governance activities (e.g., service on the governing board and on the board's executive committee). These types of changes were more likely to be observed for system than for nonsystem hospitals. In short, there is evidence to suggest that the medical staffs of hospitals are more likely to be organized, and to be better organized, today than when our data were collected. Our findings suggest that such organization is likely to promote improved quality of care within hospitals.

Appendix A • Publications and Reports Based on the Data Bases of the Extensive Study, the Intensive Study, and the Service Intensity Study

A superscript number after the name of the author indicates whether the publication or report was based on the data base of the Intensive Study (1), the Extensive Study (2), or the Service Intensity Study (3).

TECHNICAL REPORTS

Forrest, W. H., Jr.; Brown, B. W., Jr.; Scott, W. R.; Ewy, W.; and Flood, A. B.[1,2] 1977. *Studies of the determinants of service intensity in the medical care sector.* Report to the National Center for Health Services Research. PB 287-365. Springfield, Va.: National Technical Information Service.

——.[1,2] 1978. *Impact of hospital characteristics on surgical outcomes and length of stay.* Final Report to the National Center for Health Services Research. PB 233-157. Springfield, Va.: National Technical Information Service.

Stanford Center for Health Care Research (SCHCR).[1,2] 1974. *Study of institutional differences in postoperative mortality.* Report to the National Academy of Sciences–National Research Council. PB 250-940. Springfield, Va.: National Technical Information Service.

——.[1,2] 1976. The hospital as a factor in the quality of surgical care. In *Vol. III surgery in the United States: A summary report of the study on surgical services for the United States,* ed. Quality of Surgical Care Subcommittee. Washington, D.C.: American College of Surgeons and the American Surgical Association.

DISSERTATIONS AND THESES

Alexander, J. A.[1] 1980. Structural determinants of professional role orientations: The case of hospital staff nurses. Ph.D. diss., Stanford University.

Comstock, D. E.[1] 1975. Technology and context: A study of hospital patient care units. Ph.D. diss., Stanford University.

Flood, A. B.[1] 1976. Professions and organizational performance: A study of medical staff organization and quality of care in short term hospitals. Ph.D. diss., Stanford University.

Garrison, L. P., Jr.[1] 1981. Studies in the economics of surgery. Ph.D. diss., Stanford University.

Rundall, T. G.[1] 1976. Life change and recovery from surgery. Ph.D. diss., Stanford University.

Schoonhoven, C. B.[1] 1976. Organizational effectiveness: A contingency analysis of surgical technology and hospital structure. Ph.D. diss., Stanford University.

Sharp, K.[1] 1986. Organizational determinants of quality surgical care. Ph.D. diss., University of Illinois at Urbana-Champaign. Forthcoming.

Yergan, J.[3] 1982. Influence of source of payment or race on service intensity and outcomes in hospitals. Master's thesis, University of Washington.

PUBLICATIONS AND PRESENTATIONS

Alexander, J. A.[1] 1982. *The organizational structure of hospital patient care units: Effects on nursing professionalism.* Ann Arbor: University of Michigan Research Press.

―――.[1] 1984. Organizational foundations of nursing roles: An empirical assessment. *Soc. Sci. Med.* 18(12): 1045–52.

Bloom, J. R., and Alexander, J. A.[1] 1982. Team nursing: Professional coordination or bureaucratic control? *J. Health Soc. Behav.* 23: 84–95.

Brown, B. W., Jr.[1,2] 1980. Statistical problems in comparing outcomes of low incidence. In *Health care delivery in anesthesia,* ed. R. A. Hirsh, W. H. Forrest, Jr., F. Orkin, and H. Wollman. Philadelphia: George F. Stickley Co.

Comstock, D. E.[1] 1980. Dimensions of influence in organizations. *Pacific Sociol. Rev.* 23: 67–84.

Comstock, D. E., and Schrager, L. S.[1] 1979. Hospital services and community characteristics: The physicians as mediator. *J. Health Soc. Behav.* 20: 89–97.

Comstock, D. E., and Scott, W. R.[1] 1977. Technology and the structure of subunits: Distinguishing individual and workgroup effects. *Admin. Sci. Q.* 22: 177–201. Chapter 2 is an edited version of this article.

Ewy, W.[2] 1980a. Hospital death and morbidity studies—a national sample. In *Health care delivery in anesthesia,* 49–56. *See* Brown 1980.

―――.[2] 1980. Important patient control variables in outcomes of surgery and anesthesia. In *Health care delivery in anesthesia,* 85–92. *See* Brown 1980.

Flood, A. B.[1] 1980. Hospital organization and outcomes of care. In *Health care delivery in anesthesia,* 105–118. *See* Brown 1980.

―――.[2] 1985. The effects of teaching on patient care and costs in hospitals. Paper presented at the annual meeting of the American Public Health Association, Washington, D.C., November.

Flood, A. B.; Ewy, W.; Scott, W. R.; Forrest, W. H., Jr., and Brown, B. W., Jr.[3] 1979. The relationship between intensity and duration of medical services and outcomes for hospitalized patients. *Med. Care* 17(11): 1088–1102. Chapter 7 is an edited version of this article.

Flood, A. B., and Scott, W. R.[1] 1978. Professional power and professional effectiveness: The power of the surgical staff and the quality of surgical care in hospitals. *J. Health Soc. Behav.* 19: 240–54. Chapter 9 is an edited version of this article.

Flood, A. B.; Scott, W. R.; and Ewy, W.[2] 1984a. Does practice make perfect? Part I: The relation between hospital volume and outcomes for selected diagnostic categories. *Med. Care* 22(2): 99–114. The first section of chapter 11 is an edited version of this article.

————.[2] 1984b. Does practice make perfect? Part II: The relation between volume and outcomes and other hospital characteristics. *Med. Care* 22(2): 115–125. The second section of chapter 11 is an edited version of this article.

————.[2] 1984c. Reply to David Dranove. *Med. Care* 22(10): 967–69. An edited version is incorporated into chapter 11.

Flood, A. B.; Scott, W. R.; Ewy, W.; and Forrest, W. H., Jr.[1] 1982. Effectiveness in professional organizations: The impact of surgeons and surgical staff organizations on the quality of care in hospitals. *Health Serv. Res.* 17: 341–66. Chapter 8 is an edited version of this article.

Flood, A. B., Swartz, H. M.; Sharp, K.; Bonello, J. C.; and Forrest, W. H., Jr.[1] 1985a. Patient factors affecting the decision to operate for biliary tract disease. Paper, University of Illinois College of Medicine.

————.[1] 1985b. A comparison between preoperative and postoperative diagnoses for biliary tract disease. Paper, University of Illinois College of Medicine.

Forrest, W. H., Jr.[1] 1980. Outcome—the effect of the provider. In *Health care delivery in anesthesia,* 137–42. *See* Brown 1980.

Rundall, T. G.[1] 1978. Life changes and recovery from surgery. *J. Health Soc. Behav.* 19: 418–27.

Schoonhoven, C. B.[1] 1981. Problems with contingency theory: Testing assumptions hidden within the language of contingency "theory." *Admin. Sci. Q.* 26: 349–77.

Schoonhoven, C. B.; Scott, W. R.; Flood, A. B.; Forrest, W. H., Jr.[1] 1980. Measuring the complexity and uncertainty of surgery and postsurgical care. *Med. Care* 18 (9): 893–915.

Scott, W. R.[1] 1977. Effectiveness of organizational effectiveness studies. In *New perspectives on organizational effectiveness,* ed. P. Goodman and H. Pennings, 63–95. San Francisco: Jossey-Bass.

————.[3] 1979. Measuring outputs in hospitals. In *Measurement and interpretation of productivity,* ed. National Academy of Sciences Panel to Review Productivity Statistics.

Scott, W. R., and Flood, A. B. 1984. Hospital costs and quality of care: A review of the literature. *Med. Care Rev.* 41 (4): 213–61.

Scott, W. R.; Flood, A. B.; and Ewy, W.[3] 1979. Organizational determinants of services, quality and cost of care in hospitals. *Milbank Mem. Fund Q.* 57: 234–64. Chapter 10 is an edited version of this article.

Scott, W. R.; Flood, A. B.; Ewy, W.; and Forrest, W. H., Jr.[1] 1978. Organizational effectiveness and the quality of surgical care in hospitals. In *Environments and organizations,* ed. M. Meyer and Associates, 290–305. San Francisco: Jossey-Bass.

Scott, W. R.; Flood, A. B.; Ewy, W.; Forrest, W. H., Jr.; and Brown, B. W., Jr.[1] 1976. Utilizing outcomes to assess the quality of surgical care. Paper presented at the annual meetings of the American Institute for Decision Sciences, San Francisco, November. Incorporated into chapter 6.

Scott, W. R.; Forrest, W. H., Jr.; and Brown, B. W., Jr.[1] 1976. Hospital structure and postoperative mortality and morbidity. In *Organizational research in hospitals,* ed. S. Shortell and M. Brown, 72–89. An *Inquiry* Book. Chicago: Blue Cross Association.

Stanford Center for Health Care Research (SCHCR).[1,2] 1976. Comparison of hospitals with regard to outcomes of surgery. *Health Serv. Res.* 11: 112–27.

Yergan, J.; Flood, A. B.; LoGerfo, J. P.; and Diehr, P.[3] N.d. Relationship between patient race and the intensity of hospital services. Research paper, School of Medicine, University of Washington, Seattle.

————. N.d. Relationship between source of insurance and hospital services. Research Paper, School of Medicine University of Washington, Seattle.

COMMENTARIES

Donabedian, A. 1984. Volume, quality, and the regionalization of health care services. *Med. Care* 22(2): 95–97.

Dranove, D. 1984. Letter to the editor. *Med. Care* 22(10): 967.

May, J. J. 1983. Commentary on the management implications of effectiveness in professional organizations: The impact of surgeons and surgical staff organizations on the quality of care. *Health Serv. Res.* 18: 1–6.

Neuhauser, D. 1983. Hospital effectiveness. *Health Serv. Res.* 18: 13–15.

Ross, A. Applying the conclusions of the Flood study to the hospital practice world. *Health Serv. Res.* 17: 373–77.

Rundall, T. G. 1983. Effectiveness in professional organizations. *Health Serv. Res.* 18: 7–12.

Rutkow, I. M. 1982. The surgical decision-making process: Determinants of surgical rates. *Health Serv. Res.* 17: 379–85.

Shortell, S. M. 1982. Improving organizational effectiveness: A comment on effectiveness in professional organizations. *Health Serv. Res.* 17: 367–72.

Appendix B • Hospitals in the Intensive Study

Cincinnati General Hospital (now University of Cincinnati Medical Center), Cincinnati, Ohio

Harlan Appalachian Regional Hospital, Harlan, Kentucky

Lowell General Hospital, Lowell, Massachusetts

Memorial Hospital of Alamance County, Inc., Burlington, North Carolina

Memorial Hospital of Natrona County, Casper, Wyoming

Mercy Hospital (now Wilkes-Barre Mercy Hospital), Wilkes-Barre, Pennsylvania

Middlesex General Hospital (now Middlesex General University Hospital), New Brunswick, New Jersey

Porter Memorial Hospital, Denver, Colorado

St. Luke's Hospital, Bethlehem, Pennsylvania

St. Luke's Hospital Medical Center, Phoenix, Arizona

St. Mary's Hospital, Philadelphia, Pennsylvania

St. Vincent Hospital, Worcester, Massachusetts

South Coast Community Hospital (now South Coast Medical Center), South Laguna, California

Swedish Medical Center, Englewood, Colorado

Warren Hospital, Phillipsburg, New Jersey

Watts Hospital (closed October, 1976), Durham, North Carolina

West Hudson Hospital, Kearny, New Jersey

References

Abelson, R. P., and Tukey, J. W. 1959. Efficient conversion of nonmetric information into metric information. In *The quantitative analysis of social problems*, ed. E. R. Tufte, 407–17. Reading, Mass: Addison-Wesley.

Aday, L. A., and Andersen, R. 1974. A framework for the study of access to medical care. *Health Serv. Res.* 9:208–20.

Aday, L. A.; Andersen, R.; and Fleming, G. V. 1980. *Health care in the U.S.: Equitable for whom?:* Beverly Hills: Sage.

Aiken, M., and Hage, J. 1968. Organizational interdependence and intraorganizational structure. *Am. Sociol. Rev.* 33:912–30.

Aldrich, H. E. 1972. Technology and organizational structure: A reexamination of the findings of the Aston group. *Admin. Sci. Q.* 17:26–43.

Alexander, J. A., and Cobbs, D. L. 1984. More work needed on MD-multi relationships. *Hospitals* 16:54–58.

Alker, H. R., Jr. 1969. A typology of ecological fallacies. In *Quantitative ecological analysis in the social sciences*, ed. M. Dogan, 69–86. Cambridge, Mass.: MIT Press.

Allison, R. F. 1976. Administrative responses to prospective reimbursement. *Top. Health Care. Financ.* 3:97–111.

American College of Surgeons and the American Surgical Association (ACASA). 1976. *Surgery in the United States: A report on the study on surgical services in the United States.* Chicago: American College of Surgeons and the American Surgical Association.

American Hospital Association (AHA). 1973. *Guide to the health care field.* Chicago.

———. 1974a. *Guide to the health care field.* Chicago.

———. 1974b. Status of multihospital systems. *Hospitals* 48:61–63.

———. 1983. *Hospital statistics: 1983 edition.* Chicago.

———. 1985. *Multihospital system data book.* Chicago.

American Medical Association (AMA). 1973. *Consolidated list of hospitals with approved graduate training programs.* Chicago.

Andersen, R., and May, J. J. 1972. Factors associated with the increasing cost of hospital care. *Ann. Am. Acad. Polit. Social Sci.* 399:62–72.

Anderson, O. W., and Shields, M. C. 1982. Quality measurement and control in physician decision making: The state of the art. *Health Serv. Res.* 17:125–55.

Anesthesiology. 1963. New classification of physical status. *Anesthesiology* 24:111.

Arnold, D. J. 1970. 28,621 cholecystectomies in Ohio: Results of a survey in Ohio hospitals. *Am. J. Surg.* 119:714–17.

Ashley, J. S. A.; Howlett, A.; and Morris, J. N. 1971. Case-fatality of hyperplasia of the prostate in two teaching and three regional-board hospitals. *Lancet* 2(7737)(11 December): 1308–11.

Barnes, B. A. 1977. Discarded operations: Surgical innovation by trial and error. In *Costs, risks, and benefits of surgery*, ed. J. P. Bunker, B. A. Barnes, and F. Mosteller, 109–23. New York: Oxford University Press.

Bayer, R.; Callahan, D.; Fletcher, J.; Hodgson, T.; Jennings, B.; Monsees, D.; Sieverts, S.; and Veatch, R. 1983. The care of the terminally ill: Morality and economics. *N. Engl. J. Med.* 309:1490–94.

Becker, M. H.. and Maiman, L. A. 1983. Models of health-related behavior. In *Handbook of health, health care, and the health professions*, ed. D. Mechanic, 539–68. New York: Free Press.

Becker, S. W., and Neuhauser, D. 1975. *The efficient organization.* New York: Elsevier Press.

Becker, S. W.; Shortell, S. M.; and Neuhauser, D. 1980. Management practice and hospital lengths of stay. *Inquiry* 17:318–30.

Bell, G. D. 1967. Determinants of span of control. *Am. J. Sociol.* 73:100–109.

Bergner, M. 1985. Measurement of health status. *Med. Care* 23(5): 696–722.

Berry, R. E., Jr. 1967. Returns to scale in the production of hospital services. *Health Serv. Res* 2:123–39.

———. 1970. Product heterogeneity and hospital cost analysis. *Inquiry* 12:7–75.

Biggs, E. L. 1977. Accountability in corporation managed and traditionally managed nonprofit hospitals. Ph.D. diss., Pennsylvania State University.

Biggs, E. L.; Kralewski, J.; and Brown, G. 1980. A comparison of contract-managed and traditionally-managed non-profit hospitals. *Med. Care* 18(2): 585–96.

Blalock, H. M., Jr. 1963. *Causal inferences in non-experimental research.* Chapel Hill: University of North Carolina Press.

———. 1967. Status inconsistency, social mobility, status integration and structural effects. *Am. Sociol. Rev.* 32:790–800.

———. 1970. *Social statistics.* 2d ed. New York: McGraw-Hill.

Blau, P. M. 1968. Structural effects. *Am. Sociol. Rev.* 25:178–93.

Blau, P. M., and Schoenherr, R. 1971. *The structure of organizations.* New York: Basic Books.

Bloom, B. S., and Peterson, O. L. 1973. End results, cost, and productivity of coronary care units. *N. Engl. J. Med.* 288:72–78.

Blumberg, M. S., and Gentry, D. W. 1978. Routine hospital charges and intensity of care: A cross section analysis of fifty states. *Inquiry* 15:58–73.

Boice, J. L., and McGregor, M. 1983. Effect of residents' use of laboratory tests on hospital costs. *J. Med. Educ.* 58:61–64.

Brook, R. H. 1973. *Quality of care assessment: A comparison of five methods of peer review.* HRA-74-3100. Washington, D.C.: Bureau of Health Services Research and Evaluation.

Brook R. H., and Appel, F. A. 1973. Quality-of-care assessment: Choosing a method for peer review. *N. Engl. J. Med.* 288:1323–29.

Brook, R. H.; Appel, F. A.; Avery, C.; Orman, M.; and Stevenson, R. L. 1971. Effectiveness of inpatient follow-up care. *N. Engl. J. Med.* 285:1509–14.

Brook, R. H.; Davies-Avery, A.; Greenfield, S.; Harris, L. J.; Lelah, T.; Solomon, N. E.; and Ware, J. E., Jr. 1977. Assessing the quality of medical care using outcome measures: An overview of the method. *Med. Care* 15(9) (suppl.): 1–165.

Brook, R. H., and Lohr, K. A. 1985. Efficacy, effectiveness, variations, and quality: Boundary-crossing research. *Med. Care* 23(5): 710–22.

Brook, R. H., and Williams, K. N. 1976. Evaluation of the New Mexico–peer review system, 1971–1973. *Med. Care* 14(12)(suppl.): 1–122.

Brown, L. D. 1983. *Politics and health care organizations: HMOs as federal policy.* Washington, D.C.: Brookings Institution.

Brown, M., and Lewis, H. L. 1976. *Hospital management systems: Multi-unit organization and delivery of health care.* Germantown, Md.: Aspen Systems Corporation.

Brown, M., and McCool, B. 1980. *Multihospital systems strategies for organization and management.* Rockville, Md.: Aspen Systems Corporation.

Brown, R. E., ed. 1972. *Economies of scale in the health services industry: Proceedings of an invitational seminar.* HRA-74-3100. Washington, D.C.: National Center for Health Services Research and Development.

Bucher, R., and Stelling, J. 1969. Characteristics of professional organizations. *J. Health Soc. Behav.* 10:3–16.

Bunker, J. P.; Forrest, W. H., Jr.; Mosteller, F.; and Vandam, L. D. 1969. *The National Halothane Study.* Washington, D.C.: National Institute of General Medical Sciences.

Burns, T., and Stalker, G. M. 1961. *The management of innovation.* London: Tavistock.

Carr, W. J., and Feldstein, P. J. 1967. The relationship of cost to hospital care. *Inquiry* 4:45–65.

Chassin, M. R. 1982. Costs and outcomes of medical intensive care. *Med. Care* 20(2): 165–79.

Child, J. 1973. Predicting and understanding organization structure. *Admin. Sci. Q.* 18:168–85.

———. 1974. Managerial and organizational factors associated with company performance: Part I. *J. Manage. Studies* 11:175–89.

———. 1975. Managerial and organizational factors associated with company performance: Part II. *J. Manage. Studies* 12:12–27.

Child, J., and Mansfield, R. 1972. Technology, size, and organization structure. *Sociology* 6:369–93.

Clendenning, M. K.; Wolfe, H.; Shuman, L. J.; and Huber, G. A. 1976. The effect of a target date based utilization review program on LOS. *Med. Care* 14(9): 751–64.

Codman, E. A. 1916. *A study of hospital efficiency: The first five years.* Boston: Todd.

Cohen, H. A. 1970. Hospital cost curves with emphasis on measuring patient care output. In *Empirical studies in health economics,* ed. H. E. Klarman, 279–93. Baltimore: Johns Hopkins Press.

Cohen, H. S. 1973. Professional licensure, organizational behavior, and the public interest. *Milbank Mem. Fund Q.* 51:73–88.

Cohen, S. N.; Flood, A. B.; Himmelberger, D. U.; Mangini, R. J.; and Moore, T. N. 1980. *Development, implementation and evaluation of the monitoring and evaluation of drug interactions by a pharmacy oriented reporting system (MEDIPHOR)*. HS00739. Final Report to National Center for Health Services Research. Springfield, Va.: National Technical Information Service.

Colditz, G.; Tuden, R.; and Oster, G. 1985. Post-operative complications: A major source of cost savings to hospitals. Paper presented at the annual meeting of the American Public Health Association, Washington, D.C., November.

Commission on Professional and Hospital Activities (CPHA). 1968. *Hospital adaptation of ICDA*. Ann Arbor.

———. 1969. *Cholecystectomy mortality: A study from PAS and MAP*. Ann Arbor.

———. 1970. Cholecystectomy mortality. *PAS Reporter* 8(20 April).

———. 1975. *Length of stay in PAS hospitals, by operation, United States*. Ann Arbor.

———. 1977. *Hospital mortality—PAS hospitals, U.S., 1974–75*. Ann Arbor.

Comstock, D. E. 1980. Dimensions of influence in organizations. *Pacific Sociol. Rev.* 23:67–84.

Comstock, D. E., and Schrager, L. S. 1979. Hospital services and community characteristics: The physician as mediator. *J. Health Soc. Behav.* 20:89–97.

Comstock, D. E., and Scott, W. R. 1977. Technology and the structure of subunits: Distinguishing individual and workgroup effects. *Admin. Sci. Q.* 22:177–201. Chapter 2 is an edited version of this article.

Conklin, J. E.; Lieberman, J. V.; Barnes, C. A.; and Louis, D. Z. 1984. Disease staging: Implications for hospital reimbursement and management. *Health Care Financ. Rev.* 6(November): 13–22.

Cooney, J. P., and Alexander, T. L. 1975. *Multihospital system: An evaluation, parts 1– 4*. Chicago: Health Services Research Center of the Hospital Research and Educational Trust and Northwestern University.

Corn, R. F. 1980. Quality control of hospital discharge data. *Med. Care* 18(4): 416–26.

Cummings, K. M.; Becker, M.; and Maile, M. C. 1980. Bringing the models together: An empirical approach to combining variables used to explain health actions. *J. Behav. Med.* 3(June): 123–45.

Dagnone, A. 1967. A study of multiple unit hospital systems. Thesis, Program in Hospital Administration, University of Toronto.

Davis, J. A.; Spaeth, J. L., and Huson, C. 1961. A technique for analyzing the effects of group composition. *Am. Sociol. Rev.* 26:215–25.

De-Nour, A. K. 1982. Psychosocial adjustment to illness scale (PAIS): A study of chronic hemodialysis patients. *J. Psychosom. Res.* 26:11–22.

DiMatteo, M. R.,and DiNicola, D. D. 1982. *Achieving patient compliance: The psychology of the medical practitioner's role*. New York: Pergamon Press.

Dobson, A. 1978. PSROs: Their current status and their impact to date. *Inquiry* 15:113–28.

Donabedian, A. 1966. Evaluating the quality of medical care. *Milbank Mem. Fund Q.* 44:166–203.

———. 1978. The quality of medical care. In *Health care: Regulation, economics, ethics, practice*, ed. P. Abelson, 12–20. Washington, D.C.: American Association for the Advancement of Science.

———. 1980. *The definition of quality and approaches to its assessment: Vol. 1:*

Explorations in quality assessment and monitoring. Ann Arbor: Health Administration Press.

———. 1981. Advantages and limitations of explicit criteria for assessing the quality of health care. *Milbank Mem. Fund Q.* 59:99–106.

———. 1982. *The criteria and standards of quality.* Ann Arbor: Health Administration Press.

———. 1984. Volume, quality, and the regionalization of health care services. *Med. Care* 22(2): 95–97.

Donabedian, A.; Wheeler, J. R. C.; and Wyszewianski, L. 1982. Quality, cost, and health: An integrative model. *Med. Care* 20(10): 975–92.

Dornbusch, S. M., and Scott, W. R. 1975. *Evaluation and the exercise of authority.* San Francisco: Jossey-Bass.

Drake, D. 1980. The cost of hospital regulation. In *Regulating health care,* ed. A. Levin, 45–59. New York: Academy of Political Science.

Dranove, D. 1984. Letter to the editor. *Med. Care* 22(10): 967.

Dripps, R. D.; Lamont, A.; and Eckenhoff, J. E. 1961. The role of anesthesia in surgical mortality. *JAMA* 178:261–66.

Duckett, S. J., and Kristofferson, S. M. 1978. An index of hospital performance. *Med. Care* 16(5): 400–407.

Dyck, F. J.; Murphy, F. A.; Murphy, J. K.; Road, D. A.; Boyd, M. S.; Osborne, E.; De Vlieger, D.; Korchinski, B.; Ripley, C.; Bromley, A. T.; and Innes, P. B. 1977. Effect of surveillance on the number of hysterectomies in the province of Saskatchewan. *N. Engl. J. Med.* 296:1326–28.

Eckles, J. E., and Root, J. G. 1970. *A methodology for quantitative evaluation of health care with application to post-surgical care in the U.S. Air Force hospitals.* RM-6374-PR. Santa Monica, Calif.: Rand.

Eddy, D. 1980. *Screening for cancer: Theory, analysis, and design.* Englewood Cliffs, N.J.: Prentice Hall.

Edwards, S. 1972. *Demonstration and evaluation of integrated health care facilities.* 4 vols. Chicago: Hospital Research and Educational Trust and Northwestern University.

Enthoven, A. C. 1980. *Health plan: The only practical solution to the soaring cost of medical care.* Reading, Mass.: Addison-Wesley.

Enthoven, A. C., and Noll, R. G. 1984. The new prospective payment system for Medicare reimbursement: A solution to rising federal expenditures on health? Paper, Stanford University Graduate School of Business.

Eraker, S. A., and Sox, H. C. 1981. Assessment of patients' preferences for therapeutic outcomes. *Med. Decis. Making* 1:29–30.

Ermann, D., and Gabel J. 1984. Multihospital systems: Issues and empirical findings. *Health Aff.* 3(Spring): 50–64.

Etzioni, A. 1964. *Modern organizations.* Englewood Cliffs, N.J.: Prentice-Hall.

———, ed. 1969. *The semi-professions and their organization.* New York: Free Press.

Federation of American Hospitals. 1982. *Directory of investor-owned hospitals and hospital management companies.* Little Rock.

Feldstein, M. S. 1967. *Economic analysis for health service efficiency.* Amsterdam: North Holland.

———. 1971. *The rising cost of hospital care.* Washington, D.C.: Information Resources Press for the National Center for Health Services Research and Development.

———. 1981. *Hospital costs and health insurance*. Cambridge, Mass.: Harvard University Press.

Feldstein, P. J. 1970. Comment on hospital cost curves with emphasis on measuring patient care output. In *Empirical studies in health economics*, ed. H. E. Klarman, 294–96. Baltimore: Johns Hopkins Press.

———. 1983. *Health care economics*. 2d ed. New York: John Wiley & Sons.

Fernow, L. C.; McColl, I.; and Thurlaw. S. C. 1981. Measuring the quality of clinical performance with hernia and myocardial infarction patients, controlling for patient risk. *Med. Care* 19(3): 273–80.

Fetter, R. B.; Mills, R. E.; Riedel, D. C., and Thompson, J. D. 1977. The application of diagnostic specific cost profiles to cost and reimbursement control in hospitals. *J. Med. Syst.* 1(2): 137–49.

Fetter. R. B.; Shin, Y.; Freeman, J. L.; Averill, R. F., and Thompson, J. D. 1980. Casemix definition by diagnosis-related groups. *Med. Care* 18(2)(suppl.): 1–53.

Fine, J., and Morehead, M. A. 1971. Study of peer review of inhospital patient care with the aid of a manual. *N.Y. State J. Med.* 71(15 August): 1963–73.

Fineberg, H.; Scadden, D.; and Goldman, L. 1984. Care of patients with a low probability of acute infarction: Cost effectiveness of alternatives to coronary-artery unit admissions. *N. Engl. J. Med.* 310:1301–7.

Fleiss, J. L. 1981. *Statistical methods for rates and proportions*. 2d ed. New York: John Wiley & Sons.

Fleming, G. V. 1981. Hospital structure and consumer satisfaction. *Health Serv. Res.* 16:43–64.

Flood, A. B. 1976. Professionals and organizational performance: A study of medical staff organization and quality of care in short term hospitals. Ph.D. diss., Stanford University.

Flood, A. B.; Ewy, W.; Scott, W. R.; Forrest, W. H., Jr.; and Brown, B. W., Jr. 1979. The relationship between intensity and duration of medical services and outcomes for hospitalized patients. *Med. Care* 17(11): 1088–1102. Chapter 7 is an edited version of this article.

Flood, A. B., and Scott, W. R. 1978. Professional power and professional effectiveness: The power of the surgical staff and the quality of surgical care in hospitals. *J. Health Soc. Behav.* 19:240–54. Chapter 9 is an edited version of this article.

Flood, A. B.; Scott. W. R.; and Ewy, W. 1984a. Does practice make perfect? Part I: The relation between hospital volume and outcomes for selected diagnostic categories. *Med. Care* 22(2): 98–114. The first section of chapter 11 is an edited version of this article.

———. 1984b. Does practice make perfect? Part II: The relation between volume and outcomes and other hospital characteristics. *Med. Care* 22(2): 115–25. The second section of chapter 11 is an edited version of this article.

———. 1984c. Reply to David Dranove. *Med. Care* 22(10): 967–69. An edited version is incorporated into chapter 11.

Flood, A. B.; Scott, W. R.; Ewy, W.; and Forrest, W. H., Jr. 1982. Effectiveness in professional organizations: The impact of surgeons and surgical staff organizations on the quality of care in hospitals. *Health Serv. Res.* 17:341–66. Chapter 8 is an edited version of this article.

Flood, A. B.; Swartz, H. M.; Sharp, K.; Bonello, J. C.; and Forrest, W. H., Jr. 1985a. Patient factors affecting the decision to operate for biliary tract disease. Paper, University of Illinois College of Medicine.

———. 1985b. A comparison between preoperative and postoperative diagnoses for biliary tract disease. Paper, University of Illinois College of Medicine.

Forrest, W. H., Jr.; Brown, B. W., Jr.; Scott, W. R.; Ewy, W.; and Flood, A. B. 1977. *Studies of the determinants of service intensity in the medical care sector.* Report to the National Center for Health Services Research. PB 287-365. Springfield, Va.: National Technical Information Service.

———. 1978. *Impact of hospital characteristics on surgical outcomes and length of stay.* Final Report to the National Center for Health Services Research. PB 233-157. Springfield, Va.: National Technical Information Service.

Freidson, E. 1970. *Profession of medicine: A study of the sociology of applied knowledge.* New York: Dodd, Mead & Co.

———. 1973. Professions and the occupational principle. In *The professions and their prospects,* ed. E. Freidson, 19–38. Beverly Hills: Sage.

———. 1975. *Doctoring together: A study of professional social control.* New York: Elsevier.

Freidson, E., and Rhea, B. 1963. Processes of control in a company of equals. *Social Problems* 11:119–31.

Friedlander, F., and Pickle, H. 1968. Components of effectiveness in small organizations. *Admin. Sci. Q.* 13:289–304.

Fuchs, V. R. 1974. *Who shall live? Health, economics, and social choice.* New York: Basic Books.

Galbraith, J. 1973. *Designing complex organizations.* Reading, Mass.: Addison-Wesley.

Garber, A. M.; Fuchs, V. R.; and Silverman, J. F. 1984. Casemix, costs and outcomes: Differences between faculty and community services in a university hospital. N. Engl. J. Med. 310:1231–37.

Garg, M. I.; Elkhatib, M.; Kleinberg, W. M.; and Mulligan, J. L. 1982. Reimbursing for residency training: How many times? *Med. Care* 20(7): 719–26.

Georgopoulos, B. S., and Mann, F. C. 1962. *The community general hospital.* New York: MacMillan.

Gertman, P. M., and Lowenstein, S. 1984. A research paradigm for severity of illness: Issues for the diagnosis-related group system. *Health Care Financ. Rev.* 6(November): 79–84.

Gertman, P. M.; Monheit, A. C.; Anderson, J. J.; Eagle, B. J.; and Levenson, D. K. 1979. Utilization review in the United States: Results from a 1976–1977 national survey of hospitals. *Med. Care* 17(8)(suppl.): 1–148.

Gibbs, J. P., and Martin, W. T. 1962. Urbanization, technology and the division of labor: International patterns. *Am. Sociol. Rev.* 17:667–77.

Gibson, R. M. 1979. National health expenditures, 1978. *Health Care Financ. Rev.* 1(1): 1–36.

Gibson, R. M., and Waldo, D. R. 1982. National health expenditures, 1981. *Health Care Financ. Rev.* 4(September): 1–35.

Ginsburg, P. B. 1978. Impact of the economic stabilization program on hospitals: An analysis with aggregate data. In *Hospital cost containment*, ed. M. Zubkoff, I. E. Raskin, and R. S. Hanft, 293–323. New York: Prodist.

Ginsburg, P. B., and Koretz, D. M. 1979. *The effect of PSROs on health care costs: Current findings and future evaluations*. Washington, D.C.: Congressional Budget Office.

Goldfarb, M. G.; Hornbrook, M. C.; Kelly, J. V., and Monheit, A. C. 1980. Health care expenditures. In *Health United States 1980*. PHS 81-1232. Washington, D.C.: Office of Health Research, Statistics and Technology.

Goldman, L.; Sayson, R.; Robbings, S.; Cohn, L. H.; Bettmann, M.; and Weisberg, M. 1983. The value of the autopsy in three medical eras. *N. Engl. J. Med.* 308:1000–1005.

Goldsmith, J. C. 1981. *Can hospitals survive? The new competitive health care market*. Homewood, Ill.: Dow Jones–Irwin.

Gonnella, J. S., ed. 1982. *Clinical criteria for disease staging*. Santa Barbara: Systemetrics.

Gonnella, J. S., and Goran, M. J. 1975. Quality of patient care—a measurement of change: The staging concept. *Med. Care* 13(6): 467–73.

Gonnella, J. S.; Hornbrook, M. C.; and Louis, D. Z. 1984. Staging of disease: A case-mix measurement. *JAMA* 251:637–44.

Goode, W. J. 1957. Community within a community: The professions. *Am. Sociol. Rev.* 22:194–200.

Goodman, P., and Pennings, H., eds. 1977. *New perspectives on organizational effectiveness*. San Francisco: Jossey-Bass.

Goran, M. J. 1979. The evolution of the PSRO hospital review system. *Med. Care* 17(5)(suppl.): 1–47.

Goran, M. J.; Roberts, J. S.; Kellogg, M.; Fielding, J.; and Jessee, W. 1975. The PSRO hospital review system. *Med. Care* 13(4)(suppl.): 1–32.

Gordon, T.; Kannel, W.; and Halperin, M. 1979. Predictability of coronary heart disease. *J. Chronic Dis.* 32:427–40.

Goss, M. E. W. 1961. Influence and authority among physicians in an outpatient clinic. *Am. Sociol. Rev.* 26:39–50.

———. 1970. Organizational goals and quality of medical care: Evidence from comparative research on hospitals. *J. Health Soc. Behav.* 11:255–68.

Goss, M. E. W.; Battistella. R. M.; Colombotos, J.; Freidson, E.; and Riedel, D. C. 1977. Social organization and control in medical work: A call for research. *Med. Care* 15(1): 1–10.

Goss, M. E. W., and Reed, J. 1974. Evaluating the quality of hospital care through severity-adjusted death rates: Some pitfalls. *Med. Care* 12(3): 202–13.

Graham, J. B.; and Paloucek, F. P. 1963. Where should cancer of the cervix be treated? *Am. J. Obstet. Gynecol.* 84:405–9.

Gray, B. H., ed. 1983. *The new health care for profit*. Washington, D.C.: National Academy Press.

Greenfield, S.; Cretin, S.; Worthman, L. G.; Dorey, F. J.; Soloman, N. E.; and Goldberg, G. A. 1981. Comparison of a criteria map to a criteria list in quality-of-care assessment for patients with chest pain: The relation of each to outcome. *Med. Care* 19(3): 255–72.

Grieco, A., and Long, C. J. 1984. Investigation of the Karnofsky performance status as a measure of quality of life. *Health Psychol.* 3(2): 129–42.

Griffith, J. R. 1978. *Measuring hospital performance.* An *Inquiry* Book. Chicago: Blue Cross Association.

Grimes, A. J., and Klein, S. M. 1973. The technological imperative: The relative impact of task unit, modal technology, and hierarchy on structure. *Acad. Management J.* 16:583–97.

Gross, E. 1968. Universities as organizations: A research approach. *Am. Sociol. Rev.* 33:518–44.

Gulick, L. 1937. Notes on the theory of organization. In *Papers on the science of administration,* ed. L. Gulick and L. Urwick, 15–30. New York: Institute of Public Administration, Columbia University.

Hage, J., and Aiken, M. 1969. Routine technology, social structure and organization goals. *Admin. Sci. Q.* 14:366–76.

Haley, R. W.; Culver, D. H.; White, J. W.; Morgan, W. M.; and Emori, T. G. 1975. The nationwide nosocomial infection rate: A new need for vital statistics. *Am. J. Epidemiol.* 121:159–67.

Hall, R. H. 1962. Intraorganizational structural variation: Application of the bureaucratic model. *Admin. Sci. Q.* 7:295–308.

———. 1968. Professionalization and bureaucratization. *Am. Sociol. Rev.* 33:92–104.

Hall, R. H.; Haas, J. E.; and Johnson, N. J. 1967. Organizational size, complexity, and formalization. *Am. Sociol. Rev.* 32:903–12.

Hannan, M. T. 1971. *Aggregation and disaggregation in sociology.* Lexington, Mass.: Heath-Lexington.

Hannan, M. T.; Freeman, J. H.; and Meyer, J. W. 1976. Specification of models for organizational effectiveness. *Am. Sociol. Rev.* 41:136–43.

Health Care Financing Administration. 1980. *Professional standards review organization 1979 program evaluation, health care financing research report.* HCFA 03041. Baltimore: Department of Health and Human Services.

Helbig, D. W.; O'Hare, D.; and Smith, N. W. 1972. The care component score—a new system for evaluating quality of inpatient care. *Am. J. Public Health* 62:540–46.

Hellinger, F. J. 1976. The effect of certificate-of-need legislation on hospital investment. *Inquiry* 13:187–93.

———. 1978. An empirical analysis of several prospective reimbursement systems. In *Hospital cost containment,* 370–400. *See* Ginsburg 1978.

Hendley, J. O. 1984. Tonsillectomy: Justified but not mandated in special patients. *N. Engl. J. Med.* 310:717–18.

Hendrickson, L., and Myers, J. 1973. Some sources and potential consequences of errors in medical data recording. *Methods Inf. Med.* 12:38–45.

Hetherington, R. W. 1982. Quality assurance and organizational effectiveness in hospitals. *Health Serv. Res.* 17:185–201.

Heydebrand, W. V. 1973. *Hospital bureaucracy: A comparative study of organizations.* New York: Dunellen Press.

Hickson, D. J.; Hinings, C. R.; Lee, C. A.; Schneck, R. E.; and Pennings, J. M. 1971. A strategic contingencies' theory of intraorganizational power. *Admin. Sci. Q.* 16:216–29.

Hickson, D. J.; Pugh, D. S.; and Pheysey, D. C. 1969. Operations technology and organization structure: An empirical reappraisal. *Admin. Sci. Q.* 14:378–97.

Hind, R. R.; Dornbusch, S. M.; and Scott, W. R. 1974. A theory of evaluation applied to a university faculty. *Sociol. Educ.* 47:114–28.

Holmes, T. H., and Rahe, R. H. 1967. The social readjustment rating scale. *J. Psychosom. Res.* 11:213–18.

Horn, S. D.; Bulkely, G.; Sharkey, P. D.; Chambers, A. F.; Horn, R. A.; and Schramm, C. J. 1985. Interhospital differences in severity of illness: Problems for prospective payment based on diagnosis-related groups (DRGs). *N. Engl. J. Med.* 313:20–24.

Horn, S. D., and Schumacher, D. 1982. Comparing classification methods: Measurement of variations in charges, length of stay, and mortality. *Med. Care* 20(5): 489–500.

Horn, S. D., and Sharkey, P. D. 1983. Measuring severity of illness to predict patient resource use within DRGs. *Inquiry* 20:314–21.

Horn, S. D.; Sharkey, P. D.; and Bertram, D. A. 1983. Measuring severity of illness: Homogeneous case mix groups. *Med. Care* 21(1): 14–30.

Hornbrook, M. C. 1982a. Hospital casemix: Its definition, measurement and use: Part I. The conceptual framework. *Med. Care Rev.* 39(1): 1–43.

———. 1982b. Hospital casemix: Its definition, measurement and use: Part II. Review of alternative measures. *Med. Care Rev.* 39(2): 73–123.

Howard, J., and Strauss, A., eds. 1975. *Humanizing health care.* New York: John Wiley & Sons.

Howie, J. G. 1966. Death from appendicitis and appendectomy: An epidemiological survey. *Lancet* 2(17 December): 1334–37.

Hrebiniak, L. G. 1974. *Econometric methods.* 2d ed. New York: McGraw-Hill.

Hughes, E. C. 1958. *Men and their work.* Glencoe, Ill.: Free Press.

Jeffers, J. R., and Siebert, C. D. 1974. Measurement of hospital cost variation: Casemix, service intensity and input productivity factors. *Health Serv. Res.* 9:293–307.

Johnston, J. 1972. *Econometric Methods.* 2d ed. New York: McGraw-Hill.

Jones, K. R. 1984. The influence of the attending physician on indirect graduate medical education costs. *J. Med. Educ.* 59:789–98.

Jönsson, B., and Lindgren, B. 1980. Five common fallacies in estimating the economic gains of early discharge. *Soc. Sci. Med.* 14(1): 27–33.

Joskow, P. 1981. *Controlling hospital costs: The role of government regulation.* Cambridge, Mass.: MIT Press.

Kahn, R. L. 1977. Organizational effectiveness: An overview. In *New perspectives on organizational effectiveness,* 235–46. See Goodman and Pennings 1977.

Kaplan, R. M., and Bush, J. W. 1982. Health-related quality of life measurement for evaluation research and policy analysis. *Health Psychol.* 1(1): 61–80.

Kasl, S. V., and Cobb, S. 1966. Health behavior, illness behavior, and sick role behavior. *Arch. Environ. Health* 12(February): 246–66.

Katz, D., and Kahn, R. L. 1966. *The social psychology of organizations.* New York: John Wiley & Sons.

Kelly, J. V., and Hellinger, F. 1985. Physician and hospital factors associated with mortality of surgical patients. Paper presented at the annual meeting of the American Public Health Association, Washington, D.C., November.

Kempthorne, O. 1952. *The design and analysis of experiments*. New York: John Wiley & Sons.

Khandwalla, P. N. 1974. Mass output orientation of operations technology and organizational structure. *Admin. Sci. Q.* 19:74–97.

Kinzer, D. M. 1977. *Health controls out of control: Warning to the nation from Massachusetts*. Chicago: Teach'em.

Klarman, H. E. 1969. The difference the third party makes. *J. Risk Insurance* 36(December): 553–66.

———. 1977. The financing of health care. In *Doing better and feeling worse: Health in the United States,* ed. J. H. Knowles, 215–34. New York: W. W. Norton.

Knaus, W. A.; Schroeder, S.; and Davis, D. D. 1977. Impact of new technology: The CT scanner. *Med. Care* 15(7): 533–51.

Kohl, S. G. 1955. *Perinatal mortality in New York City.* Cambridge, Mass.: Harvard University Press.

Komaroff, A. L. 1985. Quality assurance in 1984. *Med. Care* 23(5): 723–34.

Kominski, G. F.; Williams, S. V.; Mays, R. B.; and Pickens, G. T. 1984. Unrecognized redistributions of revenue in diagnosis-related group-based prospective payment systems. *Health Care Financ. Rev.* 6(November): 57–69.

Kovner, A. R. 1966. The nursing unit: A technological perspective. Ph.D. diss., University of Pittsburgh.

Kushman, J. E., and Nuckton, C. F. 1977. Further evidence on the relative performance of proprietary and nonprofit hospitals. *Med. Care* 15(3): 189–204.

Labovitz, S. 1970. The assignment of numbers to rank order categories. *Am. Sociol. Rev.* 35:515–24.

Lave, J. R. 1966. A review of the methods used to study hospital costs. *Inquiry* 3:57–81.

Lave, J. R., and Lave, L. B. 1971. The extent of role differentiation among hospitals. *Health Serv. Res.* 6:15–38.

———. 1978. Hospital cost function analysis: Implications for cost control. In *Hospital cost containment,* 538–71. *See* Ginsburg 1978.

Lawrence, P. R., and Lorsch, J. W. 1967. *Organization and environment.* Boston: Harvard University Graduate School of Business Administration.

Lazarsfeld, P. F., and Menzel, H. 1961. On the relation between individual and collective properties. In *Complex organizations: A sociological reader,* ed. A. Etzioni, 422–40. Glencoe, Ill.: Free Press.

Lebow, J. L. 1974. Consumer assessments of the quality of medical care. *Med. Care* 12(4): 328–37.

Lee, J. A.; Morrison, S. L.; and Morris, J. N. 1957. Fatality from three common surgical conditions in teaching and non-teaching hospitals. *Lancet* 273(6999)(19 October): 785–90.

Lee, P. R., and Estes, C. L. 1983. New federalism and health policy. *Ann. Am. Acad. Polit. Social Sci.* 468:88–102.

Levy, M. G.; Covaleski, M. A.; and Johnson, A. C. 1982. Intraorganizational strategic decision model in the certificate-of-need application process. *Health Care Manage. Rev.* 7(2): 25–36.

Lewin, L. S.; Derzon, R. A.; and Margulies, P. 1981. Investor-owned and non-profits differ in economic performance. *Hospitals* 55:52–58.

Lewis, C. 1974. The state of the art of quality assessment—1973. *Med. Care* 12(10): 779–806.

Lindley, D. V. 1965. *Introduction to probability and statistics from a Bayesian point of view.* Cambridge: Cambridge University Press.

Lipworth, L.; Lee, J. A.; and Morris, J. N. 1963. Case-fatality in teaching and non-teaching hospitals, 1956–59. *Med. Care* 1(1): 71–76.

Litwak, E. 1961. Models of bureaucracy that permit conflict. *Am. J. Sociol.* 67:177–84.

Lohr, K. N., and Marquis, M. S. 1984. *Medicare and Medicaid: Past, present and future.* N-2088-HHS/RC. Santa Monica, Calif.: Rand.

Longest, B. B., Jr. 1974. The relationship between coordination, efficiency and quality of care in general hospitals. *Hospital Admin.* 19(Fall): 65–86.

Luft, H. S. 1978. How do health maintenance organizations achieve their savings? *N. Engl. J. Med.* 298:1336–43.

———. 1980. The relation between surgical volume and mortality: An exploration of causal factors and alternative models. *Med. Care* 19(9): 940–59.

———. 1981a. *Health maintenance organizations: Dimensions of performance.* New York: John Wiley & Sons.

———. 1981b. Diverging trends in hospitalization: Fact or artifact? *Med. Care* 19(10): 979–94.

Luft, H. S.; Bunker, J. P.; and Enthoven, A. C. 1979. Should operations be regionalized? The empirical relation between surgical volume and mortality. *N. Engl. J. Med.* 301:1364–69.

Luft, H. S.; Hunt, S. S.; and Mearki, S. C. 1985. The volume-outcome relationship: Practice makes perfect or selective referral patterns? Paper, University of California Institute for Health Policy Studies, San Francisco.

Luke, R. D., and Modrow, R. E. 1982. Professionalism, accountability, and peer review. *Health Serv. Res.* 17:113–33.

Luke, R. D., and Thompson, M. A. 1980. Utilization of within hospital services: A study of the effect of two forms of group practice. *Med. Care* 18(3): 219–27.

Lynch, B. P. 1974. An empirical assessment of Perrow's technology construct. *Admin. Sci. Q.* 19:338–56.

Lyons, T. F., and Payne, B. C. 1974. Interdiagnosis relationships of physician performance measures. *Med. Care* 12(4): 369–74.

McAuliffe, W. E. 1978. Studies of process-outcome correlations in medical care evaluations: A critique. *Med. Care* 16(11): 907–30.

———. 1979. Measuring the quality of medical care: Process versus outcome. *Milbank Mem. Fund Q.* 57:118–52.

McCarthy, E. G., and Widmer, C. W. 1974. Effects of screening by consultants on recommended elective surgical procedures. *N. Engl. J. Med.* 291:13–31.

McClure, W. 1976. *Reducing excess hospital capacity.* Bureau of Health Planning and Resources Development. HRP 0015199. Springfield, Va.: National Technical Information Service.

McDonald, C. J. 1976. Protocol-based computer reminders: The quality of care and the non-perfectability of man. *N. Engl. J. Med.* 295:1351–55.

McGrath, J. H.; Rothman, R. A.; and Schwartzbaum, A. M. 1970. Factors associated with physician's vote on the Wilmington hospital merger. *Del. Med. J.* 42(February): 35–40.

McMahon, J. A., and Drake, D. F. 1978. The American Hospital Association perspective. *Hospital cost containment,* Association perspective. In *Hospital cost containment,* 76–102. *See* Ginsburg 1978.

McPhee, S. J., and Bottles, K. 1985. Autopsy: Moribund art or vital science? *Am. J. Med.* 78:107–13.

Madoff, R. D.; Sharpe, S. M.; Fath, J. J.; Simmons, R. L.; and Corra, F. B. 1985. Prolonged surgical intensive care: A useful allocation of medical resources. *Arch. Surg.* 120(June): 698–702.

Manning, W.; Leibowitz, A.; Goldberg, G. A.; Rogers, W. H.; and Newhouse, J. P. 1984. A controlled trial of the effect of a prepaid group practice on use of services. *N. Engl. J. Med.* 310:1505–10.

March, J. G., and Simon, H. A. 1958. *Organizations.* New York: John Wiley & Sons.

Marks, S. D.; Greenlick, M. R.; Hurtado, A. V.; Johnson, J. D., and Henderson, J. 1980. Ambulatory surgery in an HMO: A study of costs, quality of care, and satisfaction. *Med. Care* 18(2): 127–46.

Martz, E. W., and Ptakowski, R. 1978. Educational costs to hospitalized patients. *J. Med. Educ.* 53:383–86.

Mason, W. B.; Bedwell, C. L.; Zwaag, R. V., and Runyan, J. W., Jr. 1980. Why people are hospitalized: A description of preventable factors leading to admission for medical illness. *Med. Care* 18(2): 147–63.

Maxwell, R.; Day, M.; Hardie, R.; Lawrence, H.; Rendall, M.; and Walton, N. 1983. Seeking quality. *Lancet* 1(8314–15) (18 January): 45–48.

May, J. J. 1983. Commentary on the management implications of "Effectiveness in professional organizations: The impact of surgeons and surgical staff organizations on the quality of care." *Health Serv. Res.* 18:1–6.

Mechanic, D. 1962. The concept of illness behavior. *J. Chronic Dis.* 15:189–94.

Melmon, K. L. 1971. Preventable drug reactions—causes and cures. *N. Engl. J. Med.* 284:1361–67.

Meyer, J. A. 1983. *Market reforms in health care.* Washington, D.C.: American Enterprise Institute for Public Policy Research.

Mohr, L. B. 1971. Organizational technology and organizational structures. *Admin. Sci. Q.* 16:444–59.

Money, W. H.; Gilfillan, D. P.; and Duncan, R. 1976. A comparative study of multi-unit health care organizations. In *Organizational research in hospitals,* ed. S. Shortell and M. Brown, 29–61. An *Inquiry* Book. Chicago: Blue Cross Association.

Moore, W. S. 1970. Classifying morbidity. *Inquiry* 7:41–45.

Morehead, M. A., and Donaldson, R. 1964. *A study of the quality of hospital care secured by a sample of Teamster family members of New York City.* New York: Columbia University.

Morlock, L.,; Nathanson, C.; Horn, S.; and Schumacher, D. 1979. Organizational factors associated with the quality of care in 17 general acute hospitals. Paper presented at the annual meeting of the Association of University Programs in Health Administration, Toronto, Canada.

Morse, E. V.; Gordon, G.; and Moch, M. 1974. Hospital costs and quality of care: An organizational perspective. *Milbank Mem. Fund Q.* 52:315–46.

Moseley, S. K., and Grimes, R. M. 1976. The organization of effective hospitals. *Health Care Manage. Rev.* 1(3): 13–23.

Moses, L. E. 1984. The series of consecutive cases as a device for assessing outcomes of intervention. *N. Engl. J. Med.* 311:705–10.

Moses, L. E., and Mosteller, F. 1968. Institutional differences in postoperative death rates: Commentary on some of the findings of the National Halothane Study. *JAMA* 203:492–94.

Mosteller, F., and Tukey, J. W. 1977. *Data analysis and regression.* Reading, Mass.: Addison-Wesley.

National Academy of Sciences Institute of Medicine. 1976. *Assessing quality in health care: An evaluation.* Washington, D.C.

———. 1980. *Reliability of national hospital discharge survey data.* IOM80-02. Washington, D.C.

National Academy of Sciences. Panel to Review Productivity Statistics, ed. 1979. *Measurement and interpretation of productivity.* Washington, D.C.

National Center for Health Services Research. 1977. *Changes in the costs of treatment of selected illnesses, 1951—1964—1971.* HRA 77-3161. Washington, D.C.: Health Resources Administration.

National Institute of Health, Office of Medical Application of Research. 1983. Consensus conference: Critical care medicine. *JAMA* 250:798–804.

Nelson-Wernick, E.; Currey, H. S.; Taylor, P. W.; Woodbury, M.; and Cantor, A. 1981. Patient perception of medical care. *Health Care Manage. Rev.* 6(1): 65–72.

Neuhauser, D. 1971. *The relationship between administrative activities and hospital performance.* Chicago: Center for Health Administration Studies.

———. 1983. Hospital effectiveness. *Health Serv. Res.* 18:13–15.

Neuhauser, D., and Andersen, R. 1972. Structural comparative studies of hospitals. In *Organization research on health institutions,* ed. B. S. Georgopoulos, 83–114. Ann Arbor: University of Michigan Institute for Social Research.

Neumann, B. R. 1974. A financial analysis of a hospital merger: Samaritan Health Service. *Med. Care* 12(12): 983–98.

Nie, Norman H.; Hull, C. H.; Jenkins, J. G.; Steinbrenner, K.; and Bert, D. H. 1975. *Statistical package for the social sciences.* 2d ed. San Francisco: McGraw-Hill.

Palmer, R. H., and Reilly, M. C. 1979. Individual and institutional variables which may serve as indicators of quality of medical care. *Med. Care* 17(7): 693–717.

Pauly, M. V. 1970. Efficiency, incentives, and reimbursements for health. *Inquiry* 7:114–31.

———. 1978. Medical staff characteristics and hospital costs. *J. Human Resources* 13(suppl.): 77–111.

Payne, B. C. 1966. *Hospital utilization review manual.* Ann Arbor: University of Michigan Press.

Payne, B. C., and Lyons, T. F. 1972. *The episode of illness: Method of evaluating and improving personal medical care quality.* Ann Arbor: University of Michigan School of Medicine.

Payne, B. C.; Lyons, T. F.; and Neuhaus, E. 1984. Relationships of physician characteristics to performance quality and improvement. *Health Serv. Res.* 19:307–32.

Payne, B. C., and Study Staff. 1976. *The quality of medical care: Evaluation and improvement.* Chicago: Hospital Research and Educational Trust.

Perrow, C. 1961. The analysis of goals in complex organizations. *Am. Sociol. Rev.* 26:854–66.

———. 1967. A framework for the comparative analysis of organizations. *Am. Sociol. Rev.* 32:194–208.

Posner, J. R., and Lin, H. W. 1975. Effects of age on length of hospital stay in a low-income population. *Med. Care* 13(10): 855–75.

Poznanski, E. O.; Miller, E.; Salguero, C.; and Kelsh, R. C. 1978. Quality of life for long-term survivors of end-stage renal disease. *JAMA* 239:2343–47.

President's Commission for the Study of Ethical Problems in Medicine and Biomedical and Behavioral Research. 1982. *Making health care decisions: The ethical and legal implications of informed consent in the patient-practitioner relationships.* Vol. 1. Washington, D.C.: GPO.

———. 1983. *Securing access to health care: The ethical implications of differences in the availability of health services.* Vol. 1. Washington, D.C.: GPO.

Price, J. L. 1972. The study of organizational effectiveness. *Sociol. Q.* 13(Winter): 3–15.

Price, J. L., and Mueller, C. W. 1981. A causal model of turnover for nurses. *Acad. Management J.* 24:543–65.

Pugh, D. S.; Hickson, D. J.; Hinings, C. R.; and Turner, C. 1968. Dimensions of organizational structure. *Admin. Sci. Q.* 13:65–105.

———. 1969. The context of organizational structures. *Admin. Sci. Q.* 14:91–114.

Quade, D. 1967. Rank analysis of covariance. *J. Am. Statist. Assoc.* 62:1187–1200.

Rackham, J., and Woodward, J. 1970. The measurement of technical variables. In *Industrial organisation: Behavior and control,* ed. J. Woodward, 19–36. London: Oxford University Press.

Redisch, M. A. 1978. Physician involvement in hospital decision making. In *Hospital cost containment,* 217–43. *See* Ginsburg 1978.

Reeves, T. K., and Woodward, J. 1970. The study of managerial control. In *Industrial Organisation,* 37–56. *See* Rackham and Woodward 1970.

Rhee, S.-O. 1976. Factors determining the quality of physician performance in patient care. *Med. Care* 14(9): 733–50.

———. 1977. Relative importance of physician's personal and situational characteristics for the quality of patient care. *J. Health Soc. Behav.* 18:10–15.

———. 1983. Organizational determinants of medical care quality: A review of the literature. In *Organization and change in health care quality assurance,* ed. R. D. Luke, J. C. Kruger, and R. E. Modrow, 127–46. Rockville, Md.: Aspen Systems Corporation.

Rhee, S.-O.; Luke, R. D., and Culverwell, M. B. 1980. Influence of client/colleague dependence on physician performance in patient care. *Med. Care* 18(8): 829–41.

Rhee, S.-O.; Luke, R. D.; Lyons, T. F.; and Payne. B. C. 1981. Domain of practice and the quality of physician performance. *Med. Care* 19(1): 14–23.

Rhee, S.-O.; Lyons, R.; and Payne, B. C. 1978. Interrelationships of physician performances: Technical quality and utilization and implications for quality and utilization controls. *Med. Care* 16(6): 496–501.

Ro, K. K. 1969. Patient characteristics and hospital use. *Med. Care* 7(July–August): 295–312.

Roberts, W. C. 1978. The autopsy: Its decline and a suggestion for its revival. *N. Engl. J. Med.* 299:322–28.

Robinson, W. M. M. 1973. Medical staffs merge: The medical staffs of two neighboring hospitals achieved patient care at lower cost through merged medical services. *Hospitals* 47:60–64 passim.

Robinson, W. S. 1950. Ecological correlation and the behavior of individuals. *Am. Sociol. Rev.* 15:351–57.

Roemer, M. I. 1959. Is surgery safer in large hospitals? *Hosp. Management* 87(January): 35–37 passim.

———. 1961. Bed supply and hospital utilization: A natural experiment. *Hospitals* 35:36–42.

Roemer, M. I., and Friedman, J. W. 1971. *Doctors in hospitals: Medical staff organization and hospital performance.* Baltimore: Johns Hopkins Press.

Roemer, M. I.; Moustafa, A. T.; and Hopkins, C. E. 1968. A proposed hospital quality index: Hospital death rates adjusted for case severity. *Health Serv. Res.* 3:96–118.

Roos, N. P.; Ross, L. L.; and Hentelett, P. D. 1977. Elective surgical rates: Do high rates mean lower standards? *N. Engl. J. Med.* 297:360–66.

Rosen, H. M., and Feigin, W. 1982. Medical peer review and information management: The deadend phenomenon. *Health Care Manage. Rev.* 7(3): 59–66.

Rosenfeld, L. S. 1957. Quality of medical care in hospitals. *Am. J. Public Health* 47:856–65.

Rosenstock, I. M. 1966. Why people use health services. *Milbank Mem. Fund Q.* 44:94–124.

Ross, A. 1982. Applying the conclusions of the Flood study to the hospital practice world. *Health Serv. Res.* 17:373–77.

Rundall, T. G. 1978. Life changes and recovery from surgery. *J. Health Soc. Behav.* 19:418–27.

———. 1983. Effectiveness in professional organizations. *Health Serv. Res.* 18:7–12.

Rushing, W. A. 1968. Hardness of material as related to division of labor in manufacturing industries. *Admin. Sci. Q.* 13:229–45.

———. 1974. Differences in profit and nonprofit organizations: A study of effectiveness and efficiency in general short-stay hospitals. *Admin. Sci. Q.* 19:474–84.

Rutkow, I. M. 1982. The surgical decision-making process: Determinants of surgical rates. *Health Serv. Res.* 17:379–85.

Salkever, D. S. 1979. *Hospital-sector inflation.* Lexington, Mass: D. C. Heath, Lexington Books.

Salkever, D. S., and Bice, T. W. 1976. The impact of certificate-of-need controls on hospital investment. *Milbank Mem. Fund Q.* 54:185–214.

———. 1978. Certificate-of-need legislation and hospital costs. In *Hospital cost containment,* 429–60. See Ginsburg 1978.

Scheffler, R. M.; Knaus, W. A.; Wagner, D. P.; and Zimmerman, J. E. 1982. Severity of illness and the relationship between intensive care and survival. *Am. J. Public Health* 72:449–54.

Schimmel, E. M. 1964. The hazards of hospitalization. *Ann. Intern. Med.* 60:100–110.

Schoonhoven, C. B. 1981. Problems with contingency theory: Testing assumptions hidden within the language of contingency "theory." *Admin. Sci. Q.* 26:349–77.

Schoonhoven, C. B.; Scott, W. R.; Flood, A. B.; and Forrest, W. H., Jr. 1980. Measuring the complexity and uncertainty of surgery and postsurgical care. *Med. Care* 18(9): 893–915.

Schroeder, S. A., and O'Leary, D. S. 1977. Differences in laboratory use and length of stay between university and community hospitals. *J. Med. Educ.* 52:418–20.

Scitovsky, A. A., and McCall, N. 1976. Changes in the costs of treatment of selected illnesses, 1964–1971. Research Digest Series. HRA 77-3161. Washington, D.C.: National Center for Health Services Research.

Scott, W. R. 1965. Reactions to supervision in a heteronomous professional organization. *Admin. Sci. Q.* 10:65–81.

———. 1966. Professionals in bureaucracies—areas of conflict. In *Professionalization,* ed. H. M. Vollmer and D. L. Mills, 265–75. Englewood Cliffs, N.J.: Prentice-Hall.

———. 1972. Professionals in hospitals: Technology and the organization of work. In *Organization research on health institutions,* 139–58. *See* Neuhauser and Andersen 1972.

———. 1975. Organizational structure. *Ann. Rev. Sociol.* 1:1–20.

———. 1977. Effectiveness of organizational effectiveness studies. In *New perspectives on organizational effectiveness,* 63–95. *See* Goodman and Pennings 1977.

———. 1981. *Organizations: Rational, natural and open systems.* Englewood Cliffs, N.J.: Prentice-Hall.

———. 1982. Managing professional work: Three models of control for health organizations. *Health Serv. Res.* 17:213–40.

———. 1985. Conflicting levels of rationality: Regulators, managers, and professionals in the medical care sector. *J. Health Admin. Educ.* 3(2), pt. 2:113–31.

Scott, W. R.; Dornbusch, S. M.; Evashwick, C. J.; Magnani, L.; and Sagatun, I. 1972. Task conceptions and work arrangements. Stanford: Stanford Center for Research and Development in Teaching.

Scott, W. R.; Flood, A. B.; and Ewy, W. 1979. Organizational determinants of services, quality and cost of care in hospitals. *Milbank Mem. Fund Q.* 57:234–64. Chapter 10 is an edited version of this article.

Scott, W. R.; Flood, A. B.; Ewy, W.; and Forrest, W. H., Jr. 1978. Organizational effectiveness and the quality of surgical care in hospitals. In *Environments and organizations,* ed. M. Meyer and associates, 290–305. San Francisco: Jossey-Bass.

Scott, W. R.; Flood, A. B.; Ewy, W.; Forrest, W. H., Jr.; and Brown, B. W., Jr. 1976. Utilizing outcomes to assess the quality of surgical care. Paper presented at the annual meeting of the American Institute for Decision Sciences, San Francisco, November. Incorporated into Chapter 6.

Scott, W. R.; Forrest, W. H., Jr.; and Brown, B. W., Jr. 1976. Hospital structure and postoperative mortality and morbidity. In *Organizational research in hospitals, See* Money, Gilfillan, and Duncan 1976.

Scott, W. R., and Shortell, S. M. 1983. Organizational performance: Managing for efficiency and effectiveness. In *Health care management,* 418–56. *See* Shortell and Kaluzny 1983.

Sharp, K. Organizational determinants of quality surgical care. Ph.D. diss., University of Illinois at Urbana-Champaign. 1986.

Shortell, S. M. 1982. Improving organizational effectiveness: A comment on effectiveness in professional organizations. *Health Serv. Res.* 17:367–72.

Shortell, S. M.; Becker, S. W.; and Neuhauser, D. 1976. The effects of management practices on hospital efficiency and quality of care. In *Organizational research in hospitals,* 90–112. *See* Money, Gilfillan, and Duncan 1976.

Shortell, S. M., and Kaluzny, A. D., eds. 1983. *Health care management: A text in organizational theory and behavior.* New York: John Wiley & Sons.

Shortell, S. M., and LoGerfo, J. P. 1981. Hospital medical staff organization and quality of care: Results for myocardial infarction and appendectomy. *Med. Care* 19(10): 1041–55.

Shortell, S. M.; Morrisey, M. A.; and Conrad, D. A. 1985. Economic regulation and hospital behavior: The effects on medical staff organization and hospital-physician relationships. *Health Serv. Res.* 20:597–628.

Simon, H. A. 1964. On the concept of organizational goal. *Admin. Sci. Q.* 9:1–22.

Simpson, J. E. 1977. Length of stay. *Lancet* 1(801D)(5 March): 531–33.

Simpson, J. H. 1972. Technology, autonomy and structure. Ph.D. diss., Stanford University.

Singer, D. E.; Carr, P. L.; Mulley, A. G.; and Thibault, G. E. 1983. Rationing intensive care—Physician responses to a resource shortage. *N. Engl. J. Med.* 309:1155–60.

Sloan, F. A.; Feldman, R. D.; and Steinwald, A. B. 1983. Effects of teaching on hospital costs. *J. Health Econom.* 2(March): 1–28.

Sloan, F. A.; Perrin, J. M.; and Valvona, J. 1985. In-hospital mortality of surgical patients: Is there an empirical basis for standard setting?: Paper, Vanderbilt University Institute for Public Policy.

Sloan, F. A., and Steinwald, A. B. 1980a. *Hospital labor markets.* Lexington, Mass.: D. C. Heath, Lexington Books.

———. 1980b. *Insurance, regulation, and hospital costs.* Lexington, Mass.: D. C. Heath, Lexington Books.

Smith, H. L. 1955. Two lines of authority are one too many. *Mod. Hospital* 84:59–64.

Smits, H. L.; Fetter, R. B.; and McMahon, L. F., Jr. 1984. Variation in resource use within diagnosis-related groups: The severity issue. *Health Care Financ. Rev.* 6(November): 71–78.

Somers, H. M., and Somers, A. R. 1961. *Doctors, patients, and health insurance.* Garden City, N.Y.: Doubleday.

———. 1967. *Medicare and the hospitals.* Washington, D.C.: Brookings Institution.

Stanford Center for Health Care Research (SCHCR). 1974. *Study of institutional differences in postoperative mortality.* A Report to the National Academy of Sciences–National Research Council. Springfield. Va.: National Technical Information Service (PB 250 940).

———. 1976. Comparisons of hospitals with regard to outcome of surgery. *Health Serv. Res.* 11:112–27.

Starkweather, D. B. 1981. *Hospital mergers in the making.* Ann Arbor. Mich.: Health Administration Press.

Starr, P. 1982. *The social transformation of American medicine.* New York: Basic Books.

State of Maryland Commission. 1964. *Report of the State of Maryland Commission to study hospital costs.* Baltimore.

Steers, R. M. 1977. *Organizational effectiveness: A behavioral view.* Santa Monica, Calif.: Goodyear.

Stigler, G. 1958. The economies of scale. *J. Law Econom.* 1(October): 54–71.

Studnicki, J. C. 1979. Multihospital systems: A research perspective. *Inquiry* 16:315–22.

Studnicki, J. C.; Stevens, E.; and Knisely, L. 1985. Impact of a cybernetic system of feedback to physicians on inappropriate hospital use. *J. Med. Educ.* 60:454–60.

Suchman, E. A. 1965. Social patterns of illness and medical care. *J. Health and Human Behav.* 6:2–16.

———. 1967. *Evaluative research.* New York: Russell Sage Foundation.

Sugimoto, T. 1985. Cost effectiveness analysis of elective surgical procedures as preventive measures: The case of incidental appendectomy. Paper presented at the annual meetings of the American Public Health Association, Washington, D.C., November.

Sullivan, D. F. 1966. Conceptual problems in developing an index of health. *National Center for Health Statistics,* 2d ser., no. 17.

Sullivan, R. J., Jr.; Estes, E. H., Jr.; Stopford, W.; and Lester, A. J. 1980. Adherence to explicit strategies for common medical conditions. *Med. Care* 18(4): 388–99.

Tancredi, L. R., and Barondess, J. A. 1978. The problem of defensive medicine. In *Health care,* 37–40. *See* Donabedian 1978.

Tannenbaum. A. S. 1968. *Control in organizations.* New York: McGraw-Hill.

Tannenbaum, A. S., and Bachman, J. 1964. Structural versus individual effects. *Am. J. Sociol.* 69:585–95.

Thompson, J. D. 1967. *Organizations in action.* New York: McGraw-Hill.

Thompson, J. D.; Fetter, R. D.; and Mross, C. D. 1975. Case mix and resource use. *Inquiry* 12:300–312.

Treat, T. F. 1976. The performance of merging hospitals. *Med. Care* 14(3): 199–209.

Trussell, R. E.; Morehead, M.; and Ehrlich, J. 1962. *The quantity, quality, and costs of medical and hospital care secured by a sample of Teamster families in the New York Area.* New York: Columbia University.

Udy, S. H., Jr. 1965. The comparative analysis of organizations. In *Handbook of organizations,* ed. J. G. March, 682–707. Chicago: Rand McNally.

U.S. Bureau of the Census. 1962. *U.S. census of population: 1960. Vol. 1, Characteristics of the population.* Washington, D.C.

———. 1970. *U.S. census of housing block statistics.* Washington, D.C.

———. 1973a. *County and city data book, 1972.* Washington, D.C.

———. 1973b. *U.S. census of population: 1970. Vol. 1, Characteristics of the population.* Washington, D.C.

U.S. Department of Health, Education, and Welfare. 1971. *Health manpower: A county and metropolitan area data book,* Washington, D.C.: GPO.

Vacanti, C. J.; Van Houten, R. J.; and Hill, R. C. 1970. A statistical analysis of the relationship of physical status to postoperative mortality in 68,388 cases. *Anesth. Analg.* 49(4): 564–66.

Van de Ven, A., and Delbecq, A. 1974. A task contingent model of work-unit structure. *Admin. Sci. Q.* 19:183–97.

Verba, S., and Nie, N. J. 1972. *Participation in America: Political democracy and social equality.* New York: Harper & Row.

Vuori, H. 1980. Optimal and logical quality: Two neglected aspects of quality of health services. *Med. Care* 18(10): 975–85.

Wagner, D. P., and Draper, E. A. 1984. Acute physiology and chronic health evaluation

(APACHE II) and Medicare reimbursement. *Health Care Financ. Rev.* 6(November): 91–105.

Walker, S. H., and Duncan, D. B. 1967. Estimation of the probability of an event as a function of several independent variables. *Biometrika* 54:167–79.

Wallace, C. 1984. HCFA's next target will be reform of physician reimbursement: Davis. *Modern Healthcare* 14:23.

Wedel, K.; Katz, A. J.; and Weick A. 1979. *Social services by government contract.* New York: Praeger.

Weisman, C. S.; Alexander, C. S.; and Chase, G. A. 1981. Determinants of hospital staff nurse turnover. *Med. Care* 19(4): 431–43.

Wennberg, J. E.; Blowers, L.; Parker, P.; and Gittelsohn, A. M. 1977. Changes in tonsillectomy rates associated with feedback and review. *Pediatrics* 59:821–26.

Wennberg, J. E., and Gittelsohn, A. 1973. Small area variations in health care delivery. *Science* 182(14 December): 1102–8.

———. 1982. Variations in medical care among small areas. *Sci. Am.* 246(1): 120–34.

White, W. D. 1982. The American hospital industry since 1900: A short history. In *Advances in health economics and health services research,* ed. R. M. Scheffler, 143–70. Greenwich, Conn.: JAI Press.

Wilensky, G. R., and Rossiter, L. F. 1983. Relative importance of physician induced demand. *Milbank Mem. Fund Q.* 61:52–77.

Wolinsky, F. D., and Kurz, R. S. 1984. How the public chooses and views hospitals. *Hosp. Health Serv. Admin.* 29(6): 58–67.

Wood, A. P. 1984. Hospital occupancy down, physicians adapting to DRGs. *Int. Med. News* 17(19): 1ff.

Woodward, J. 1965. *Industrial Organisation: Theory and practice.* New York: Oxford University Press.

World Health Organization (WHO) 1958. Constitution of the World Health Organization, Annex I. In *First ten years of the W.H.O.* Geneva.

Wyszewianski, L.; Wheeler, J. R. C.; and Donabedian, A. 1982. Market-oriented cost-containment strategies and quality of care. *Milbank Mem. Fund Q.* 60:518–50.

Yale Law J. 1954. The American Medical Association: Power, purpose, and politics in organized medicine. *Yale Law J.* 63:938–1022.

Yates, J. W.; Chalmer, B.; and McKegney, F. P. 1980. Evaluation of patients with advanced cancer using Karnofsky performance status. *Cancer* 45:2220–24.

Young, W. W. 1984. Incorporating severity of illness and comorbidity in case-mix measurement. *Health Care Financ. Rev.* 6(November): 23–31.

Young, W. W.; Swinkola, R. B.; and Zorn, D. M. 1982. The measurement of hospital case mix. *Med. Care* 20(5): 501–12.

Yuchman, E., and Seashore, S. E. 1967. A system resource approach to organizational effectiveness. *Am. Sociol. Rev.* 32:891–903.

Zuckerman, H. S. 1979. Multi-institutional systems: Their promise and performance. In *Multi-institutional hospital systems,* ed. H. S. Zuckerman and L. E. Weeks, 3–51. Chicago: Hospital Research and Educational Trust.

Name Index

Subject Index

ABOUT THE AUTHORS

Ann Barry Flood is on the faculty of the Medical Humanities and Social Sciences Program of the College of Medicine and the Department of Health and Safety Studies at the University of Illinois at Urbana-Champaign. W. Richard Scott is professor of sociology with an appointment in the School of Medicine at Stanford University. His previous books include *Organizations: Rational, Natural, and Open Systems.*